Color Atlas of Chemical Peels

Antonella Tosti • Pearl E. Grimes
Maria Pia De Padova
Editors

Color Atlas of Chemical Peels

Second Edition

Springer

Editors
Prof. Dr. Antonella Tosti
University of Miami
Leonard M. Miller School of Medicine
Department of Dermatology and Cutaneous Surgery
Miami, FL
USA
atosti@med.miami.edu

Dr. Maria Pia De Padova
Ospedale Privato Nigrisoli
Bologna
Italy
mdepadova@gmail.com

Pearl E. Grimes, MD
Institute of Southern California
Division of Dermatology
Los Angeles, CA
USA
raz@pearlgrimesmd.com

ISBN 978-3-662-49982-5 e-ISBN 978-3-642-20270-4
DOI 10.1007/978-3-642-20270-4
Springer Heidelberg Dordrecht London New York

Softcover reprint of the hardcover 2nd edition 2012

Printed on acid-free paper

Springer is part of Springer Science+Business Media (www.springer.com)

Preface to the Second Edition

We revised and extended the materials of the first edition, adding new interesting cases. We also investigated the state of the art of the most updated procedure, working on new materials, new compounds and techniques. We also extended the side effects section, highlighting the importance of the correct algorithm to follow in order to reduce the chance of complications.

We believe that the book will be of great value also for those readers who already have the previous edition.

Chemical peels are very effective in a variety of different skin conditions and are easy to perform with minimal and controllable side effects. This book teaches step by step how to select and perform the best peeling for each single indication.

Bologna, Italy — Antonella Tosti
Los Angeles, CA, USA — Pearl E. Grimes
Bologna, Italy — Maria Pia De Padova

Preface to the First Edition

This Atlas is an easy-to-understand book that gives the reader fact-based information about when and how to perform chemical peels.

Authors' experiences in cosmetic dermatology give rise to a guide for anyone interested in learning more about cosmetology.

The book provides information about each single chemical peel, fully explained in terms of its properties, formulations, indications, performing technique, advantages and disadvantages.

It also reviews different dermatological disorders showing step-by-step the procedure for the best peeling with which to treat them.

This is an up-to-date book which will help the clinician improve his skill in this field.

Bologna, Italy — Antonella Tosti
Los Angeles, CA, USA — Pearl E. Grimes
Bologna, Italy — Maria Pia De Padova

Contents

Part III How to Choose the Best Peeling for the Patient

Part IV Management of Complications

Part V Management of the Patient

Part I

Types of Chemical Peels

1 Types of Chemical Peels: Advantages/Disadvantages, an Illustrated Algorithm

Maria Pia De Padova and Antonella Tosti

1.1 Advantages/Disadvantages

1.1.1 Summary

- Glycolic acid
- Jessner's solution
- Pyruvic acid
- Resorcinol
- Salicylic acid
- Trichloroacetic acid
- Tretinoin
- Malic acid
- Deep chemical peels
- Combinations peels: Salicylic acid + trichloroacetic acid

1.1.2 Glycolic Acid 30–70%

1.1.2.1 Advantages

- Very mild erythema
- Mild desquamation
- Short postoperative period
- Useful in photodamage

1.1.2.2 Disadvantages

- Penetration often not uniform
- Neutralization is mandatory
- High risk of overpeel if time of application is too long or the skin is inflamed
- Cautious application in patients with active acne

1.1.3 Jessner's Solution

1.1.3.1 Advantages

- Excellent safety profile
- Can be used in all skin types
- Substantial efficacy with minimal "down time"
- Utilized for combination peels as it enhances the penetration of other agents
- Can be used in active acnes
- Can be used in postinflammatory hyperpigmentation and melasma

1.1.3.2 Disadvantages

- Concerns regarding resorcinol toxicity, including thyroid dysfunction
- Manufacturing variations
- Instability with exposure to light and air
- Excessive exfoliation in some patients

1.1.4 Pyruvic Acid

1.1.4.1 Advantages

- Homogeneous penetration with uniform erythema (Fig. 1.1)
- Mild desquamation

M.P. De Padova
Ospedale Privato Nigrisoli, Bologna, Italy
e-mail: mdepadova@gmail.com

A. Tosti (✉)
Department of Dermatology and Cutaneous Surgery, Miller School of Medicine, University of Miami, US
e-mail: atosti@med.miami.edu

A. Tosti et al. (eds.), *Color Atlas of Chemical Peels*,
DOI 10.1007/978-3-642-20270-4_1, © Springer-Verlag Berlin Heidelberg 2012

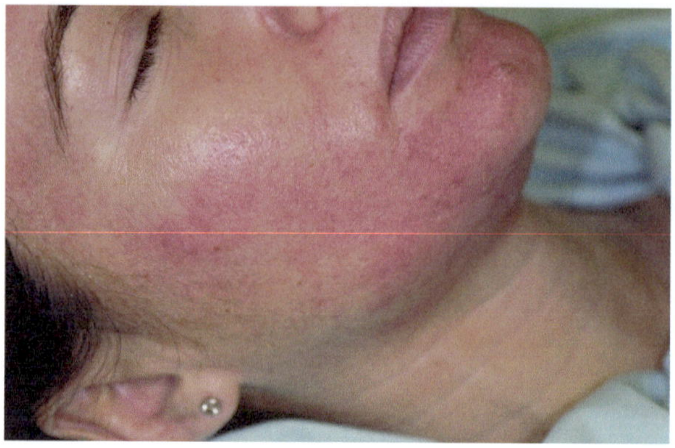

Fig. 1.1 Homogeneous erythema following peeling with pyruvic acid 50%

- Short postoperative period
- Can be used in all skin types
- Can be used in active acnes
- Can be used in postinflammatory hyperpigmentation and melasma

1.1.4.2 Disadvantages

- Intense stinging and burning sensation during the application
- Neutralization is mandatory
- Pungent and irritating vapors for the upper respiratory mucosa

1.1.5 Resorcinol

1.1.5.1 Advantages

- Easy to perform
- Not painful (the burning sensation during the peeling is usually mild)
- Homogeneous penetration
- Can be used in active acnes
- Can be used in postinflammatory hyperpigmentation and melasma

1.1.5.2 Disadvantages

- Intense dark desquamation in the postpeel period
- Not recommended for dark-skinned individuals
- Resorcinol may be a sensitizer and cause thyroid dysfunction, cardiac arrhythmia, and methemoglobinemia

1.1.6 Salicylic Acid

1.1.6.1 Advantages

- Established safety profile in all skin types
- Formation of white precipitate allows to verify if application is homogeneous (Fig. 1.2)
- Salicylic acid has an anesthetic effect that is useful in combination peelings
- Can be used in active acnes
- Can be used in postinflammatory hyperpigmentation and melasma

1.1.6.2 Disadvantages

- Intense stinging and burning sensation during the application
- Minimal efficacy in patients with significant photodamage

1.1.7 Trichloroacetic Acid

1.1.7.1 Advantages

- Low cost
- Uniformity of application
- Penetration can be easily evaluated by the color of frost (Fig. 1.3)

1.1.7.2 Disadvantages

- Stinging and burning sensation during the application
- High concentrations are not recommended in skin types V–VI
- Can cause hypo/hyperpigmentation

1.1.8 Tretinoin

1.1.8.1 Advantages

- Painless
- Easy to perform
- Short postoperative period

1.1.8.2 Disadvantage

- Can cause intense erythema

1.1.9 Malic Acid

1.1.9.1 Advantages

- Short postoperative period
- Can be used in all skin types

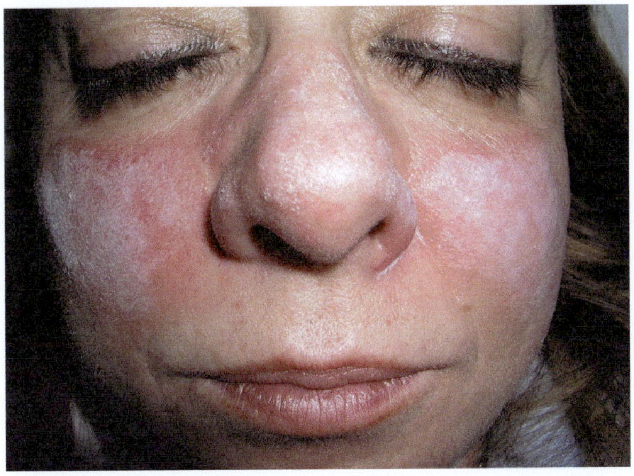

Fig. 1.2 Formation of white precipitate after peeling with salicylic acid 25%

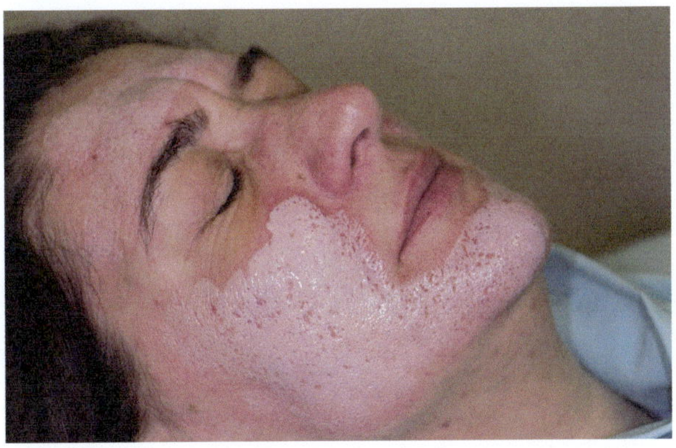

Fig. 1.3 Peeling with TCA 25%: Development of white frosting indicates penetration in the papillary dermis

1.1.9.2 Disadvantage

- Minimal efficacy

1.1.10 Deep Chemical Peels

1.1.10.1 Advantages

- Improves severe photodamage
- Improves perioral wrinkles
- Improves atrophic acne scars

1.1.10.2 Disadvantages

- Requires sedation and cardiovascular monitoring
- Not recommended in skin types IV to VI
- Cardiotoxicity
- Can cause hypo/hyperpigmentation

1.1.11 Combination Peels: Salicylic Acid + TCA

1.1.11.1 Advantages

- Can be used in all skin types
- Most beneficial in treating melasma and postinflammatory hyperpigmentation

1.1.11.2 Disadvantages

- Risk of overpeeling
- Can cause hypo/hyperpigmentation

1.2 How to Choose the Best Peeling for the Patient

1.2.1 Summary

- Acne
- Actinic keratoses
- Dark skin
- Melasma
- Photoaging
- Postinflammatory hyperpigmentation
- Rosacea
- Solar lentigos

1.2.2 Acne

Acute phase	
Comedonal acne	Salicylic acid 25% Pyruvic acid 40–60% Jessner's solution Unna Paste Glycolic acid 70%
Mild/moderate inflammatory acne	Salicylic acid 25–30% Pyruvic acid 40–60% Jessner's solution Unna Paste
Severe nodulo-cystic acne	Pyruvic acid 40–60%
Superficial post-acne scars	Pyruvic acid 40–60% Trichloroacetic acid 25–50% Salicylic acid 25% + trichloroacetic acid 25–30%
Medium-deep post-acne scars	Phenol 45–80% Trichloroacetic acid >40%

1.2.3 Actinic Keratosis

- Trichloroacetic acid >30%
- Pyruvic acid 50–60%
- Salicylic acid 25% + trichloroacetic acid 25–30%

1.2.4 Dark Skin

- Salicylic acid 20–30%
- Jessner's solution
- Glycolic acid 20–70%
- Trichloroacetic acid 10–30%

1.2.5 Melasma

- Salicylic acid 25%
- Salicylic acid 25% + trichloroacetic acid 10–25%
- Glycolic acid 50–70%
- Pyruvic acid 40–50%
- Trichloroacetic acid 15–20%
- Resorcinol
- Jessner's solution

1.2.6 Photoaging

Mild to moderate	Glycolic acid 50–70% Trichloroacetic acid 30–50% Salicylic acid 30% Salicylic acid 25% + trichloroacetic acid >25%
Severe	Glycolic acid 70% + trichloroacetic acid 35% Jessner's solution + trichloroacetic acid 35% Phenol 88%

1.2.7 Postinflammatory Hyperpigmentation

- Salicylic acid 30%
- Salicylic acid 25% + trichloroacetic acid 10–25%
- Glycolic acid 50–70%
- Pyruvic acid 40–50%
- Trichloroacetic acid 15–25%
- Resorcinol
- Jessner's solution

1.2.8 Rosacea

Erythrosis	Salicylic acid 15–25% Pyruvic acid 40%
Papulopustular rosacea	Salicylic acid 25–30% Pyruvic acid 40%

1.2.9 Solar Lentigos

- Trichloroacetic acid >25%
- Salicylic acid 25% + trichloroacetic acid 25–30%
- Pyruvic acid 50–70%
- Phenol 60–80%

Part II

Modalities of Application

2 Glycolic Acid

Gabriella Fabbrocini, Maria Pia De Padova, and Antonella Tosti

2.1 History

In a study of more than 60 substances chosen for their possible antikeratinogenic properties, Van Scott and Yu [1] found that the most effective drug belongs to the group of alpha-hydroxy acids. A three-times-a-day application of citric, glycolic, lactic, malic, pyruvic, and glucuronic acid, for instance, gave excellent results in all forms of ichthyosis except epidermolytic hyperkeratosis. The substances were applied at 5% strength in a hydrophilic ointment, though the base was a matter of the patient's preference. Sustained remission was obtained as long as the treatment continued. The use of these agents has been extended to other hyperkeratotic conditions. Glycolic acid became available in the late 1980s as a peeling agent.

2.2 Chemical Background

Glycolic acid is an alpha-hydroxy acid, soluble in alcohol, derived from fruit and milk sugars. It can be produced with ethylene glycol–oxidizing microorganisms such as *Pichia naganishii* AKU 4267 and *Rhodotorula* sp. 3 Pr-126. Under optimized conditions, they form 105 g/L and 110 g/L of glycolic acid (corrected molar conversion yields 88.0% and 92.2%) during a 120-h reaction, respectively [2].

G. Fabbrocini (✉)
Section of Dermatology, Department of Systematic Pathology, University of Naples Federico II, Via Sergio Pansini 5, 80133, Napoli, Italy
e-mail: gafabbro@unina.it

M.P. De Padova
Ospedale Privato Nigrisoli, Bologna, Italy
e-mail: mdepadova@gmail.com

A. Tosti
Department of Dermatology and Cutaneous Surgery, Miller School of Medicine, University of Miami, US
e-mail: atosti@med.miami.edu

2.3 Properties

It has been shown that glycolic acid has a keratolytic, germinative layer and a fibroblast-stimulating action. Reported studies have shown its anti-inflammatory effects and anti-oxidant action. It acts by thinning the stratum corneum, promoting epidermolysis, dispersing basal layer melanin and epidermal and dermal hyaluronic acid and collagen gene expression that increases through an elevated secretion of IL-6 [3].

Glycolic acid acts both on epidermis and derma. We can summarize this effect in this box:

Effect on epidermis

- Exfoliation of superficial layers of the stratum corneum through an alteration of corneocyte cohesion ≠ from a keratolytic action
- Regeneration of new epidermal tissues:
  - Increase of epidermal thickness (increased turn over)
  - Improvement of GDE structure
  - Increase of the GAG physiological production
  - Less cellular alteration
  - Less melanin "compact areas"

Effects on derma

- Increase of dermal thickness

A. Tosti et al. (eds.), *Color Atlas of Chemical Peels*,
DOI 10.1007/978-3-642-20270-4_2, © Springer-Verlag Berlin Heidelberg 2012

- Fibroblasts-stimulating action
- Improvement in the collagen fibers production: Derma appears more dense
- Better quality of elastic fibers that appears longer, sharper, and less fragmented
- Improvement in the GAG physiological production (hyaluronic acid)

It is unknown how a superficial peel working on epidermis could have effects on derma too. It has been proposed that this process could be based on growing factors as keratinocytes TGF-β and their transduction signals. This is a new research field on the science of chemical peels.

2.4 Formulations

The absorption of glycolic acid in human skin is pH-, strength-, and time-dependent. Seventy percent glycolic acid solutions are commonly used as superficial chemical peeling agents; the pH of these solutions ranges from 0.08 to 2.75. Peeling solutions with a pH below 2 have demonstrated the potential to induce crusting and necrosis, which has not been seen with the partially neutralized solutions with a pH above 2 [4]. The higher concentration acid (70%) created more tissue damage than the lower concentration (50%) compared to solutions with free acid. An increase of transmembrane permeability coefficient is observed with a decrease in pH, providing a possible explanation for the effectiveness of glycolic acid in skin treatment.

2.5 Indications

Glycolic acid has been recognized as an important adjunctive therapy in a variety of conditions including photodamage, acne, rosacea, striae albae pseudofolliculitis barbae, hyperpigmentation disorders, actinic keratoses, fine wrinkles, lentigines, melasma, and seborrheic keratoses [5]. Moreover, it can reduce UV-induced skin tumor development and it has been proposed as a therapeutic modality against skin exfoliative conditions such as ichthyosis, xeroderma, and psoriasis. In postmenopausal women, a cream containing 0.01% estradiol and 15% glycolic acid, applied to one side of the face for 6 months, induces a significant improvement in reversing markers (rete peg pattern, epidermal thickness) of skin aging [6].

Glycolic acid chemical peels are an effective treatment for all types of acne, inducing rapid improvement and restoration of normal-looking skin. In these patients, glycolic acid is more widely used than Jessner's solution, considering the equal treatment effect but a reduced exfoliation in glycolic acid [7]. Although the treatment of atrophic acne scars is difficult and generally unsatisfactory, many clinical studies have been performed to investigate the efficacy of glycolic acid in the treatment of acne vulgaris. It is now widely used to treat many defects of the epidermis and papillary dermis in a variety of strengths, ranging from 20% to 70%, depending on the condition being treated [8].

The most important clinical indications (Acne and photoaging) are listed in this box:

Skin Photoaging (Glogau Grading I and II)
- Improvement of skin brightness
- Improvement of dyschromia
- Improvement of fine superficial wrinkling
- Improvement of skin texture
- Improvement of collagen deposition

2.5.1 Acne

Comedonic acne	As a complement in the acne microsurgery
Seborrheic acne	Improvement of skin texture
Acne scarring	Clinical reduction
Pigmentations	Clinical reduction
Postinflammatory erythema	Clinical reduction
Smoker skin	Improvement of skin appearance

2.6 Contraindications

Glycolic acid peels are contraindicated in contact dermatitis, pregnancy, and in patients with glycolate hypersensitivity. Moreover, they can increase skin sensitivity to ultraviolet light.

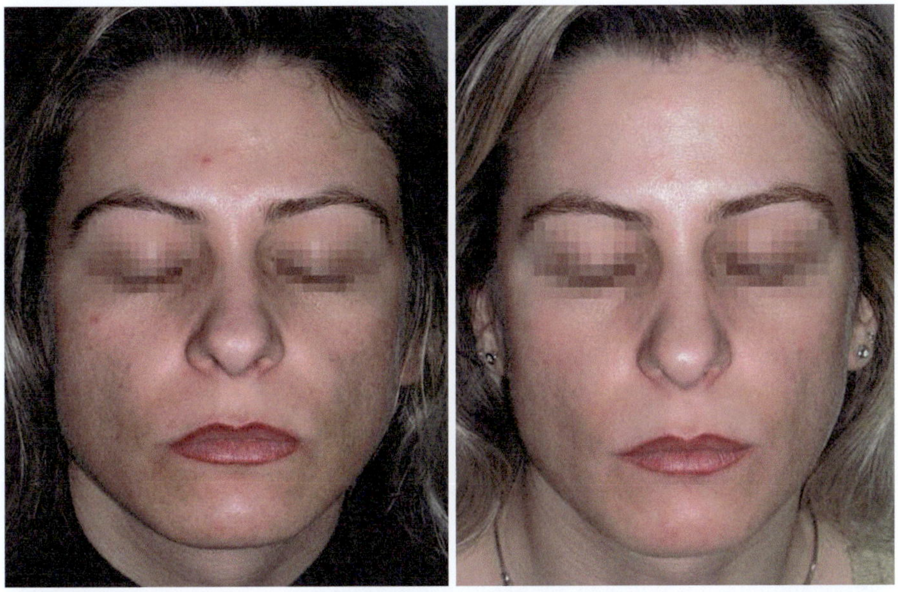

Fig. 2.1 Patient with photodamage: before and after treatment with glycolic acid

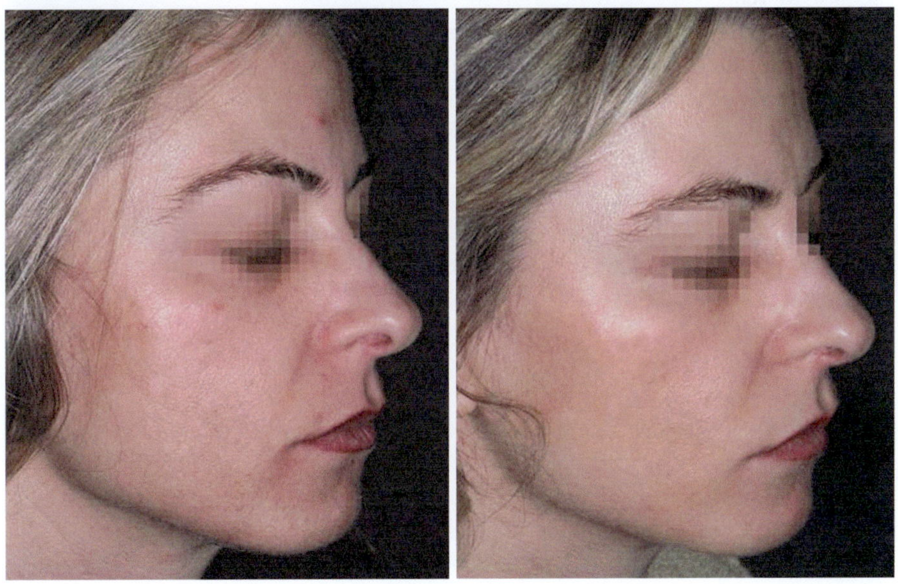

Fig. 2.2 Patient with photodamage: before and after treatment with glycolic acid.

2.7 Peeling Preparation

Patients with photodamage can apply a lotion containing 25% glycolic acid for 6 months. In such cases, an increase in total skin thickness of approximately 25% was reported, accompanied by an increased thickness of viable epidermis and dermis, an increased content of acid mucopolysaccharides, a greater collagen density, and an improved quality of the elastic fibers. This could be defined as self-treatment. However, a better efficiency in peeling can be achieved with a concentration of 50–70% of glycolic acid and, for maximum benefit, glycolic acid peels are combined with retinoids and other antioxidants. Some studies have evaluated the efficacy of a cream containing 4% hydroquinone and 2% glycolic acid used alone or with salicylic acid in reversing actinic damage on the neck and upper chest for 12 weeks; salicylic acid peelings are performed every 3 weeks. This treatment induces a 33–71% improvement in cases of photodamage (Figs. 2.1a, b and 2.2a, b), hyperpigmentation, texture problems, fine lines, dryness, tone, and clarity [9].

Other studies have demonstrated that the application of 50% glycolic acid peels mildly improves photoaging of the skin. Generally, for a light peeling, glycolic acid (50%) was applied topically for 5 min to one side of the face, forearms, and hands, once weekly for 4 weeks. The improvement observed was significant and included decrease in rough texture and fine wrinkling, fewer solar keratoses, and a slight lightening of solar lentigines. Histology showed thinning of the stratum corneum, granular layer enhancement, and epidermal thickening. Longer treatment intervals may result in collagen deposition as suggested by the measured increase in mRNA.

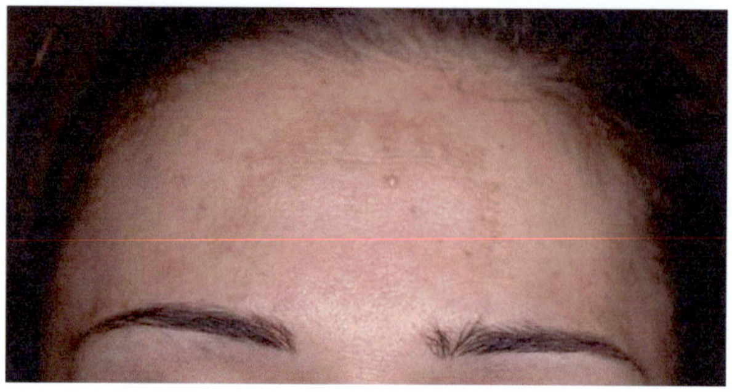

Fig. 2.3 Patient with melasma of the forehead

2.8 Peeling Technique

Before applying glycolic acid, the skin is cleaned with alcohol to reduce the acid neutralized by oily skin. Glycolic acid is applied in any cosmetic unit order, rapidly covering the entire face within about 20 s with a large cotton applicator. A starting application time for weekly or monthly applications with 50% or 70% unbuffered glycolic acid is generally in the range of 3 min, and the time is increased with subsequent peels. Neutralizers with sodium bicarbonate marketed to the physician have no advantage over water rinsing as long as all acid is removed thoroughly from all rhytidis and cosmetic units. Glycolic acid applied simultaneously with TCA represents another technique for a medium-depth peel. Several weeks prior to a peel, the skin may be prepared with topical tretinoin or glycolic acid, and immediately prior to the peel, the skin may be degreased with a variety of agents. Some studies demonstrated that glycolic acid-trichloroacetic acid peels, called combination medium-depth peeling, are usually performed as a single procedure to remove actinic keratoses, mild rhytidis,or pigmentary dyschromias or to flatten depressed scars. These peelings can be repeated approximately every 6 or 12 months based on the amount of actinic damage still remaining or recurring after the peel or for continued scar effacement. The classic peel for this depth category was the 50% TCA peel.

Since TCA in higher concentrations tends to produce increased scarring and hypopigmentation, 70% glycolic acid solution was applied to the entire face of patients and diluted with water after 2 min. This was followed by the sequential application of EMLA cream (lidocaine 2.5% and prilocaine 2.5%) or ELA-Max cream (lidocaine 4%) to selected areas on the face for 30 min without occlusion. These agents were then removed and 35% TCA was applied to the entire face [10].

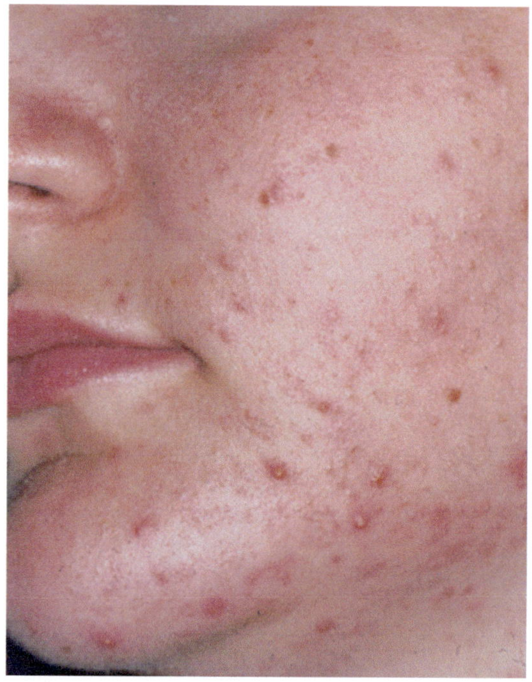

Fig. 2.4 Patient with comedonic-inflammatory acne

Patients with melasma (Fig. 2.3) applied topical sunscreens (sun protection factor 15) and 10% glycolic acid lotion at night for 2 weeks. They were then treated with 50% glycolic acid facial peels once a month for 3 consecutive months. At regular intervals and at the end of the follow-up period (3 months) after the last peel, the degree of improvement in pigmentation was assessed by measuring MASI (Melasma Area and Severity Index) [11]. In patients with acne (Fig. 2.4), the chemical peels were performed with a 70% glycolic

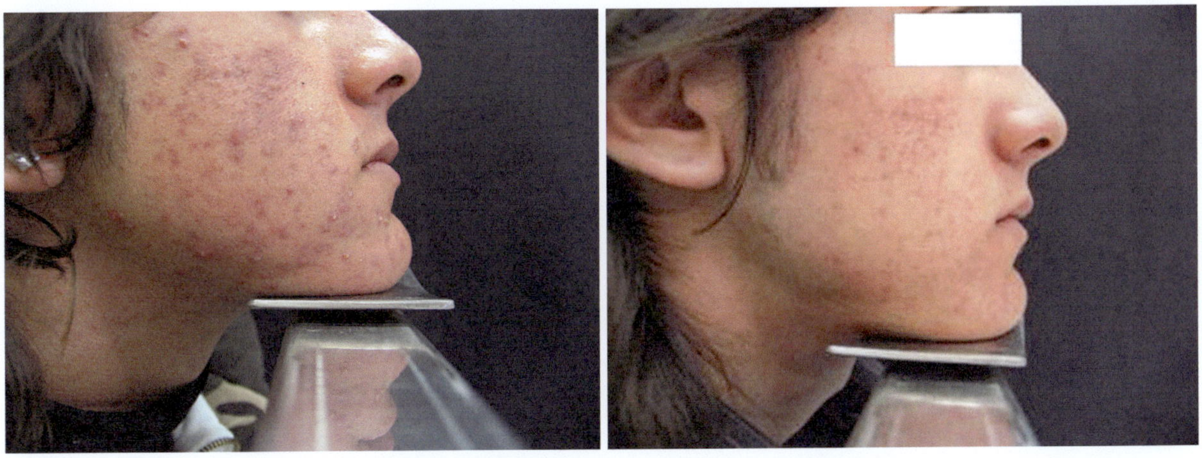

Fig. 2.5 Papulo-pustolar acne: pre and post treatment with glycolic acid

acid solution, for 2–8 min. The number and frequency of the applications depended on the intensity of the clinical response. The most rapid improvement was observed in comedonic acne, in the papulo-pustular forms. An average of six applications were necessary (Fig. 2.5a, b). Although nodular-cystic forms required eight to ten applications, a significant improvement of the coexisting post-acne superficial scarring was noted. The procedure was well tolerated and patient compliance was excellent [12]. In the treatment of atrophic acne scars (Fig. 2.6), repetitive glycolic acid peels (at least six times) at 70% concentration are necessary to obtain evident improvement. Long-term daily use of low-strength products may also have some useful effects on scars and may be recommended for patients who cannot tolerate the peeling procedure [13] (Fig. 2.7a, b). Patients of varying skin types (I–V) having striae distensae alba on the abdomen or thighs can apply topical 20% glycolic acid daily to the entire treatment area. In addition, these patients apply 10% *L*-ascorbic acid, 2% zinc sulfate, and 0.5% tyrosine to half of the treatment area and 0.05% tretinoin emollient cream to the other half of the treatment area. The creams are applied on a daily basis for 12 weeks. Improvement is evaluated at 4 and 12 weeks with increased elastin content within the reticular and papillary dermis [14]. Pseudofolliculitis barbae is a foreign-body inflammatory reaction surrounding ingrown facial hair, which results from shaving. Topical application of glycolic acid lotion is an effective therapy and allows the patient to resume a daily shaving regimen [15]. In patients with scalp psoriasis, a combination of a 10% glycolic acid scalp lotion is used as well as a 0.1% betamethasone scalp application, applied twice daily without any bandage for a period of 8 weeks [16]. To obtain a global management of the patient that is performing chemical peels and to obtain a good home compliance between peelings session, new gel formulations at Ph ~ 1 have been proposed, using xanthan gum as solidifying agent. With this process we can obtain a good formulation to apply an uniform acid layer, that cannot drain. There are concentration variable of 30–70% glycolic acid.

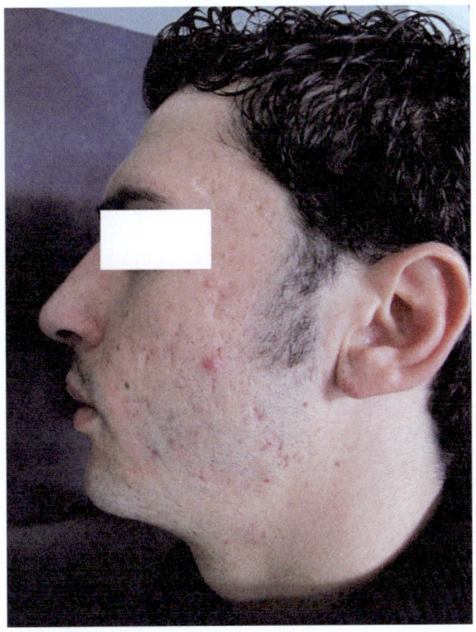

Fig. 2.6 Patient with atrophic acne scars

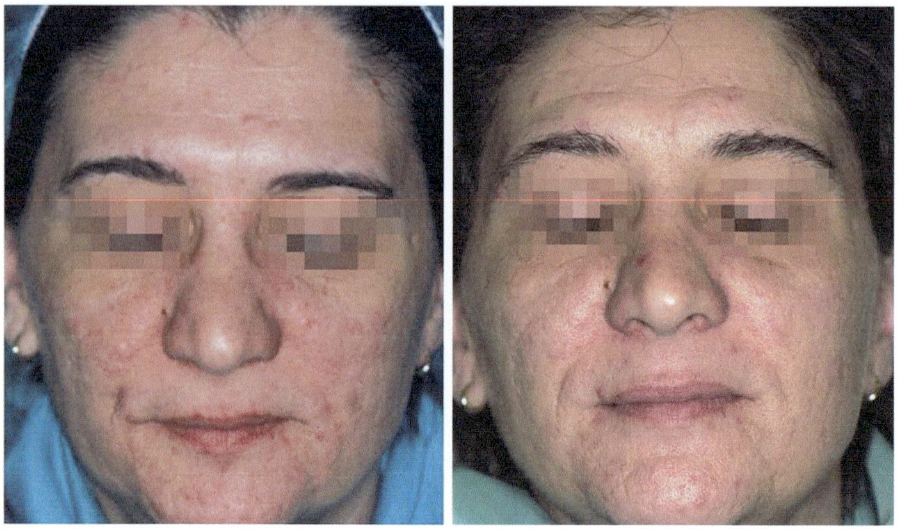

Fig. 2.7 Long-term daily use of low-strength products in patients who cannot tolerate the peeling procedure: before and after treatment

The most important advantages of this technique are:

- This is a formulation that facilitates the glycolic acid skin permeability, thanks to the propylene glycol.
- The commercial mould based on serviettes allows to control the glycolic acid dose that we apply on the skin.
- The commercial mould enriched with alcohol allows to purify skin with an uniform application of the acid on the face.

2.9 Post-peeling Care and Complications

Following the peel, the skin is carefully observed for any complications such as hyperpigmentation and infection. Results are maintained with serial peels and by using at-home tretinoin or glycolic acid, as well as by sun avoidance.

2.10 Disadvantages

Through the patient's history and physical examination, the physicians will identify any specific factor such as medications, prior procedures, and medical conditions that can affect the outcome of the peel [17]. Complications of glycolic acid peel like hyperpigmentation and infection are rare. Chemical peel with glycolic acid may cause sensible irritation symptoms, characterized by stinging, burning, and itching.

A substance capable of counteracting sensory irritation is strontium nitrate at 20% concentration, which applied topically with 70% glycolic acid potently suppresses the sensation of chemically induced irritation [18]. Moreover, some studies have demonstrated that glycolic acid could cause an increase in the level of skin damage in a dose- and time-dependent manner. Lower doses (1 and 3 mg/cm^2) of glycolic acid caused erythema and eschar at most, whereas higher doses (5 and 7 mg/cm^2) of glycolic acid caused redness, edema, and necrotic ulceration. Glycolic acid also increased the thickness of the epidermal layer, reduced the organization of the stratum corneum, and eventually destroyed some parts of the epidermal layer at 7 mg/cm^2. UVB caused redness and edema and also reduced the integrity of the stratum corneum. Glycolic acid enhances UVB-induced skin damage without accompanying PGE (2) production or COX-2 protein expression. Therefore, caution should be exercised by those using glycolic acid chronically or in excessive amounts. Moreover, people with photosensitive skins and those particularly exposed to the sun should be particularly careful. However, this photosensitivity could be reversed within a week after terminating treatments [19]. Laboratory investigations have rarely shown a complex I deficiency in the mitochondrial oxidative phosphorylation of patients who had recurrent episodes characterized by nausea, vomiting, and signs of dehydration necessitating admission to the hospital. In these patients, glycolic acid was detected in blood and they were diagnosed as having ethylene glycol intoxication [3].

2.11 Side Effects

Side effects, such as temporary hyperpigmentation or irritation, are not very significant. Finally, glycolic acid is a member of the alpha-hydroxy acid family, which provides an important adjunctive therapy in a variety of skin disorders. It is widely used in chemical peels in a variety of concentrations, ranging from 20% to 70%. People of almost any skin type and color are candidates and almost any area of the body can be peeled. Glycolic acid can be applied simultaneously with TCA, which represents another technique for a medium-depth peel. Glycolic acid is also used in creams for self-treatment. Since complications such as hyperpigmentation, infection, irritation, and photosensitivity are very rare, it is well tolerated. Glycolic acid peeling is a medical procedure that requires the informed consent of the patient. The medical doctor must obtain from the patient a well-standardized formal consent that shows that all information about the medical procedure performed was explained to the patient. We include below the formal consent form submitted to the patient before the glycolic acid peeling procedure.

I, __________________, after carefully reading the information regarding the glycolic acid peeling procedure, give my informed consent to undergo glycolic acid peeling treatment.

I have been well informed about side effects that the procedure could cause.

I have been well informed of temporary effects of the therapy.

I confirm that I have informed the medical doctor about all actual pathologies of pathologies that I have had.

I confirm that I have informed the medical doctor pharmacological therapies that I am currently receiving or have received in the past.

I confirm that I want to perform the treatment of my own free will without any physical or moral conditioning and I confirm that I have the right to interrupt the therapy such as I want without the necessity of justifying my decision.

Surname and name

Date of birth

Place of birth

Address

Town

Tel

Signature of the patient

Date

I, medical doctor, ________________, confirm that I have explained with accuracy the type, aim and possible risks of the medical procedure to be performed on the patient indicated, who has given consent to begin the treatment.

Surname and name of the medical doctor

Signature of the medical doctor

Date

References

1. Van Scott EJ, Yu RJ (1974) Control of keratinization with alpha-hydroxy acids and related compounds. I. Topical treatment of ichthyotic disorders. Arch Dermatol 110: 586–590
2. Kataoka M, Sasaki M, Hidalgo AR, Nakano M, Shimizu S (2001) Glycolic acid production using ethylene glycol-oxidizing microorganism. Biosci Biotechnol Biochem 65(10): 2265–2270
3. Bernstein EF, Lee J, Brown DB, Yu R, Van Scott E (2001) Glycolic acid treatment increases type I collagen mRNA and hyaluronic acid content of human skin. Dermatol Surg 27(5):429–433
4. Becker FF, Langford FP, Rubin MG, Speelman P (1996) A histological comparison of 50% and 70% glycolic acid peels using solutions with various pHs. Dermatol Surg 22(5): 463–465
5. Moy LS, Murad H, Moy RL (1993) Glycolic acid peels for the treatment of wrinkles and photoaging. J Dermatol Surg Oncol 19(3):243–246
6. Fuchs KO, Solis O, Tapawan R, Paranjpe J (2003) The effects of an estrogen and glycolic acid cream on the facial skin of postmenopausal women: a randomized histologic study. Cutis 71(6):481–488

7. Kim SW, Moon SE, Kim JA, Eun HC (1999) Glycolic acid versus Jessner's solution: which is better for facial acne patients? A randomised prospective clinical trial of split-face model therapy. Dermatol Surg 25(4):270–273
8. Murad H, Shamban AT, Premo PS (1995) The use of glycolic acid as a peeling agent. Dermatol Clin 13(2):285–307
9. Gladstone HB, Nguyen SL, Williams R, Ottomeyer T, Wortzman M, Jeffers M, Moy RL (2000) Efficacy of hydroquinone cream (USP 4%) used alone or in combination with salicylic acid peels in improving photodamage on the neck and upper chest. Dermatol Surg 26(4):333–337
10. Koppel RA, Coleman KM, Coleman WP (2000) The efficacy of ELMA versus ELA-Max for pain relief in medium-depth chemical peeling: a clinical and histopathologic evaluation. Dermatol Surg 26(1):61–64
11. Javaheri SM, Handa S, Kaur I, Kumar B (2001) Safety and efficacy of glycolic acid facial peel in Indian women with melasma. Int J Dermatol 40(5):354–357
12. Atzori L, Brundu MA, Orru A, Biggio P (1999) Glycolic acid peeling in the treatment of acne. J Eur Acad Dermatol Venereol 12(2):119–122
13. Erbagci Z, Akcali C (2000) Biweekly serial glycolic acid peels vs. long-term daily use of topical lowstrength glycolic acid in the treatment of atrophic acne scars. Int J Dermatol 39(10):789–794
14. Ash K, Lord J, Zukowski M, McDaniel DH (1998) Comparison of topical therapy for striae alba (20% glycolic acid/ 0,05% tretinoin versus 20% glycolic acid/ 10% L-ascorbic acid). Dermatol Surg 24(8):849–856
15. Perricone NV (1993) Treatment of pseudofolliculitis barbae with topical glycolic acid: a report of two studies. Cutis 52(4):232–235
16. Kostarelos K, Teknetzis A, Lefaki I, Ioannides D, Minas A (2000) Double-blind clinical study reveals synergistic action between alpha-hydroxy acid and betamethasone lotions towards topical treatment of scalp psoriasis. J Eur Acad Dermatol Venereol 14(1):5–9
17. Tung RC, Bergfeld WF, Vidimos AT, Remzi BK (2000) Alpha-hydroxy acid-based cosmetic procedures. Guidelines for patient management. Am J Clin Dermatol 1(2): 81–88
18. Zhai H, Hannon W, Hahn GS, Pelosi A, Harper RA, Maibach HI (2000) Strontium nitrate suppresses chemically induced sensory irritation in humans. Contact Dermat 42(2):98–100
19. Parks KS, Kim HJ, Kim EJ, Nam KT, Oh JH, Song CW, Jung HK, Kim DJ, Yun YW, Kim HS, Chung SY, Cho DH, Kim BY, Hong JT (2002) Effects of glycolic acid on UVB-induced skin damage and inflammation in guinea pigs. Skin Pharmacol Appl Skin Physiol 15(4):236–245

3 Salicylic Acid

Pearl E. Grimes

3.1 History

P.G. Unna, a German dermatologist, was the first to describe the properties and use of salicylic acid. It has since been used for many decades as a keratolytic agent in concentrations of 3–6%. Salicylic acid is frequently utilized in topical acne preparations because of its comedolytic effects. In addition, it facilitates the penetration of other topical agents.

3.2 Chemical Background/Properties

Salicylic acid (ortho-hydroxybenzoic acid) is a beta-hydroxy acid agent (Fig. 3.1). It is a lipophilic compound which removes intercellular lipids that are covalently linked to the cornified envelope surrounding cornified epithelioid cells [1]. Due to its antihyperplastic effects on the epidermis, multiple investigators have used salicylic acid as a peeling agent [2–4]. Recently, histologic assessments using salicylic acid peels in hairless mice reported loss of cornified cells followed by activation of epidermal basal cells and underlying fibroblasts. These findings suggest that salicylic acid peeling can alter the underlying dermal tissue without directly wounding the tissue or causing inflammation [5]. Salicylic acid has also been shown to have anti-inflammatory and antimicrobial properties. When used in combination with benzoic acid in Whitfield's ointment, it has fungicidal properties.

Fig. 3.1 Chemical structure

Salicylic acid

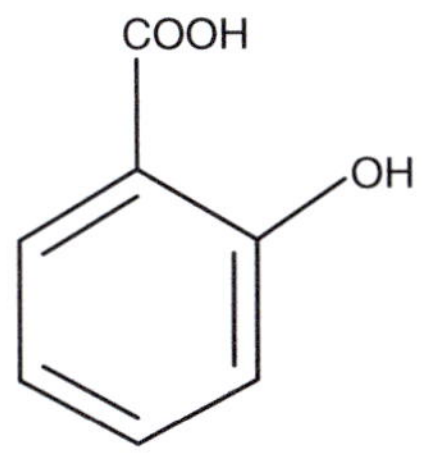

3.3 Formulations

A variety of formulations of salicylic acid have been used as peeling agents. These include 50% ointment formulations (Table 3.1) [2, 3]; as well as 10–30% ethanol formulations (Tables 3.1 and 3.2) [4, 6]. More recently, a variety of commercial formulations of salicylic acid are currently available.

3.4 Indications

The efficacy of salicylic acid peeling has been assessed in several studies. Fifty percent salicylic acid ointment peeling was first used by Aronsohn to treat 81 patients who had freckles, pigmentation, and aging changes of the hands [3]. He reported excellent results. Subsequently, Swinehart [2] successfully used a methyl-salicylate-buffered, croton oil-containing, 50% salicylic acid ointment paste for treatment of lentigines,

P.E. Grimes
Division of Dermatology, Department of Medicine, David Geffen School of Medicine, University of California—Los Angeles, Vitiligo and Pigmentation Institute of Southern California, 5670 Wilshire Blvd., Suite 650, Los Angeles, CA 90036, USA
e-mail: pegrimesmd@earthlink.net

A. Tosti et al. (eds.), *Color Atlas of Chemical Peels*,
DOI 10.1007/978-3-642-20270-4_3,

Table 3.1 Formulations of salicylic acid: salicylic acid ointment

Salicylic acid powder USP 50%
Methyl salicylate, 16 drops
Aquaphor 112 g

From Swinehart [2]

Table 3.2 Formulations of salicylic acid: salicylic acid solutions

Salicylic acid peel (%)	Weight of salicylic acid powder (g)	Amount of ethyl alcohol 95% (cc)
10	10	100
20	20	100
30	30	100
40	40	100
50	50	100

From Draelos [6]

pigmented keratoses, and actinically damaged skin of the dorsal hands and forearms. After pretreatment with topical tretinoin and localized TCA 20%, the 50% salicylic acid paste was applied to the affected area and occluded for 48 h. Following dressing removal, peeling and desquamation occurred and was relatively complete by the tenth day. Overall results were described as excellent. Despite these results, salicylic acid peeling did not move into the arena of popular peeling techniques until the mid-1990s. Kligman and Kligman [4] ushered salicylic acid into the current arena of superficial peeling agents. They treated 50 women with mild-to-moderate photodamage, reporting improvement in pigmented lesions, surface roughness, and reduction in fine lines.

Grimes [7] reported substantial efficacy and minimal side effects in 25 patients treated with 20% and 30% salicylic acid peels in darker racial-ethnic groups. Conditions treated included acne vulgaris, melasma, and post-inflammatory hyperpigmentation.

Thirty-five Korean patients with facial acne were treated biweekly for 12 weeks with 30% salicylic acid peels [8]. Both inflammatory and non-inflammatory lesions were significantly improved. In general, the peel was well tolerated with few side effects.

In a randomized, split-face study of 10 patients with skin types IV to VI showing post-inflammatory hyperpigmentation, salicylic acid peels were found to be a safe treatment in dark skin. Treatment was judged effective by the patients, but efficacy ratings by blinded scores fell short of significance. Quality-of-life measurements showed a trend toward improvement after treatment [9].

Ahn and Kim [10] used colorimetry to assess the whitening effect of biweekly 30% salicylic acid peels in Korean patients with acne and post-inflammatory pigmentation. After 3 months, there were significant improvements in colorimetric parameters, reflecting a reduction in hyperpigmentation.

Kodali [11], in a prospective, randomized split-face study, assessed the efficacy of 20% and 30% salicylic acid peels in 20 Latin American women with melasma. Salicylic acid peels were applied to one side while both sides were treated with hydroquinone 4%. Although both sides of the face had significant reduction in pigment, there were no differences between the peeled and unpeeled side with all outcome measures suggesting that salicylic acid did not improve outcomes versus hydroquinone monotherapy in patients with melasma.

Oresajo et al. [12] compared the efficacy of glycolic acid to that of a novel derivative of salicylic acid, capryloyl salicylic acid (LHA). In this split-face study, 50 female subjects with mild-to-moderate facial hyperpigmentation and fine lines and wrinkles were randomized and the GA was applied to one side of the face and the LHA to the other side. Patients were treated with increasing concentrations of each agent (LHA, 5–10% and GA 20–50%). Forty-four subjects completed the study at 12 weeks. Forty-one percent of the LHA treated areas versus 30% of the GA-treated areas demonstrated a significant reduction in fine lines and wrinkles. In addition, 40% of the LHA areas showed a significant reduction in pigment compared to 34% of the GA-treated subjects albeit there were no statistically significant differences between the GA and LHA outcomes [12].

Given the aforementioned findings, indications for salicylic acid peels include acne vulgaris (inflammatory and non-inflammatory lesions), acne rosacea, melasma, post-inflammatory hyperpigmentation, freckles, lentigines, mild-to-moderate photodamage, and texturally rough skin.

3.5 Contraindications

In general, there are few contraindications to salicylic acid chemical peeling. Salicylic acid peels are well tolerated in all skin types (Fitzpatrick's I through VI) and all racial-ethnic groups. General contraindications include salicylate hypersensitivity/allergy; unrealistic patient expectations; active inflammation/dermatitis or infection at the salicylic acid peeling site; acute viral infection; pregnancy; and isotretinoin therapy within 3–6 months of the peeling procedure. The author has performed more than 1,000 salicylic acid peels without observing any evidence of salicylate allergy/hypersensitivity following a salicylic acid peel.

3.6 Patient Preparation

Peel preparation varies with the condition being treated. Regimens differ for photodamage, hyperpigmentation (melasma and post-inflammatory hyperpigmentation), and acne vulgaris [13]. In addition, there are special issues to be considered when treating darker racial-ethnic groups (see Chapter 3). A detailed history and cutaneous examination should be performed in all patients prior to chemical peeling. Standardized photographs are taken of the areas to be peeled including full-face frontal and lateral views.

Use of topical retinoids (tretinoin, tazarotene, retinol formulations) for 2–6 weeks prior to peeling thins the stratum corneum, and enhances epidermal turnover [14]. Such agents also reduce the content of epidermal melanin and expedite epidermal healing. Retinoids also enhance the penetration of the peeling agent. They should be discontinued several days prior to the peeling procedure. Retinoids can be resumed postoperatively after all evidence of peeling and irritation subsides. In contrast to photodamage, when treating conditions such as melasma, acne, and post-inflammatory hyperpigmentation, as well as darker skin types, retinoids should be discontinued 1 or 2 weeks before peeling or even eliminated from the prep to avoid post-peel complications such as excessive erythema, desquamation, and post-inflammatory hyperpigmentation.

Topical alpha-hydroxy acid or polyhydroxy acid formulations can also be used to prep the skin. In general, they are less aggressive agents in impacting peel outcomes. The skin is usually prepped for 2–4 weeks with a formulation of hydroquinone 4% or higher compounded formulations (5–10%) to reduce epidermal melanin [15]. This is extremely important when treating the aforementioned dyschromias. Although less effective, other topical bleaching agents include azelaic acid, ascorbic acid, niacinamide, kojic acid, arbutin, and licorice (see Chapter 14). Patients can also resume use of topical bleaching agents postoperatively after peeling and irritation subsides.

When treating acne vulgaris, topical and systemic therapies (if indicated) are initiated 2–4 weeks prior to peeling. Topical antibiotics and benzoyl peroxide–based products can be used daily and discontinued 1 or 2 days prior to peeling. However, unless a deeper peel is desired, retinoids should be discontinued 7–14 days prior to salicylic acid peeling. Broad-spectrum sunscreens (UVA and UVB) should be worn daily (see Chapter 14).

3.7 Peeling Technique

Despite some general predictable outcomes, even superficial chemical peeling procedures can cause hyperpigmentation and undesired results. Popular standard salicylic acid peeling techniques involve the use of 20% and 30% salicylic acid in an ethanol formulation. Salicylic acid peels are performed at 2–4 week intervals. Maximal results are achieved with a series of 3–6 peels.

The author always performs the initial peel with a 20% concentration to assess the patients' sensitivity and reactivity. Before treatment, the face is thoroughly cleansed with alcohol and/or acetone to remove oils. The peel is then applied with 2×2 wedge sponges, 2×2 gauge sponges, or cotton-tipped applicators. Cotton-tipped swabs can also be used to apply the peeling agent to periorbital areas. A total of 2–3 coats of salicylic acid are usually applied. The acid is first applied to the medial cheeks working laterally, followed by application to the perioral area, chin, and forehead. The peel is left on for 3–5 min. Most patients experience some mild burning and stinging during the procedure. After 1–3 min, some patients experience mild peel-related anesthesia of the face. Portable handheld fans substantially mitigate the sensation of burning and stinging.

A white precipitate, representing crystallization of the salicylic acid, begins to form at 30 s to 1 min following peel application (Fig. 3.2). This should not be confused with frosting or whitening of the skin which represents protein agglutination. Frosting usually indicates that the patient will observe some crusting and peeling following the procedure (Fig. 3.3a–d). This may be appropriate when treating photodamage. However, the author prefers to have minimal to no

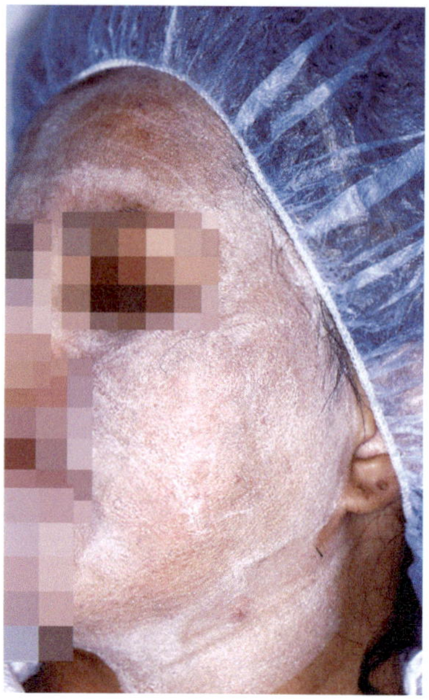

Fig. 3.2 Salicylic acid precipitate

frosting when treating other conditions. After 3–5 min, the face is thoroughly rinsed with tap water, and a bland cleanser such as Cetaphil is used to remove any residual salicylic acid precipitate. A bland moisturizer is applied after rinsing. My favorites are Cetaphil, Purpose, Theraplex (Figs. 3.4a, b, 3.5a, b and 3.6a, b).

3.8 Post-peeling Care and Complications

Bland cleansers and moisturizers are continued for 48 h or until all post-peel irritation subsides. Patients are then able to resume the use of their topical skin care regimen including topical bleaching agents, acne medications, and/or retinoids. Post-peel adverse reactions such as excessive desquamation and irritation are treated with low to high potency topical steroids. Topical steroids are extremely effective in resolving post-peel inflammation and mitigating the complication of post-inflammatory hyperpigmentation. In the author's experience, any residual post-inflammatory hyperpigmentation resolves with use of topical hydroquinone formulations following salicylic acid peeling.

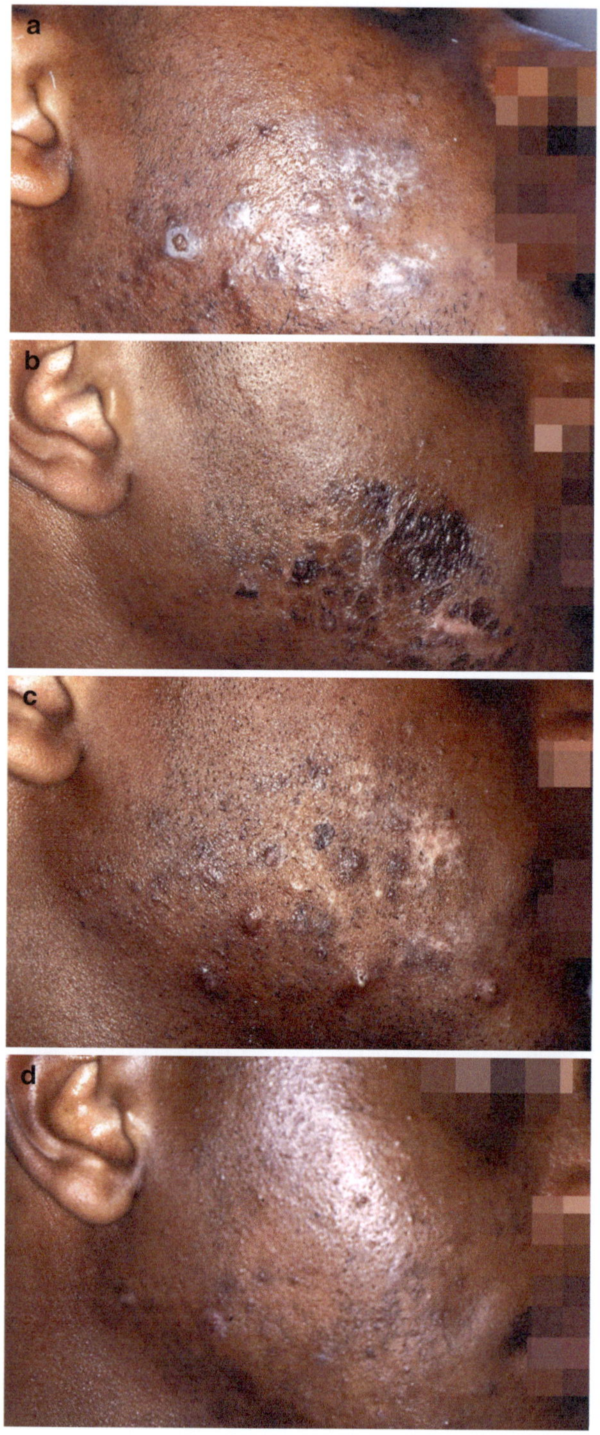

Fig. 3.3 (**a**) Frosting after salicylic acid. (**b**) Crusting 48 h later. (**c**) Resolution of crusting in 3–4 days. (**d**) Complete clearing of hypopigmentation by day 7–10

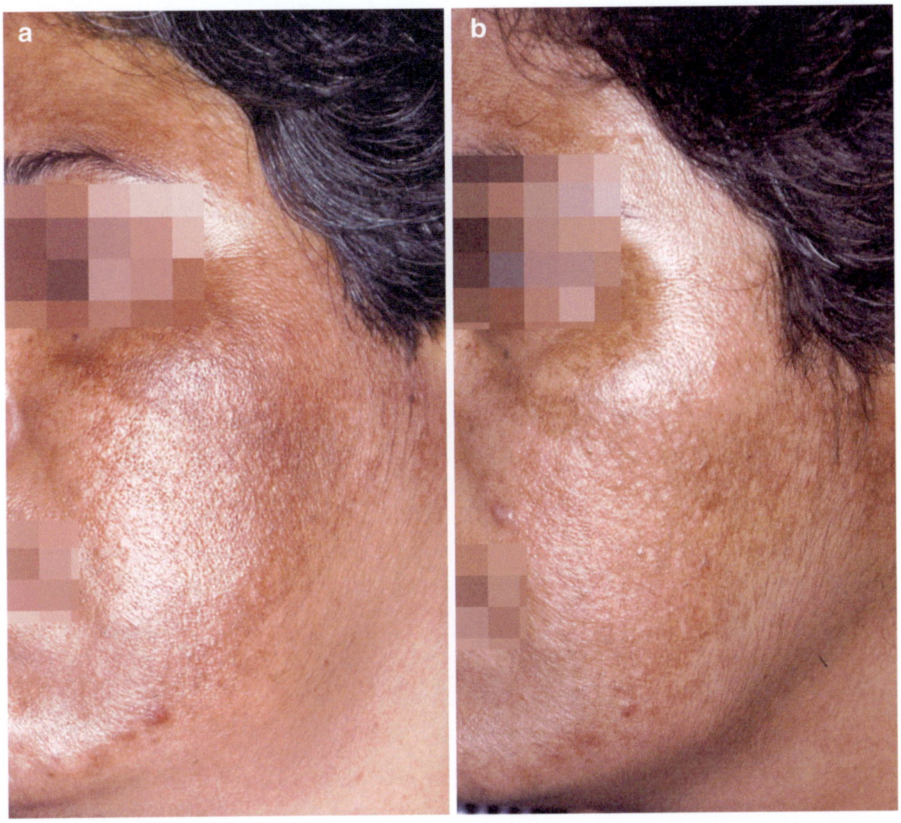

Fig. 3.4 (**a**, **b**) Melasma before and after a series of five salicylic acid peels and 4% hydroquinone

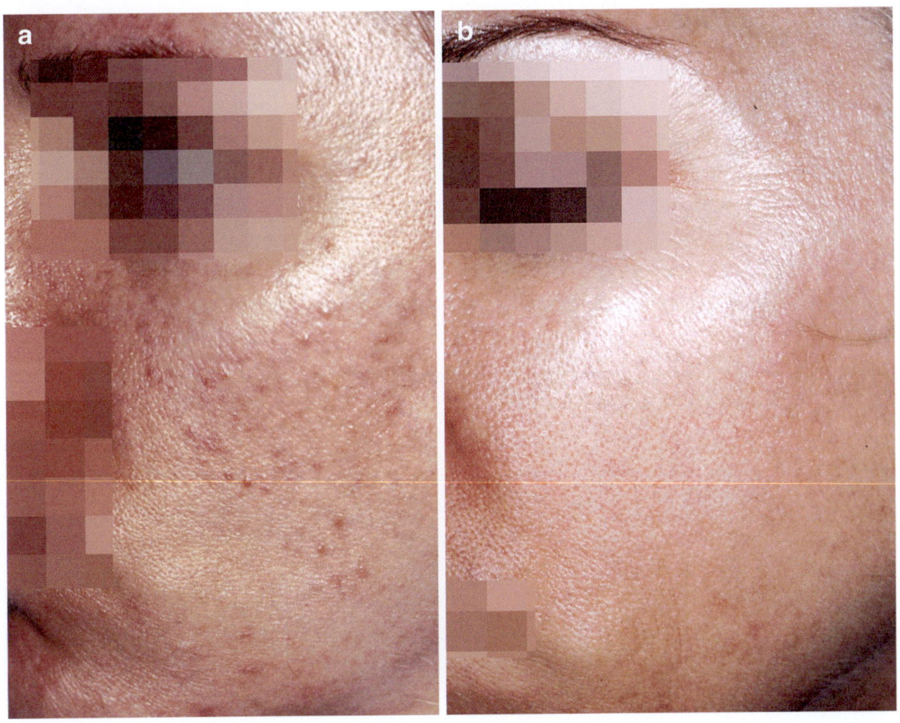

Fig. 3.5 (**a**, **b**) Acne vulgaris before and after four salicylic acid peels

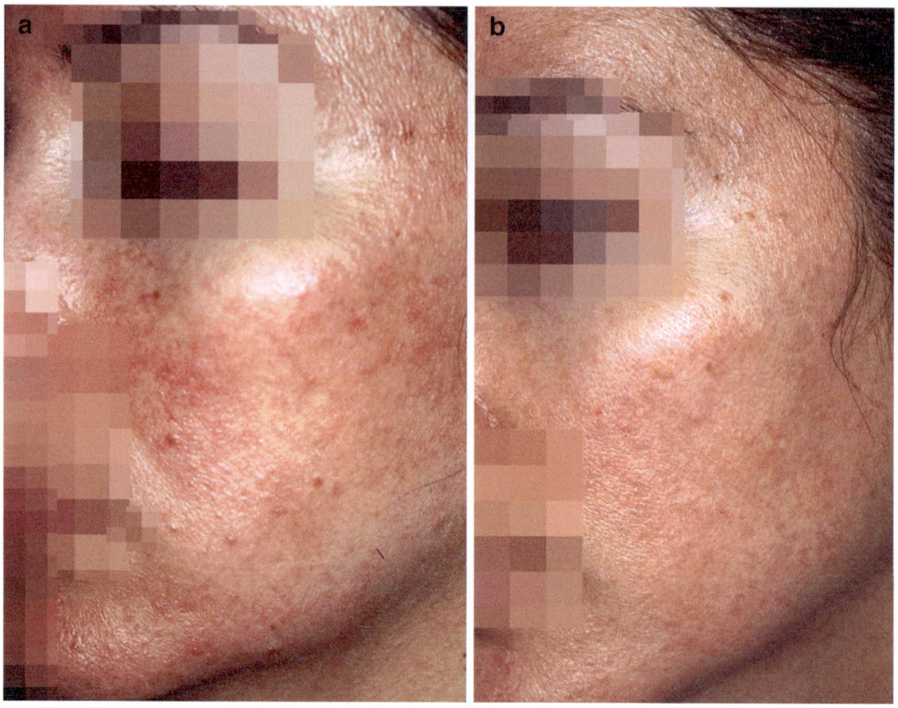

Fig. 3.6 (**a**, **b**) Acne rosacea before and after three salicylic acid peels, moderate improvement

3.9 Advantages

The key benefits of salicylic acid peeling include:

- An established safety profile in patients with skin types I through VI.
- It is an excellent peeling agent in patients with acne vulgaris.
- Given the appearance of the white precipitate, uniformity of application is easily achieved.
- After several minutes, the peel can induce an anesthetic effect whereby increasing patient tolerance.

3.10 Disadvantages

- Limited depth of peeling
- Minimal efficacy in patients with significant photodamage

3.11 Side Effects

Side effects of salicylic acid peeling are mild and transient. In a series of 35 Korean patients, 8.8% had prolonged erythema that lasted more than 2 days [8]. Dryness occurred in 32.3%, responding to frequent applications of moisturizers. Intense exfoliation occurred in 17.6%, clearing in 7–10 days. Crusting was noted in 11.7%. There were no cases of persistent postinflammatory hyperpigmentation or scarring. In a series of 25 patients comprising 20 African Americans and 5 Hispanics, 16% experienced mild side effects [4]. One patient experienced temporary crusting and hypopigmentation which cleared in 7 days. Three patients had transient dryness and hyperpigmentation which resolved in 7–14 days.

Salicylism, or salicylic acid toxicity, is characterized by rapid breathing, tinnitus, hearing loss, dizziness, abdominal cramps, and central nervous system reactions. It has been reported with 20% salicylic acid applied to 50% of the body surface, and it has also been reported with use of 40% and 50% salicylic acid paste preparations [2]. The author has peeled more than 1,000 patients with the current 20% and 30% marketed ethanol formulations and has observed no cases of salicylism.

Patient's Informed Consent

I, ________________, hereby consent to having my ____________ (site) treated with SALICYLIC ACID CHEMICAL PEELING. The peel will be performed to improve the overall appearance of the skin at the site of treatment. Salicylic acid peels are used to improve acne vulgaris, hyperpigmentation (dark spots), rough texture, oily skin, and photodamage (sun damage).

The procedure involves first having the peel site prepped with alcohol, acetone, or other pre-peel cleansing agents. The peeling agent is applied for 3–5 min followed by cleaning with tap water and a bland cleanser.

In general, salicylic acid peels are extremely well tolerated. However, the procedure can cause swelling, redness, crusting, dryness, and obvious peeling of the face which could last for up to 7–10 days.

I understand that there is a small risk of developing permanent darkening after the procedure. There is a rare chance that the peel could cause: undesirable pigment loss at the treated site, or the condition being treated could worsen after the peeling procedure; or a scar could develop. In addition, there is a small chance that a bacterial infection could develop, or the peel could also trigger a flare of a pre-existing Herpetic infection at the treated site. In addition, there have been uncommon cases of allergic reactions to salicylates (the active peel ingredient). The benefits and side effects of the procedure have been explained to me in detail. All of my questions have been answered.

- I am in stable health.
- I have not used isotretinoin in the past 6 months.
- I have no allergies to salicylic acid.
- I am not pregnant.

Outcomes are not guaranteed

_______________________________   ____________

Signature of Patient   Date

____

Patient Name (Please Print)

_______________________________   ____________

Witness   Date

Disclaimer The author has no financial interest in any of the products or equipment mentioned in this chapter.

References

1. Lazo ND, Meine JG, Downing DT (1995) Lipids are covalently attached to rigid corneocyte protein envelope existing predominantly as beta-sheets: a solid state nuclear magnetic resonance study. J Invest Dermatol 105:296–300
2. Swinehart JM (1992) Salicylic acid ointment peeling of the hands and forearms. Effective nonsurgical removal of pigmented lesions and actinic damage. J Dermatol Surg Oncol 18:495–498
3. Aronsohn RB (1984) Hand chemosurgery. Am J Cosmet Surg 1:24–28
4. Kligman D, Kligman AM (1998) Salicylic acid peels for the treatment of photoaging. Dermatol Surg 24:325–328
5. Imayama S, Ueda S, Isoda M (2000) Histologic changes in the skin of hairless mice following peeling with salicylic acid. Arch Dermatol 136:1390–1395

6. Draelos ZD (2000) Atlas of cosmetic dermatology. Churchill Livingstone, New York, pp 94–97
7. Grimes PE (1999) The safety and efficacy of salicylic acid chemical peels in darker racial-ethnic groups. Dermatol Surg 25:18–22
8. Lee HS, Kim IH (2003) Salicylic acid peels for the treatment of acne vulgaris in Asian patients. Dermatol Surg 29:1196–1199
9. Joshi SS, Boone SL, Alam M et al (2009) Effictiveness, safety, and effect on quality of life of topical salicylic acid peels for treatment of postinflammatory hyperpigmentation in dark skin. Dermatol Surg 35:638–644
10. Ahn HH, Kim IH (2006) Whitening effect of salicylic acid peels in Asian patients. Dermatol Surg 32:372–375
11. Kodali S (2010) A prospective, randomized, split-face, controlled trial of salicylic acid peels in the treatment of melasma in Latin American women. J Am Acad Dermatol 63: 1030–1035
12. Oresajo C, Yatskayer M, Hansenne I (2008) Clinical tolerance and efficacy of capryloyl salicylic acid peel compared to a glycolic acid peel in subjects with fine lines/wrinkles and hyperpigmented skin. J Cosmet Dermatol 7:259–262
13. Brody HJ (1997) Chemical peeling, 2nd edn. Mosby, St Louis
14. Bhawan J, Olsen E, Lufrano L, Thorne EG, Schwab B, Gilchrest BA (1996) Histologic evaluation of the long term effects of tretinoin on photodamaged skin. J Dermatol Sci 11:177–182
15. Jimbow K, Obata H, Pathak MA et al (1974) Mechanism of depigmentation by hydroquinone. J Invest Dermatol 62:436–449

Pyruvic Acid

4

Maria Pia De Padova and Antonella Tosti

4.1 History

Pyruvic acid is a carboxylic acid having a keto group at the α position of the aliphatic carbon atom (α-keto acid). Because of its low pKa and its small dimension, it penetrates rapidly and deeply through the skin and is considered a potent chemical peel agent.

Pyruvic acid has keratolytic, antimicrobial, sebostatic properties, and stimulates formation of collagen and elastic fibers.

Sixty percent pyruvic acid in ethanol was first utilized by Griffin, who suggested a combination of 5 cc. of pyruvic acid with eight drops of an emulsifying agent (such as polyethylene laurel ether) and one drop of crotonoil to obtain an epidermolytic inflammatory agent with an effect similar to Baker's phenol formula.

Pyruvic acid is utilized as a medium chemical peeling agent, in concentrations ranging from 40% to 70%. Possible applications include photoaging, pigmentary disorders, active and microcystic acne, and superficial scarring. It is an effective and safe peeling agent.

Pathological studies by Moy et al. showed that the effects of pyruvic acid on the dermis are similar to those of trichloroacetic acid.

4.1.1 Properties

- α-keto-acid (CH_3-CO-COOH)
- Converts physiologically into lactic acid
- Soluble in water and alcohol
- Keratolytic action
- Desmoplastic properties
- Increases collagen, elastic fiber, and glycoprotein production
- Anti-microbial activity
- Sebostatic properties
- Activity related to its concentration, solvent used, and time and number of applications

4.2 Formulations

- 40% pyruvic acid solution/gel
- 50% pyruvic acid solution/gel
- 60% pyruvic acid solution

4.3 Indications

- Active acne, especially microcystic acne (Fig. 4.1, 4.8, 4.9)
- Oily skin
- Mild acne scars
- Flat warts
- Mild to moderate photoaging (Fig. 4.10)
- Rosacea (papulo-pustular)
- Melasma

M.P. De Padova
Ospedale Privato Nigrisoli,
Bologna, Italy
e-mail: mdepadova@gmail.com

A. Tosti (✉)
Department of Dermatology and Cutaneous Surgery,
Miller School of Medicine, University of Miami, US
e-mail: atosti@med.miami.edu

A. Tosti et al. (eds.), *Color Atlas of Chemical Peels*,
DOI 10.1007/978-3-642-20270-4_4, © Springer-Verlag Berlin Heidelberg 2012

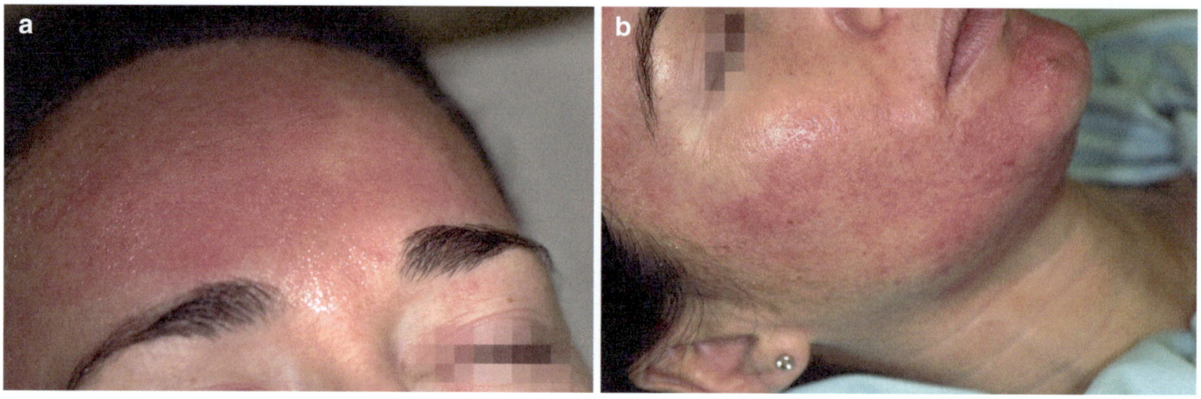

Fig. 4.1 Microcystic acne

4.4 Contraindications

- History of recurrent herpes simplex virus infection
- Autoimmune skin disorders
- Pregnancy
- Isotretinoin treatment in the previous 3 months
- Keloids and hypertrophic scars

4.4.1 Peeling Preparation (Home Treatment)

- Acne, oily skin, and photoaging: prescribe topical products containing 2–3% pyruvic acid, or 5–15% glycolic acid, or1–2% salicylic acid, or 0.05% tretinoin for 3 weeks before the procedure to reduce thickness of the stratum corneum and improve uniform penetration of the pyruvic acid. This treatment should be interrupted 3 days before the procedure.
- Rosacea: prescribe topical products containing 2–3% pyruvic acid, or 1–2% salicylic acid, or 0.05% tretinoin for 3 weeks before the procedure to reduce thickness of the stratum corneum and improve uniform penetration of the pyruvic acid. This treatment should be interrupted 3 days before the procedure. Treatment with topical metronidazole or azelaic acid can be maintained.
- Photoaging and melasma: also add topical bleaching agents (4% topical hydrochinone) to decrease the risk of post-inflammatory hyperpigmentation.

4.5 Peeling Technique (Figs. 4.2–4.7)

- Before peeling the skin should be cleaned with alcohol or acetone to remove the hydrolipidic film and obtain optimal penetration.
- Solution application:
  The modality of application depends on formulation. Liquid formulations are better applied using a fan brush; gel products can be applied with cotton tipped applicators or gloved fingers.
  - Apply the liquid formulation in two to three layers and neutralize with 10% sodium bicarbonate solution when erythema appears. Products with a disposable brush applicator are now available.
  - For gel products a gentle scrub for 1–3 min permits to obtain optimal penetration.
- Apply the solution to small areas and neutralize each area before progressing to the next area.
- A small fan should be used during the application of pyruvic acid to avoid inhaling the vapors.
- Moisturizing creams and sun screens must be applied after the peel.
- Three to five peeling sessions are needed at 3-week intervals.

4.6 Post-peeling Care

- Apply a moisturizing cream containing a sunblock and inform the patient to avoid sun exposure, to wash skin with great gentleness, avoid scrubbing, and to avoid self-prescription of medicines and/or cosmetics.

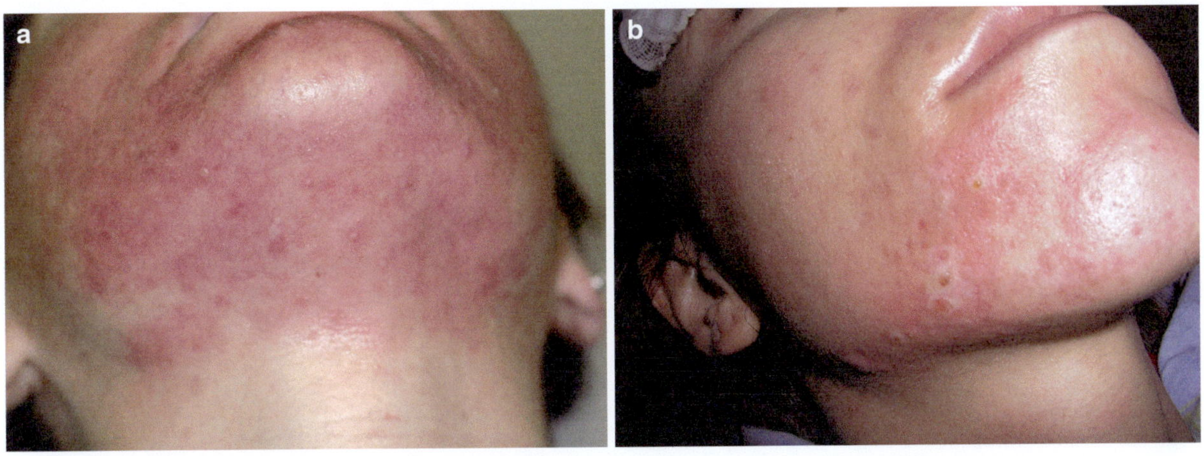

Fig. 4.2 Peeling procedure in a patient with microcystic acne

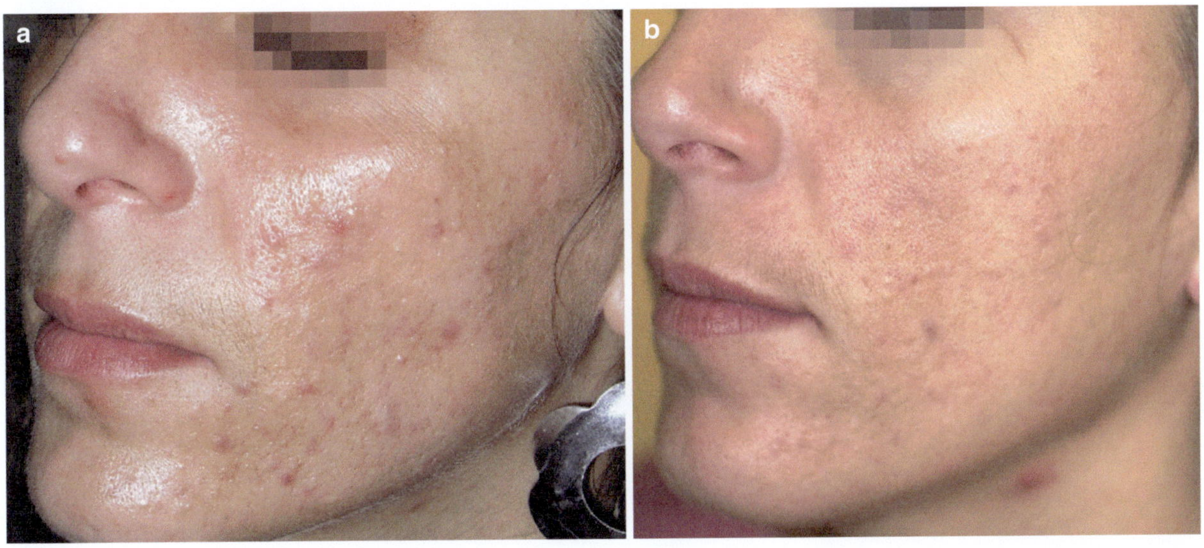

Fig. 4.3 Peeling procedure in a patient with microcystic acne

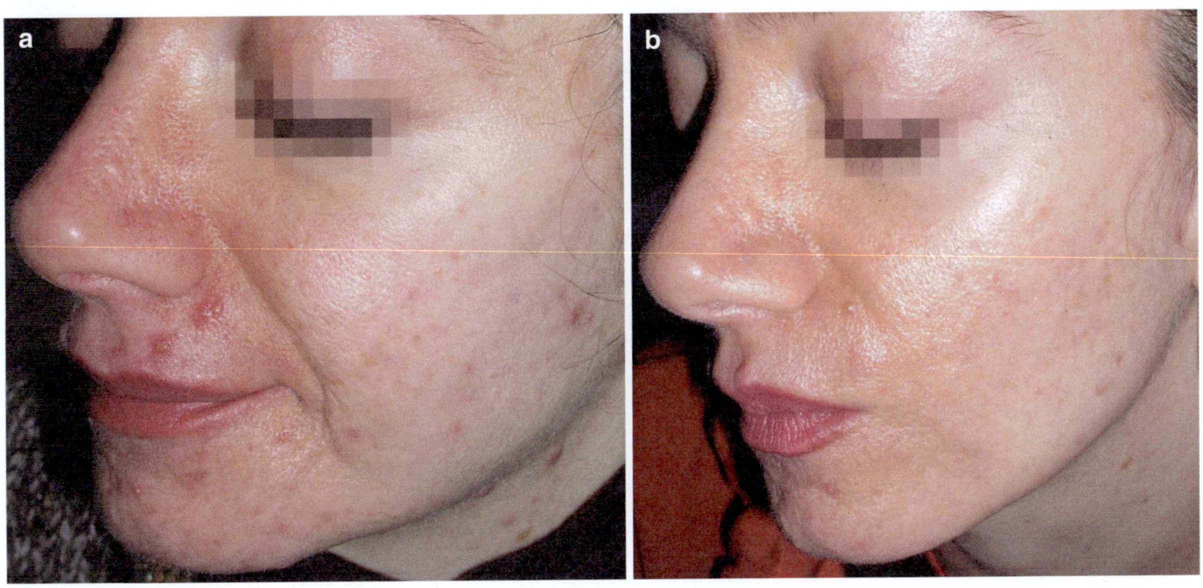

Fig. 4.4 Peeling procedure in a patient with microcystic acne

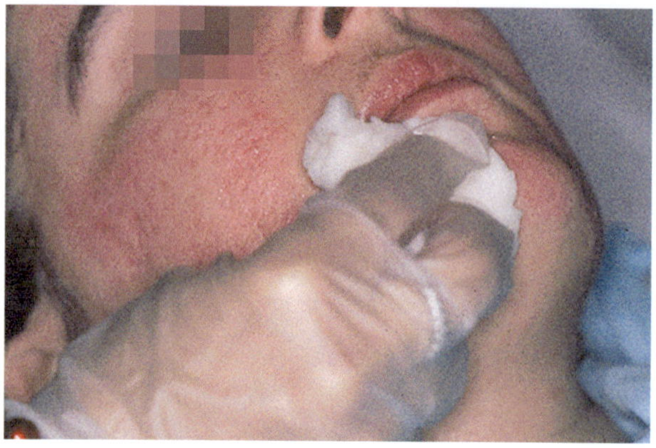

Fig. 4.5 Peeling procedure in a patient with microcystic acne. Note in Fig. 4.5 the neutralization with sodium bicarbonate

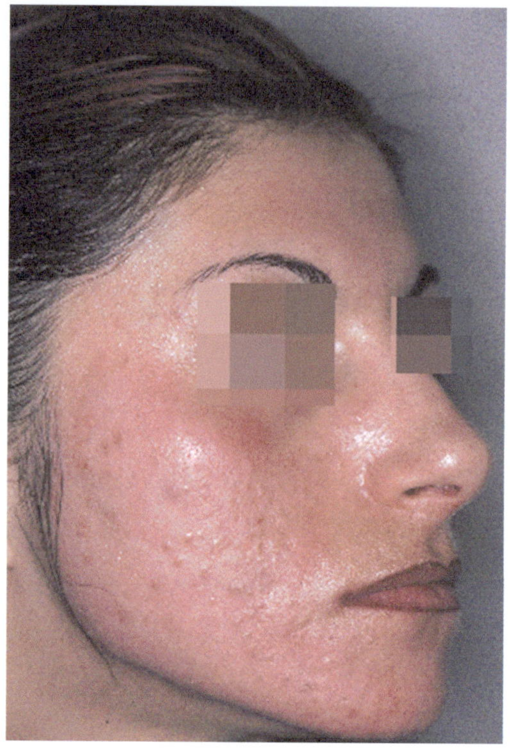

Fig. 4.7 Peeling procedure in a patient with microcystic acne

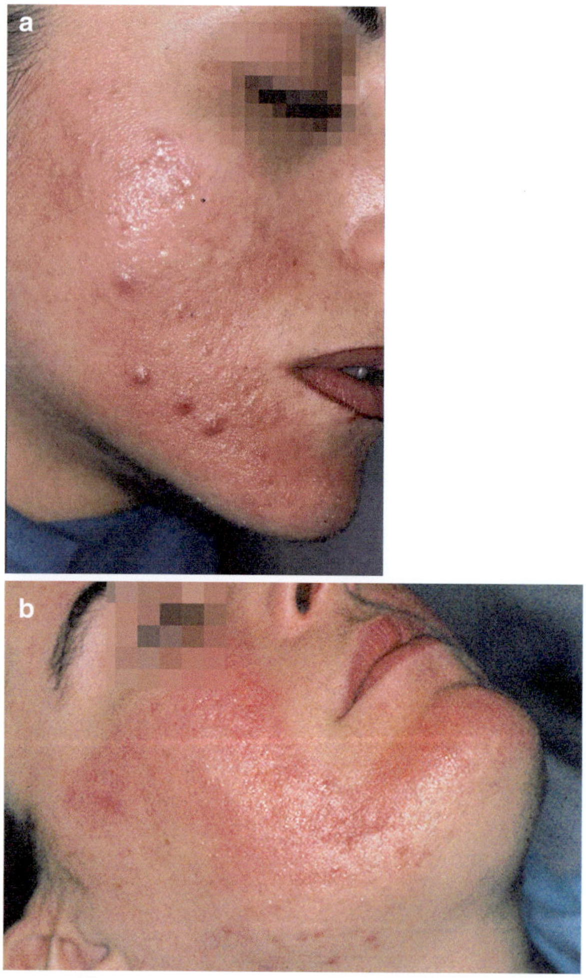

Fig. 4.6 Peeling procedure in a patient with microcystic acne

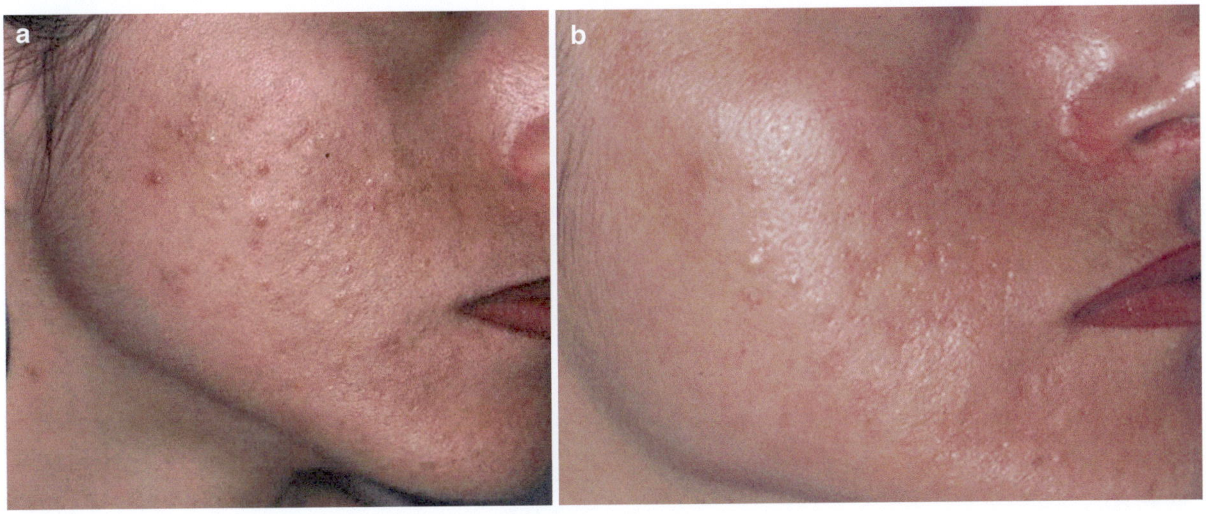

Fig. 4.8 (**a**, **b**) Before and after chemical peeling with 50% pyruvic acid

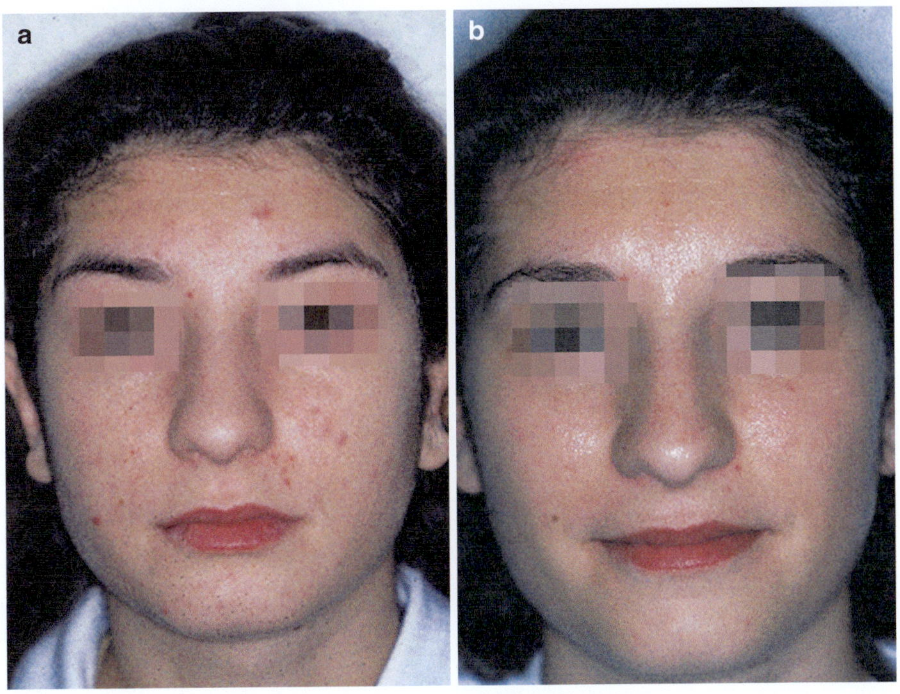

Fig. 4.9 (**a**, **b**) Before and after chemical peeling with 50% pyruvic acid

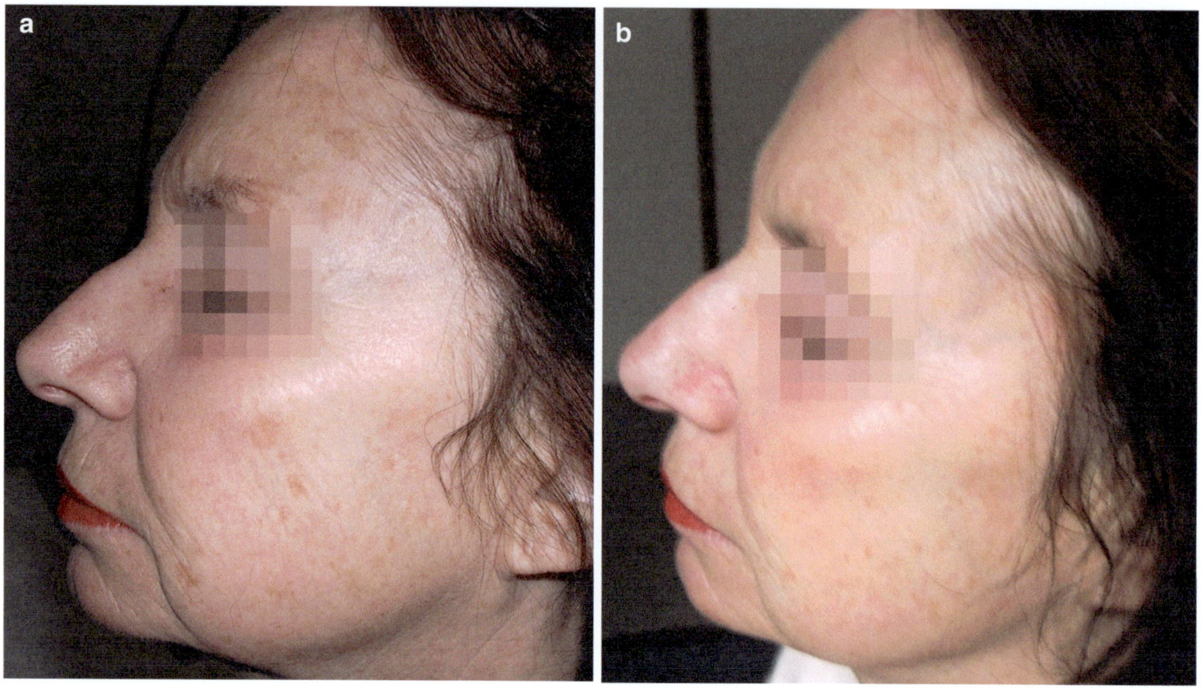

Fig. 4.10 (**a**, **b**) Photodamage with wrinkles and solar lentigo before and after peeling

- When reepithelization is complete the patient can reassume application of topical products to prepare the skin for the next procedure.

4.7 Side Effects

- Crusting in areas of inflamed or thinner skin.

4.8 Advantages

- Very mild erythema.
- Mild desquamation.
- Short post-operative period.
- Can be used in Fitzpatrick skin type III and IV.

4.9 Disadvantages

- Intense stinging and burning sensation during the application.
- Pungent and irritating vapors for the upper respiratory mucosa.

4.10 Results

- Improves skin texture, skin color, fine wrinkles, and reduces hyperpigmented lesions.
- Reduces active acne and rosacea lesions and seborrhea. Accelerates efficacy of topical and systemic acne therapy.
- Reduces pigmentation in patients with melasma.

Patient's Informed Consent

I hereby request and authorize Dr. ____________________, M.D., to have the procedure known as a Pyruvic acid peel. I understand that the peel is not a "cure all" for my skin problems, and I have had the opportunity to ask questions about the risks and benefits of a peel and all my questions have been answered to my satisfaction.

The effect and nature of the treatment to be given, as well as possible alternative methods of treatment, have been fully explained to me.

I acknowledge that during the procedure pyruvic acid in an alcoholic solution will be applied for 1–5 min on my face and that I can experience temporary nasal irritation due to the acid vapor.

I acknowledge that the procedure may cause pain and burning.

I know that my face will become red and subsequently dry and that hyperpigmented skin may occur. Crusts may occur in some areas and must be medicated with topical antibiotics. Exfoliation will then start and last about 5–10 days. An erythema may persist for 15–20 days.

I have been advised that the following conditions may arise after treatment. These conditions are uncommon and usually not serious, but may appear at any time because of circumstances beyond the Doctor's control:

a. A darkening (hyperpigmentation) of the skin or blotchiness may occur at any time up to 3 months following treatment. This is usually due to excess sun or heat exposure. Special medication may be prescribed for this and will usually clear the condition completely. Occasionally, further treatment may be required, consisting of a second procedure. Persons with dark complexions undergoing treatment are advised that a blotchy complexion may arise which will usually even out over a period of 3–6 months.

I have been advised that exposure to sun must be avoided at all costs for a period of 6 months. No sunbathing is permitted for 6 months. To do so would encourage blotchy skin pigmentation requiring further treatment.

You should not have a Pyruvic Peel if you are:

- Pregnant or are trying to become pregnant or breastfeeding
- Affected by a skin condition including but not limited to: psoriasis, systemic lupus erythematosus, active Herpes infection, open sores or bites, non-healing sores, eczema, erysipelas, sun burns, chemical or electrical burns, frostbite, facial surgery in the last 3 months including facelifts or eyelid surgery, or active skin infections.
- Taking or have taken oral isotretinoin in the last 3 months.
- Unwilling to comply with the Pre-Peel or Post-Peel instructions. I understand my identity will be protected.

_____I understand that a cold sore or herpes infection during the healing phase of the peel can cause a severe infection with possible scarring and I have been counseled and/or premedicated to prevent or lessen this possibility.

_____I understand that sun exposure, even a small amount, can have an adverse effect on the outcome of the peel and I will avoid direct sun exposure as long as I can after the peel.

_____I understand to keep my eyes closed during the procedure to prevent accidental spillage of the peeling agent into my eyes. Such an event can cause a severe corneal ulceration and may require treatment by an eye specialist.

_____I understand that there is a risk of bacterial infection after the peel and have been told how to best prevent this.

_____I understand that there is a risk of scarring both from the peeling agent and any resulting infection and how to take steps to prevent this.

_____I understand that some stinging and other sensations will occur during the peel and will last up to several minutes.

_____I understand that there is a chance for an allergic reaction to medications used before or after the peel.

_____I recognize that the practice of medicine and therefore the performance of this procedure is not an exact science, and acknowledge that no guarantees or assurances have been made to me concerning the results of this procedure.

I give my permission that my before and after pictures will be used for:

□ Educational purposes only

□ Patients demonstration

□ Medical congresses and medical articles

The operation has been explained to me and I fully understand the nature of the procedure and the risks involved. I acknowledge and understand that no expressed or implied warranty has been given to me.

Date_________ Signature _____________

Disclaimer The authors have no financial interest in any of the products or equipment mentioned in this chapter.

Bibliography

Berardesca E, Cameli N, Primavera G et al (2006) Clinical and instrumental evaluation of skin improvement after treatment with a new 50% pyruvic acid peel. Dermatol Surg 32(4): 526–531

Cotellessa C, Manunta T, Ghersetich I, Brazzini B, Lotti T, Peris K (2004) The use of pyruvic acid in the treatment of acne. J Eur Acad Dermatol Venereol 18(3):275–278

Fabbrocini G, De Padova MP, Tosti A (2009) Chemical peels: what's new and what isn't new but still works well. Facial Plast Surg 25(5):329–336

Ghersetich I, Brazzini B, Lotti T (2003) Chemical peeling. In: Lotti TM, Katsambas AD (eds) European handbook of dermatological treatments, 2nd edn. Sprinter, Berlin/Heidelberg

Ghersetich I, Brazzini B, Peris K, Cotellessa C, Manunta T, Lotti T (2004) Pyruvic acid peels for the treatment of photoaging. Dermatol Surg 30(1):32–36

Griffin TD, Van Scott EJ (1991) Use of pyruvic acid in the treatment of actinic keratoses: a clinical and histopathologic study. Cutis 47:325–329

Griffin TD, Van Scott EJ, Maddin S (1989) The use of pyruvic acid as a chemical peeling agent. J Dermatol Surg Oncol 15:1316

Halasz CL (1998a) Treatment of warts with topical pyruvic acid: with and without added 5-fluorouracil. Cutis 62(6):283–285

Halasz CL (1998b) Treatment of warts with topical pyruvic acid with and without added 5-fluorouracil. Cutis 62:283–285

Moy LS, Peace S, Moy RL (1996) Comparison of the effect of various chemical peeling agents in a mini pig model. Dermatol Surg 22:429–432

Seitz JC, Whitemore CG (1988) Measurement of erythema and tanning response in human skin using a Tri-Stimulus colorimeter. Dermatologica 177:70–75

Tosson Z, Attwa E, Al-Mokadem S (2006) A pyruvic acid as a new therapeutic peeling agent in acne, melasma, and warts. EDOJ 2(2):7. http://www.edoj.org.eg/vol002/00202/07/01.htm

Trichloroacetic Acid

5

Christopher B. Harmon, Michael Hadley, and Payam Tristani

5.1 History

The use of trichloroacetic acid (TCA) as a peeling agent was first described by German dermatologist P.G. Unna in 1882. Over the past 40 years a number of innovations and applications of the TCA peel have been discovered. These discoveries include a more precise understanding of the exact depth of penetration of these agents and the ensuing histologic changes that occur. Other important advancements have been the use of TCA with a variety of other agents to achieve a deeper peel; these include the use of solid CO_2, Jessner's solution, glycolic acid, and manual dermasanding. More recently there has been promising reports of using higher strength TCA for treatment of deeper acne scarring.

5.2 Chemical Background

TCA occurs naturally as a colorless crystal and is easily formulated by mixture with distilled water. TCA is stable under normal conditions with a melting point of 54°C. It is not light sensitive; however, it is hygroscopic so the crystals should be stored in a closed container to limit its absorption of water. Once mixed, TCA has a shelf life of at least 2 years.

5.3 Chemical Formulations

TCA concentrations are correctly formulated using a weight-in-volume (W/V) method. Simply stated a 30% TCA solution is made by adding 30 g of TCA with enough water to make 100 mL solution. This should not be mistaken by adding 30 g to 100 mL of water thus yielding a weaker concentration. Other methods including a weight-in-weight formulation, used in topical ointments and creams, is not accurate. Also, dilution of existing TCA with water should not be employed as the resulting concentration is higher than one would expect. TCA is readily obtained in a number of concentrations from suppliers such as Delasco who specialize in its production.

Recently there have been a variety of suppliers with chemical peel kits claiming ease of use and increased efficacy. These proprietary kits vary from the vehicle used in delivering the TCA to having color indicators to inform the physician of a peel's completion. Caution should be used when using such kits as many times the physician loses the ability to easily assess the degree of frosting and in turn the depth and safety of the chemical peel.

5.4 Classification of Peel Depths

TCA is a chemical cauterant the application of which to the skin causes protein denaturation, so-called keratocoagulation, resulting in a readily observed white

C.B. Harmon (✉)
Department of Dermatology, University of Alabama at Birmingham, Birmingham, AL, USA
e-mail: charmon887@pol.net

M. Hadley • P. Tristani
University of Utah, Department of Dermatology, 4B454 School of Medicine, 30N 1900E Salt Lake City, UT 84132, USA

A. Tosti et al. (eds.), *Color Atlas of Chemical Peels*,
DOI 10.1007/978-3-642-20270-4_5, © Springer-Verlag Berlin Heidelberg 2012

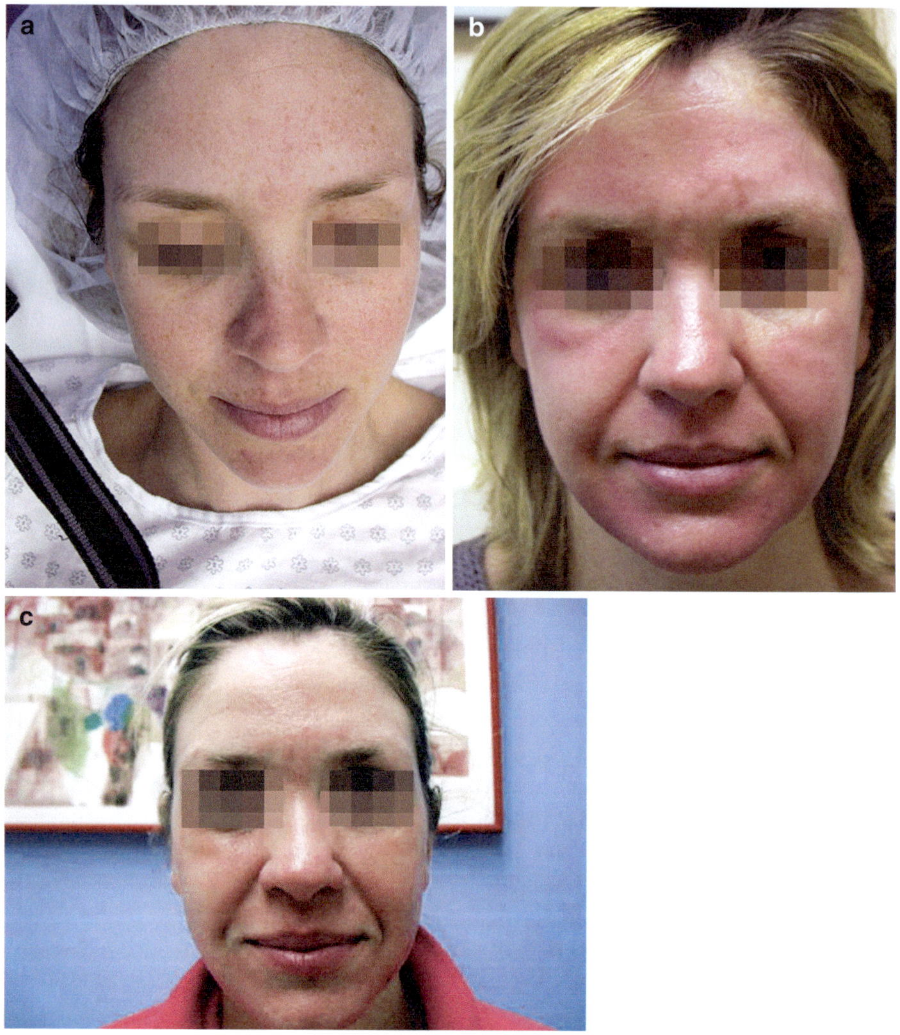

Fig. 5.1 (a–c) Medium depth chemical peel for widespread lentigines in type II skin. (a) Pre-operative, (b) 10 days status post medium-depth chemical peel, (c) 1 month status post medium-depth chemical peel

frost. The degree of tissue penetration and ensuing injury by a TCA solution is dependent on several factors, including strength of TCA used, skin preparation, and anatomic site.

Selection of appropriate strength TCA is critical when performing a peel. TCA in strengths of 10–20% results in a very light superficial peel not penetrating below the stratum granulosum; a strength of 25–35% results in a light superficial peel with penetration encompassing the full thickness of the epidermis; 40–50% results in a medium-depth peel injury to the papillary dermis; and finally, greater than 50% results in injury extending to the reticular dermis. Unfortunately the use of TCA concentrations above 35% TCA can produce unpredictable results including scarring. Therefore, the medium-depth chemical peel should only be obtained with the combination of 35% TCA and another agent such as Jessner's solution, solid CO_2, or glycolic acid. The use of TCA in strengths greater than 35% should be discouraged with the exception of deliberate destruction of isolated lesions or where intentional controlled scarring is desired such as the treatment of ice-pick scars (Fig. 5.1).

5.5 Indications

The use of TCA as a peeling agent has a wide variety of applications depending on the concentration used (Fig. 5.2). The most important principal in determining response to a peeling agent is accurately assessing the

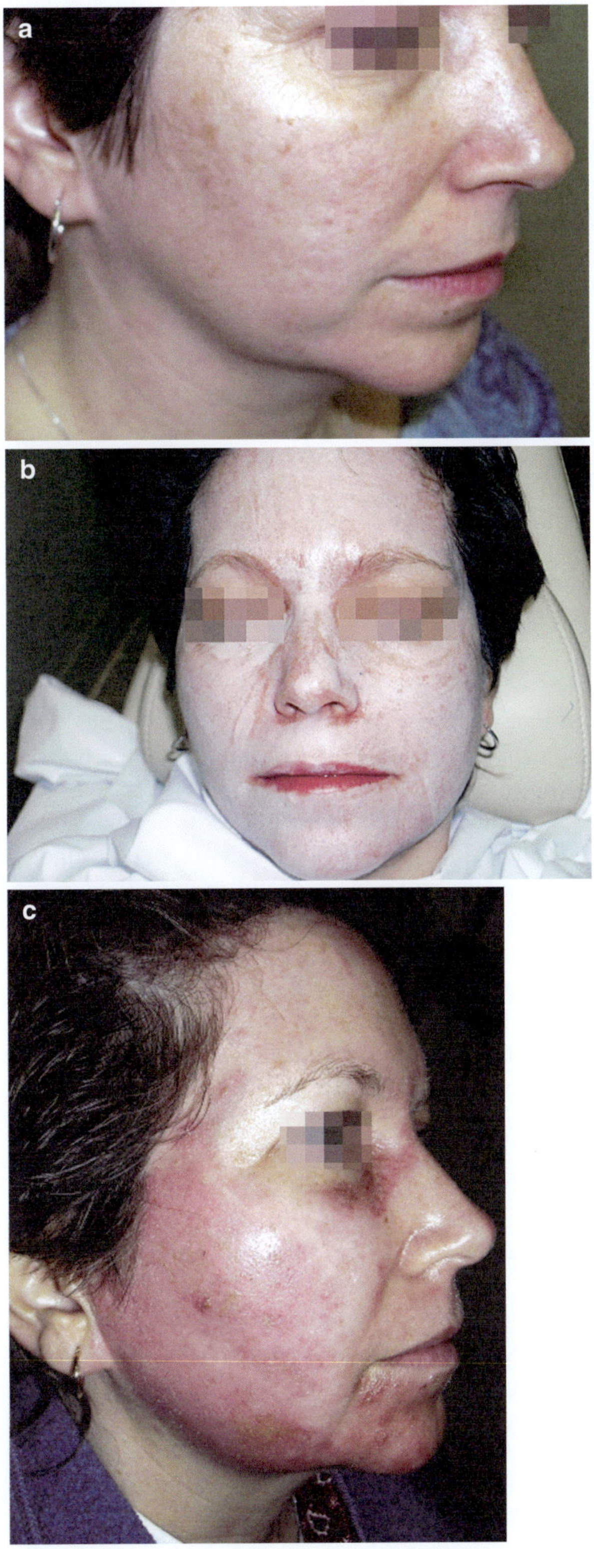

Fig. 5.2 (**a**, **b**) Medium depth chemical peel for melasma. (**a**) Pre-operative, (**b**) intraoperative – Level III frosting

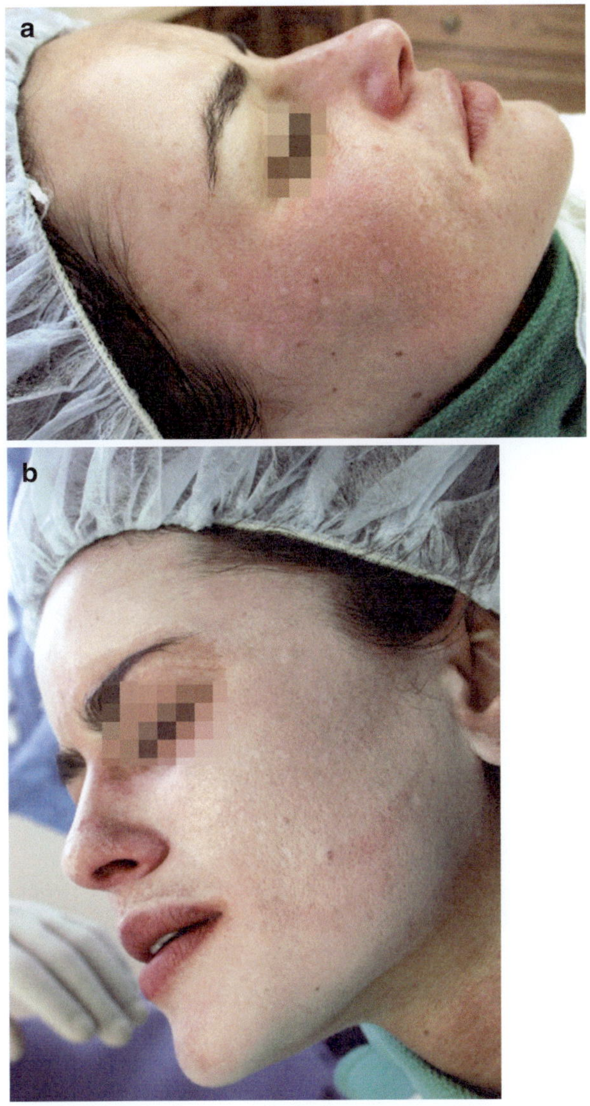

Fig. 5.3 (**a**, **b**) Medium depth chemical peel for melasma. (**a**) Pre-operative, (**b**) intraoperative – Level III frosting

depth of the condition for which treatment is intended. This principal applies to the depth of skin growths, pigmentation, and degree of wrinkling. Superficial conditions such as epidermal melasma and actinic keratoses are readily treated with chemical peeling and may only require a superficial peeling agent, whereas deeper conditions such as dermal melasma and severe wrinkling may prove difficult if not impossible to treat despite using a deeper peeling agent (Fig. 5.3). As a general rule a higher concentration TCA results in deeper penetration yielding a more thorough and longer-lasting treatment; this of course must be balanced with

Table 5.1 Indications

Indications
Epidermal growths including actinic keratoses and thin seborrheic keratoses
Mild to moderate photoaging
Pigmentary dyschromias including melasma and post-inflammatory hyperpigmentation
Pigmented lesions including lentigines and ephelides
Acne
Acne scarring

Table 5.2 Efficacy of treatment

Efficacy of treatment
Excellent to good response
Actinic keratoses
Superficial melasma
Superficial hyperpigmentation
Ephelides
Lentigines
Depressed scars (CROSS technique)
Variable response
Seborrheic keratoses
Hypertrophic keratoses
Mixed melasma
Mixed hyperpigmentation
Poor response
Thick seborrheic keratoses
Deep melasma
Deep hyperpigmentation

the lengthened downtime associated with a deeper peel. Multiple superficial chemical peels generally do not equal the efficacy of a single medium-depth peel. Still, not all conditions need to be treated with a deeper chemical peel as consideration must be given to what type of condition is being treated and most importantly what the patient's goals and tolerance are for the prescribed peel (Table 5.1).

Epidermal growths such as actinic keratosis, lentigines, or thin seborrheic keratoses can all be treated effectively with 25–35% TCA peels. Thicker epidermal growths or growths involving the dermis will be more resistant to treatment such as hypertrophic actinic keratoses and thicker seborrheic keratoses and may even be resistant to a medium-depth peel. Resistant lesions many times are best treated with a combination of a medium-depth chemical peel and other modalities such as manual dermasanding or CO_2 laser (Table 5.2).

Mild to moderate photoaging can be effectively treated with TCA peels. Mild photoaging as defined by the Glogau classification as type 1 include mild pigmentary alterations and minimal wrinkles. Often a superficial TCA peel 10–25% will be all that is necessary to make improvements with mild photoaging; this is especially true if multiple superficial peels are employed at regular intervals of 3–6 weeks. Moderate photoaging defined by Glogau as type II improves minimally with a superficial chemical peel, but can be improved with a deeper peel such as a medium-depth peel. This is truer for the pigmentary changes versus the wrinkles. While some pigmentary improvements can be made with a medium-depth peel in the advanced aging seen in Glogau types III and IV, often these individuals require a deeper peel (phenol), laser resurfacing, or a face lift to deal with the profound wrinkling encountered.

Pigmentary dyschromias can be effectively treated with chemical peeling. This can include ephelides, epidermal melasma, lentigines, and epidermal hyperpigmentation. Many times repetitive superficial peels are sufficient to deal with these conditions; however, single medium-depth peels are an important tool to utilize, particularly if there is a deeper pigmentary component. Often times a Wood's lamp can prove invaluable in assessing pigmentary levels as epidermal pigmentation is accentuated. The deeper the pigment extends into the dermis the more the effectiveness of chemical peeling diminishes. Other treatment modalities including Q switched Nd:YAG or Alexandrite lasers might prove more useful in conditions where pigment is below the papillary dermis.

One caveat in treating post-inflammatory hyperpigmentation is taking care in not being too aggressive with a peeling regimen. A medium-depth peel may produce more inflammation and a resultant worsening of hyperpigmentation in susceptible individuals. This is especially true in patients with Fitzpatrick skin types 3–6. It is better to start out with multiple superficial chemical peels in combination with bleaching agents before proceeding too soon to a medium-depth chemical peel.

The use of high-strength TCA (65–100%) for acne scarring has proven to be an exciting new application of TCA. In this technique chemical reconstruction of skin scars (CROSS technique) showed significant improvement. Specifically high-concentration TCA is focally applied to depressed or ice-pick scars and pressed hard with the wooden end of a cotton tip applicator. This induces a localized scar to occur, which over time effaces the depressed scar. Typically this requires five or six courses of treatment spread out over intervals of weeks to months.

5.6 Facial Versus Non-facial Skin

Another critical consideration when performing a peel is realizing the difference of peeling facial versus non-facial skin. As a rule non-facial skin takes much longer to heal and is at much greater risk of scarring than when using a similar concentration on the face. This is due to the higher concentration of pilosebaceous units on the face compared with non-facial sites. These units play a critical role in reepithelialization. As a result if a peel is performed on non-facial skin such as the arms, upper chest, and lower neck, one should proceed cautiously and not attempt concentrations greater than 25% TCA. Beyond the poor wound healing and higher risk of scarring, another major limitation of chemical peeling off of the face is lack of efficacy in comparison with facial peels. The remainder of this chapter is limited to peeling facial skin.

5.7 Peeling Preparation

Proper skin preparation prior to TCA peels is not only a critical component of the peeling process, but is also important in avoiding post-peel complications such as post-inflammatory hyperpigmentation. The following adjunctive agents should ideally be started 6 weeks prior to peeling. It is important for patients to fully understand the role of these agents for priming of the skin:

- Broad spectrum UVA and UVB sunscreens
- Tretinoin 0.05–0.1%, which is the most critical component of this regimen as it results in decreased stratum corneum thickness, increases the kinetics of epidermal turnover, and decreases corneocyte adhesion
- Exfoliants such as glycolic acid or lactic acid result in decreased corneocyte adhesion and stimulate epidermal growth by disrupting the stratum corneum
- Bleaching products such as hydroquinone 4–8% are particularly useful in patients with dyschromias and in patients with Fitzpatrick skin types III–VI

5.8 Peeling Technique

As with any other chemical peeling procedure, the art and science of TCA chemical peels is dependent on the proper peeling technique. TCA is a versatile peeling agent, and depending on its concentration can be used for superficial, medium, or deep chemical peels. However, the cleaning and peeling technique is essentially the same for each depth. In general for the superficial peels patients do not require any sedation; however, for medium-depth peels, a mild sedative such as diazepam 5–10 mg p.o. or ativan 0.25–0.5 mg p.o. may be used. The patient should be comfortably positioned with the head at a 30–45° angle. A topical anesthetic such as 4% lidocaine may be used prior to application of the TCA to reduce patient discomfort with burning and stinging.

Prior to the application of TCA, a thorough cleaning is of vital importance for defatting the skin to allow for even penetration of the peeling solution. The skin is first cleaned with either Hibiclens or Septisol. Subsequently either acetone or alcohol is used to remove the residual oils and scale until the skin feels dry.

After thorough cleaning, TCA is applied, using either two to four cotton-tipped applicators or folded 2×2 gauze in a predetermined sequential manner, starting from the forehead, to temples, cheeks, lips, and finally to the eyelids. It is imperative that following application to each area, the physician observes not only the degree of frosting, but also the duration to this reaction before proceeding to the next area. If the desired level of frosting is not reached within 2–3 min, an additional application of the agent should be performed. Care must be taken not to overcoat TCA as each application will result in greater depth of penetration. Patients experience a burning sensation, particularly with the higher concentrations of TCA.

If a Jessner's-35% TCA peel (Monheit) is performed, Jessner's solution is applied first prior to the TCA in an even sequential fashion from the forehead to the rest of the face, waiting 2–3 min to allow for penetration and assessment of frost. Typically this will produce a level 1 frost, erythema with faint reticulate whitening (see below). An additional one or two coats of Jessner's may be applied if a level 1 frost is not obtained. Patience must be practiced before proceeding to the application of TCA, as the physician might perform a more aggressive peel than intended if they had waited the proper time to evaluate the degree of frosting produced by the application of the chemical. Always be mindful of this lag effect.

As noted previously, TCA results in keratocoagulation or protein denaturation which is manifested by frosting of the skin. As the extent of frosting appears to correlate with the depth of penetration of

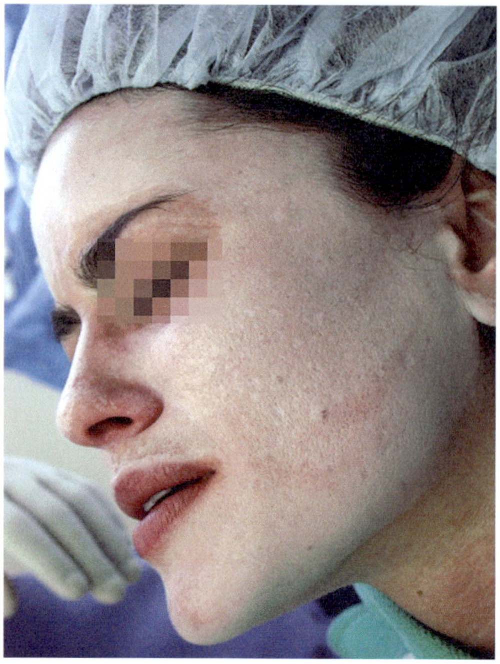

Fig. 5.4 Level II frosting

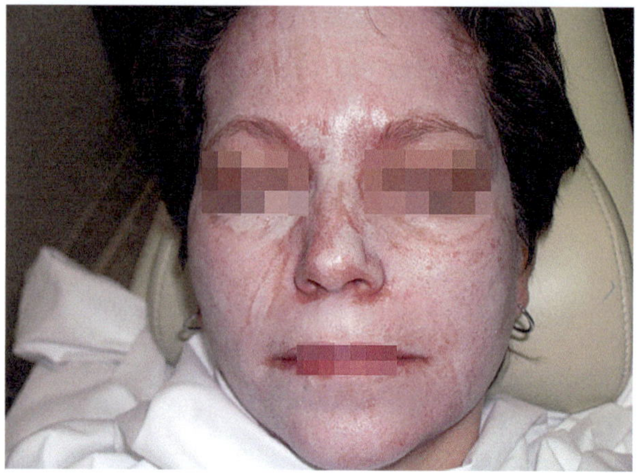

Fig. 5.5 Level III frosting

TCA, the following classification can be used as a general guideline for TCA peels. It is imperative to keep in mind, however, that the results are dependent on multiple factors including type/thickness of skin, priming of skin, and technique of application of the TCA:

- Level 1: Erythema with blotchy or wispy areas of white frosting. This indicates a superficial epidermal peel as can be achieved with TCA concentrations <30%. This peel will result in light flaking lasting 2–4 days.
- Level 2: White frosting with areas of erythema showing through. This level of peel is indicative of a full-thickness epidermal peel to the papillary dermis and can be achieved with TCA concentration of >30%.This peel will result in full exfoliation of the epidermis (Fig. 5.4).
- Level 3: Solid white frosting with no erythema. This is indicative of penetration of TCA through the papillary dermis and can also be achieved with TCA concentrations >30%, depending on the number of applications (Fig. 5.5).

TCA in concentrations of 10–25% can be used safely for superficial depth peels and in concentrations >30% can be used for medium-depth peels. However, multiple coats of even the lower concentrations of TCA can result in a deeper penetration of this agent, thus essentially resulting in a medium-depth peel. In general, use of TCA in concentrations >40% is not recommended as it results in uneven depth of penetration and a greater risk of scarring and pigmentary dyschromias.

Several areas of the face require particular consideration. Care must be taken in the periorbital area to prevent any excess TCA solution from rolling into the eye, and as such TCA should not be applied to the upper eyelid. If tearing occurs, this can be gently wicked using a cotton-tipped applicator. With areas of deeper rhytides such as in the perioral area, the wrinkled skin should be stretched and the TCA applied over the folds. In addition, TCA should be applied evenly over the lip skin to the vermillion.

Once the desired frost is achieved, the skin can be rinsed off with water, or cooled down with cool wet compresses which are applied to the skin. The wet compresses can provide a welcome relief to the burning induced by the peel. Unlike glycolic peels the water does not neutralize the peel, as the frosting indicates the end-point of the reaction; rather, it dilutes any excess TCA. The compresses can be repeated several times until the burning sensation has subsided. Subsequently, a layer of ointment such as plain petrolatum or Aquaphor is applied and post-peel instructions and what to expect are reviewed with the patient prior to discharge to home.

5.9 Post-peeling Care

Patients should be counseled with the typical phases of wound healing post peeling. With superficial TCA peels, there may be mild to moderate erythema with fine flaking of the skin, lasting up to 4 days. Some patients may experience mild edema as well. With medium-depth TCA peels, patients should be advised that the peeled skin will feel and look tight. Preexisting pigmented lesions will darken considerably, and appear grayish to brown. There is also a varying degree of erythema and edema. Edema may last several days (peaks at 48 h) and patients should elevate their head while sleeping. Frank desquamation typically begins by the third day and is accompanied by serous exudation. Reepithelialization is usually complete by the 7th to 10th day, at which time the skin appears pink.

Following the chemical peel, patients are advised to wash their skin gently twice daily with a mild nondetergent cleanser. Acetic acid soaks (0.25%, one tablespoon of white vinegar in one pint of warm water) are performed up to four times per day, and have antiseptic as well as debriding properties. In addition, a bland emollient such as plain petrolatum is applied to prevent dryness of skin and formation of crust. The patient must be advised not to vigorously rub their skin or pick at the desquamating skin, as this can lead to scarring. If patients complain of pruritus and are at risk for scratching, a mild topical steroid such as 1% hydrocortisone can be recommended. Once reepithelialization is complete, patients can use a moisturizing cream instead of the occlusive emollient. Long-term care following TCA peels is essentially the same as pre-peel priming regimen and includes use of broad-spectrum sunscreens, bleaching creams, tretinoin, or vitamin C, in combination with an exfoliating agent such as alpha-hydroxy acid. Patients should be advised that the post-peel regimen is necessary to maintain the benefits gained from the peel. Although superficial TCA peels can be repeated every 4–6 weeks, medium-depth chemical peels should not be repeated for a period of 6 months, until the phases of healing are completed.

5.10 Complications

It is of paramount importance that the dermatologic surgeon be familiar with the complications of TCA peels. These include infections (bacterial, viral, fungal), pigmentary changes, prolonged erythema, milia, acne, textural changes, and scarring. Bacterial infections include *Pseudomonas*, *Staphylococcus*, or *Streptococcus*. In general, prophylaxis with antibiotics is not indicated and strict adherence to wound care instructions will prevent this untoward complication. In patients with a history of herpes labialis, even if remote, prophylaxis with antiviral agent is necessary. Scarring is a rare, yet feared, complication of medium-depth chemical peels. Although the etiology of scarring is unknown, factors which are contributory include poor wound care, infections, uneven peeling depth, mechanical injury, and previous history of ablative procedures. Localized areas of prolonged erythema, particularly on the angle of the jaw, can be indicative of incipient scarring. Proper attention to risk factor, use of mild topical steroids for localized areas of erythema, and proper wound care and infection prophylaxis can minimize the risk of scarring. If scarring is imminent, use of higher-strength steroids (class I to II), silicone gel and/or sheaths, and pulsed-dye lasers may be beneficial. Prolonged erythema may be secondary to underlying rosacea, eczema, or use of tretinoin. Use of a mild topical steroid such as 2.5% hydrocortisone lotion is likely beneficial. Milia formation is most likely due to over occlusion and can be minimized with the use of less occlusive emollients after reepithelialization. As noted previously, use of sunscreens, bleaching agents, and tretinoin can minimize pigmentary changes which can develop post peeling.

5.11 Advantages/Disadvantages of TCA Peels

TCA peels confer several advantages for both the patient and physician. TCA is an inexpensive solution that can be easily prepared, is stable, and has a long shelf life. TCA, as opposed to peels such as Baker's phenol, does not have any systemic toxicity. In addition, as noted previously, it is a versatile agent that can be used for superficial, medium, and deep chemical peeling. The frosting reaction can be utilized as a reliable indicator for the depth of the chemical peel, making this a safe agent in the hands of the experienced dermatologist. However, TCA in concentrations >40% has an unreliable penetration depth and can result in scarring.

5.12 Conclusion

TCA is the most versatile of all the peeling agents and can be effectively used to perform superficial to medium-depth chemical peels in the treatment of a variety conditions ranging from pigmentary dyschromias to moderate photoaging. A proper understanding of the correct techniques, indications, limitations, and complications is paramount before using TCA. When performed properly, peeling with TCA can be one of the most rewarding procedures we can do for our patients.

Disclaimer The author has no financial interest in any of the products or equipment mentioned in this chapter.

Bibliography

Brody HJ (2001) Complications of chemical resurfacing. Dermatol Clin 3:427–437

Koppel RA, Coleman KM, Coleman WP (2000) The efficacy of EMLA versus ELA-Max for pain relief in medium-depth chemical peeling: a clinical and histopathologic evaluation. Dermatol Surg 26:61–64

Monheit GD (1996) Skin preparation: an essential step before chemical peeling or laser resurfacing. Cosmet Dermatol 9:9–14

Monheit GD (2001) Medium-depth chemical peels. Dermatol Clin 3:413–525

Rubin MG (1995) Manual of chemical peel: superficial and medium depth. Lippincott, Philadelphia

Deep Chemical Peels (Phenol) 6

Marina Landau

6.1 History

Since deep chemical peels are based on phenol-containing solutions, it seems that the history of this procedure starts at the moment of carbolic acid discovery in 1834 by the German chemist Friedlieb Ferdinand Runge. The name phenol had been coined in 1841 by Charles Frederick Gerhardt. Nowadays, phenol is prepared synthetically in a process that utilizes chlorobenzene as a starting point.

One hundred years ago, a New York dermatologist, chairman of New York Dermatology and Syphilology Center, George Miller MacKee began using phenol peeling at this prestigious institution. Together with his colleague, lady dermatologist Florentine L. Karp, he published their experience with 540 treatments over a 10-year period with phenol peels for post-acne scarring [1]. Among other contributors to the development of phenol-based peels at that time were Bames [2], Urkov [3], Combes and Sperber [4], Brown [5], Litton [6], etc.

Most of the credit of phenol-based peels during the late 1940s and early 1950s is attributed to lay operators. Their illegal work was probably one of the reasons for rejection and skepticism related to the procedure by medical profession in those years.

The main role in the final revival of deep chemical peeling was played by two American plastic surgeons Thomas J. Baker and Howard L. Gordon, who during 1960s medically legitimated this procedure by discussing it in national meetings and demonstrating their impressive results [7, 8].

Since then, numerous other authors, such as Stone [9], Spira [10], Hetter [11], Fintsi [12], contributed to the procedure to emerge from semiobscurity to its respectable and valued place in the field of esthetic surgery.

6.2 Chemical Background

Following the fundamental work by Gregory Hetter [11], it is now commonly accepted that in the "heart" of solutions for deep peeling is a combination of croton oil and phenol.

Phenol (C5H5OH) or carbolic acid is an aromatic hydrocarbon derived originally from coal tar, but prepared synthetically in a process that utilizes monochlorobenzene as a starting point. Ninety-eight percent phenol appears as transparent crystals, while liquefied phenol consists of 88% USP solution of phenol in water.

Other chemicals such as hydroquinone and resorcinol, widely used in cosmetic dermatology, share similar chemical structure with phenol (Fig. 6.1).

Croton oil is an extract of the seed of the plant *Croton tiglium* and has been commercially prepared as Croton resin since 1932. Its activity on the skin is related to free hydroxyl groups which cause skin vesiculation even in low doses.

Other chemicals in use in deep chemical peel formulas include septisol, water, vegetable oils (glycerin, olive, sesame).

M. Landau
Wolfson Medical Center,
56 Joshua Ben Nun Street,
Herzlia Pituach, 46763 Holon, Israel
e-mail: mlandau@zahav.net.il

A. Tosti et al. (eds.), *Color Atlas of Chemical Peels*,
DOI 10.1007/978-3-642-20270-4_6,

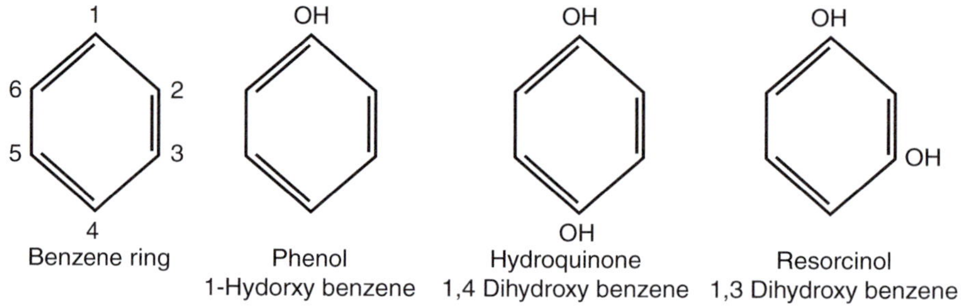

Fig. 6.1 Formulas of common benzene ring components

6.3 Formulations

All the modern phenol formulas are based and modified from a few lay peelers' formulations. Names such as Grade, Coopersmith, Kelsen, and Maschek are the origins of Baker-Gordon's, Brown's, Hetter's, Stone's, Litton's, Exoderm, and other formulas. All of them are based on the aforementioned chemical components in different concentrations (Fig. 6.2). Concentration of phenol ranges between 45% and 80% (Fig. 6.3), while concentration of croton oil is between 0.16% and 2.05% (Fig. 6.4). It is generally accepted that the role of liquid soap is to reduce the skin surface tension and to improve solution penetration. In spite of this, septisol is not included in all of the formulas. Some of the formulas contain oils. The role of the oils in the formula has not being clarified yet. Our personal experience shows that oily phenol solution penetrates the skin in more slow and controllable fashion.

So far, no controlled study has been conducted to compare clinically and histologically between the various peeling formulations. However, few ideas regarding phenol-based peeling solutions have been challenged recently. The concept of "all-or-none" effect of phenol on the skin was confronted by Gregory Hetter [11], who showed that minute amount of croton oil deepens the penetration, prolongs healing period, and improves clinical outcome of the peeling. Deeper peel can be achieved by using higher concentrations of phenol, or croton oil, or multiple applications of the solution [13].

Baker-Gordon's formula	
Phenol, USP, 88%	3 mL
Tap or distilled water	2 mL
Septisol liquid soap	8 drops
Croton oil	3 drops

Brown's formula	
Phenol	60–95%
Saponated cresol	0.3%
Olive or sesame oil	0.25%
Distilled water	ad 100%

Venner-Kellson's formula	
Concentrated Lysol	1.0 oz
Olive oil	0.5 oz
Distilled water	1.5 oz
Croton oil	10 drops
Melted losses phenol crystals	8 oz

Litton's formula	
Phenol crystals	1lb
Distilled water	8 cc
Glycerine	8 cc
Liquified phenol	4 oz
Croton oil	1 cc
Distilled water	4 oz

Fig. 6.2 Various phenol-containing formulas

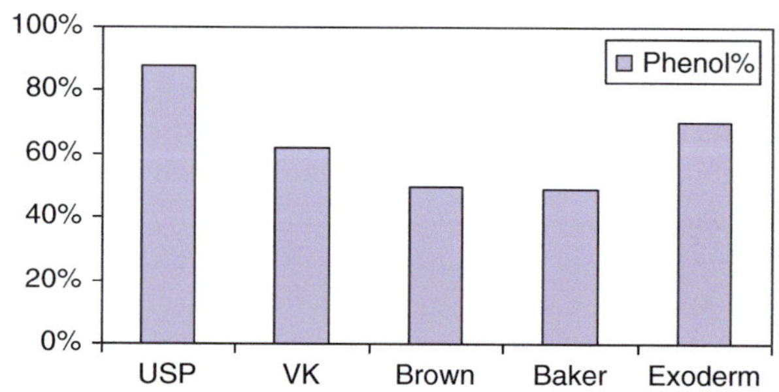

Fig. 6.3 Phenol content in various peeling solutions (*VK* Venner-Kellson)

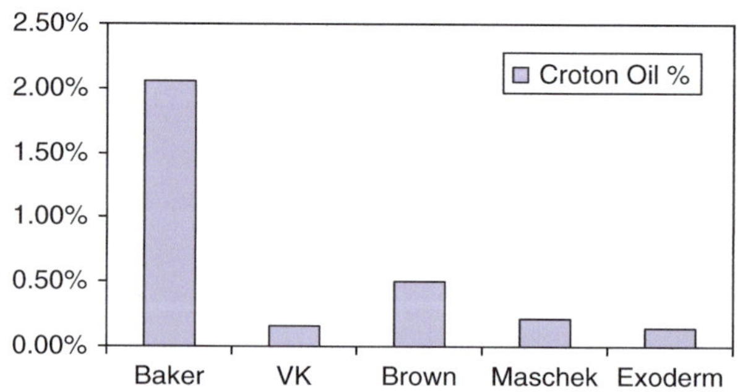

Fig. 6.4 Croton oil content in various peeling solutions (*VK* Venner-Kellson)

6.4 Histology

Biopsies obtained 48 after phenol peeling demonstrate necrosis of the epidermis, extending through the papillary dermis, surrounded by a marked inflammatory reaction [6]. Epidermal regeneration is completed within 7 days, while dermal healing usually lags behind. Histological changes in human skin induced by deep chemical peeling include newly formed band of dermis found directly beneath the epidermis consisting of horizontal compact bundles of collagen and dense network of fine elastic fibers, as well as even and uniform shape keratinocytes in epidermis. Although peeled skin tends to be hypopigmented, melanocytes are present [14]. These changes are evident even as long as 20 years after the peel [15].

6.5 Indications and Patient Selection

The main indications for deep chemical peel include: dyschromia, wrinkles, premalignant skin tumors, and acne scars.

Originally, the ideal patient for deep chemical peel is blond, blue-eyed, fair complexion woman. Our experience shows that phenol-based peel can be safely performed on olive and dark skin patients with dark eyes and hair (Fig. 6.5a, b) [16]. As long as a patient is aware and cooperative in using bleaching preparation and potent sun screens during the post-peel period, the procedure is equally effective and safe in dark skins [17].

Thick male skin is usually less responsive to deep peel, but men with severe actinic damage or acne scarring benefit significantly from the procedure.

Deep peeling can be performed on the eyelids to improve periorbital pigmentation or wrinkling or as an adjunct procedure to surgical blepharoplasty [18].

6.6 Contraindications

There are few absolute contraindications for deep peeling, mainly physical or mental instability. During pregnancy and lactation, any cosmetic intervention is

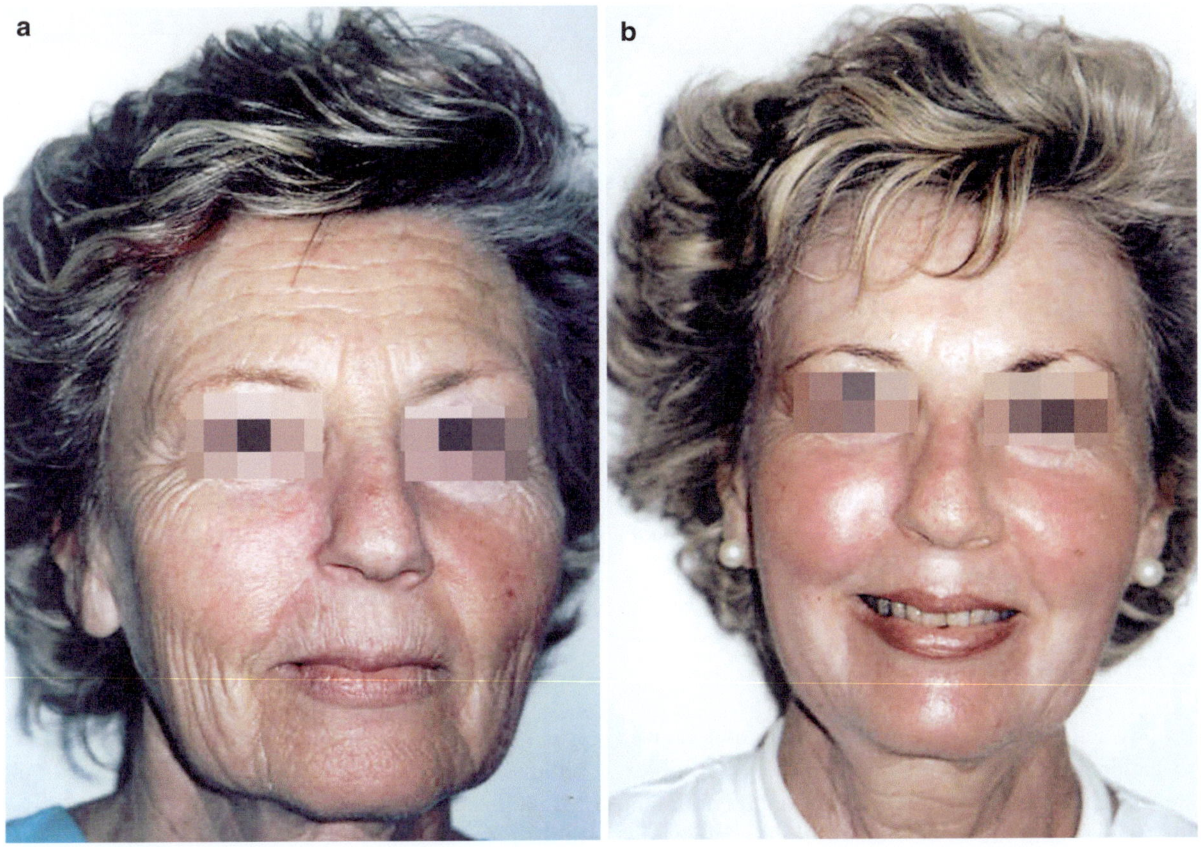

Fig. 6.5 (**a**, **b**) "Ideal" candidate for deep chemical peeling – middle-aged fair skin woman with blue eyes and blond hair and photodamage-induced wrinkling before and after deep chemical peel; (**c**, **d**) dark skin women are also possible candidates for deep chemical peels. Note the accentuation of intradermal nevus next to the left ala nasi following the peel

c d

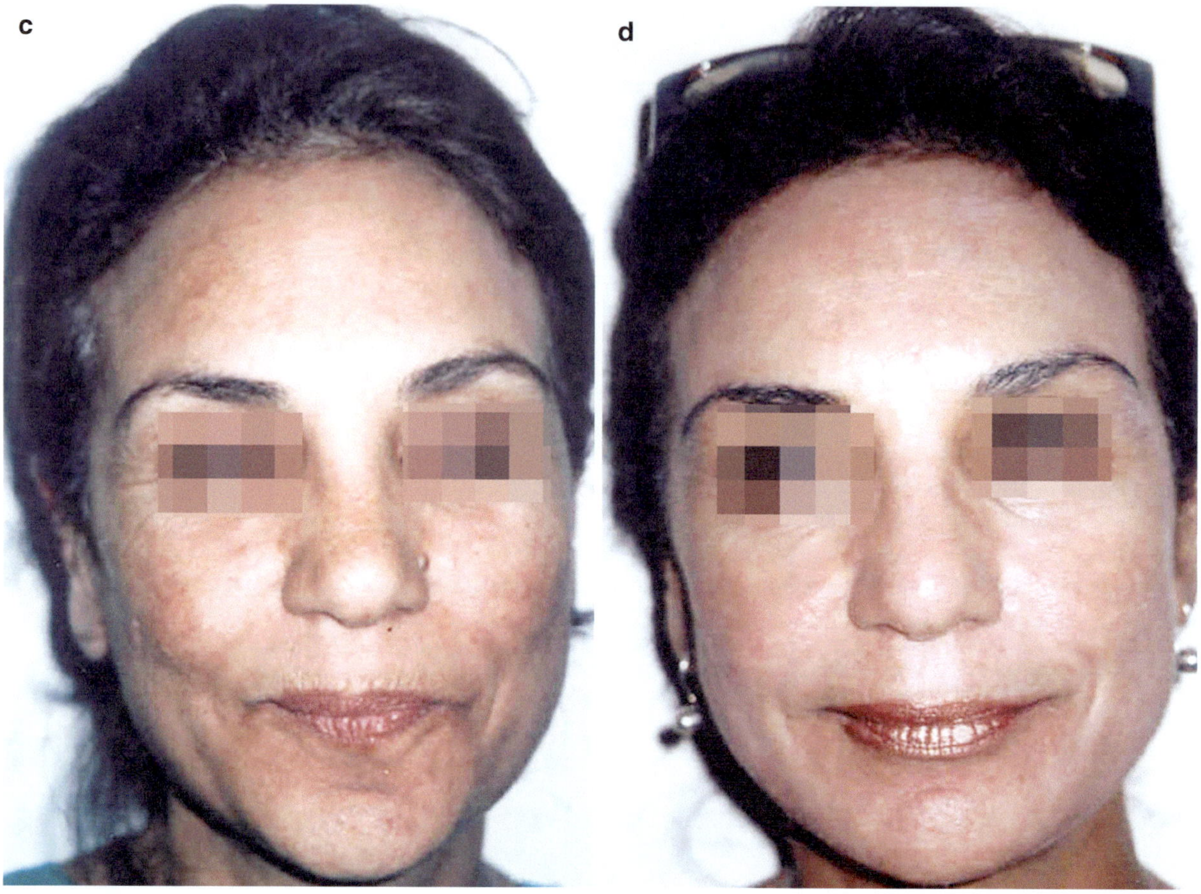

Fig. 6.5 (continued)

considered to be undesirable. We peel safely patients with hypertension, diabetes mellitus, thrombocytopenia, thyroid malfunction, etc., as long as their disease is well-controlled and stable. All patients are required to perform electrocardiogram and complete blood count prior to the procedure. Any heart disease requires special precautions and it is always recommended to work in cooperation with patient's cardiologist.

6.7 Pre-peeling Preparation

Prophylactic acyclovir, valacyclovir, or famvir is given to patients with history of recurrent herpes simplex, starting in a day before the procedure and continuing for 10 days until full re-epithelialization is achieved.

We do not use to stop any of the patient's medications including anticoagulants, aspirin, or nonsteroidal anti-inflammatory drugs. Systemic isotretinoin (Acutane) is considered to be a contraindication to any external treatment on the skin. We feel that minimal interval to peeling after stopping this medication should be 6 months in thick sebaceous skin and 1 year for thin skin patients.

According to our experience, smoking does not have any adverse effect on post-peel healing, neither on the extent of the results.

6.8 Preparation of the Skin

It is still debatable whether preparation of the skin is required for deep chemical peeling. We feel that topical retin A preparations used daily for 3–6 weeks prior to the procedure may create better and more even penetration of the peeling solution in sebaceous and hyperkeratotic skins. We did not find any benefit of this regimen in thin-skinned patients.

Standard photography and consent form are always obtained before the procedure.

6.9 Peeling Preparation

Phenol-based peel can be performed as a full-face or partial procedure. If only one cosmetic unit is peeled with phenol-based solution, it is strongly recommended to perform medium-depth peel on the rest of the facial skin. Full-face peels should be carried out under full cardiopulmonary monitoring with intravenous hydration throughout the procedure (Fig. 6.6). Intravenous sedation or regional blocks make the procedure pain-free. One day prior to the procedure, a patient is required to avoid using any cosmetics or creams. Before the peeling, meticulous degreasing of the skin is performed using oil-free acetone-soaked gauze sponges. This step is imperative to obtain even penetration of the solution into the skin.

In addition to good central ventilation, electric fan to vent the phenol fumes is important for the comfort of the staff.

6.10 Peeling Technique

Before the administration of intravenous sedation, a line inferior to the mandible is placed while a patient in sitting position to conceal a potential demarcation line (Fig. 6.7). For application of the peeling solution, cotton-tipped applicators are employed. The ready-to-use applicators come in different sizes, but usually a cotton-tip is very condense and has only limited absorption ability. Therefore, we suggest to add regular cotton to soften the tip (Fig. 6.8). The application of phenol solution is accomplished with semi-dry applicator. The usual end point is ivory-white to gray-white color of skin. The procedure starts on the forehead, and the solution is feathered into all hair-bearing areas, including scalp and eyebrows. Phenol does not affect hair growth. All the cosmetic units are gradually covered, including the earlobes and a "hidden" triangle above the ears. In the most sensitive areas, such as periorbital skin or periauricular area in postsurgical face-lift patients, we use almost dry applicator and only a single layer of the solution. In all other facial areas, after the frosting fades, additional application of peeling solution is advisable (Fig. 6.9).

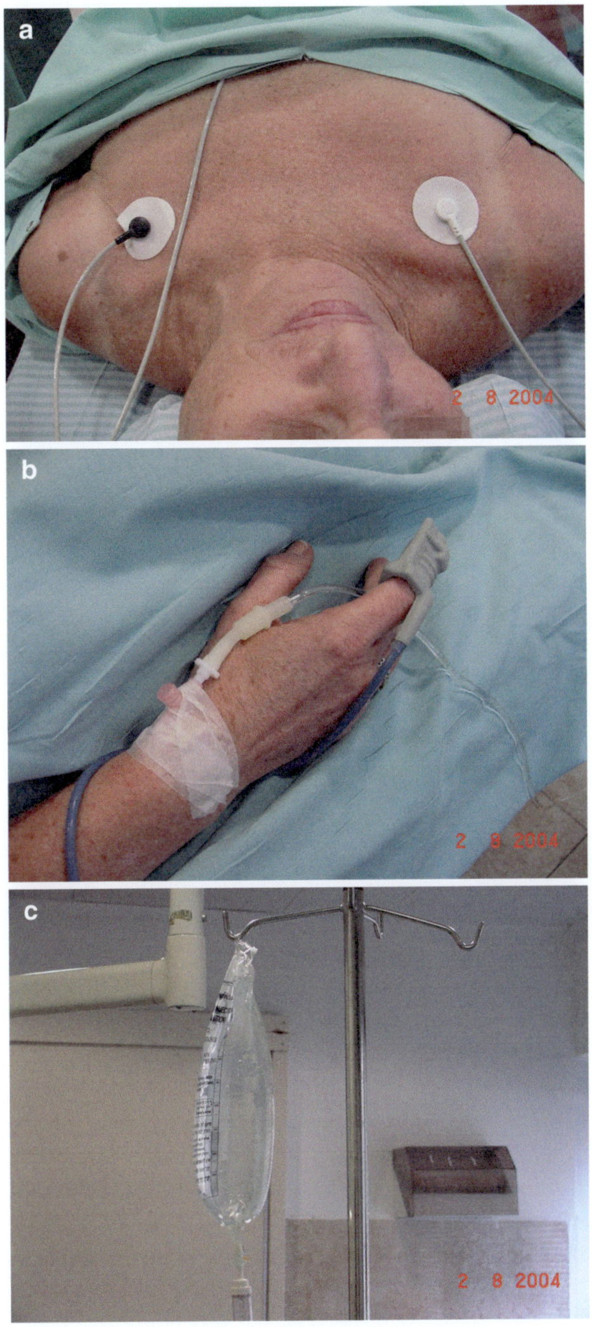

Fig. 6.6 (**a–c**) Full-face phenol-based peels are performed under cardiopulmonary monitoring with intravenous hydration

Trichloroacetic acid 25% can be applied on the neck at this stage. The entire peeling procedure should take about 60 min.

Immediately after the face is covered with the solution, waterproof zinc oxide non-permeable tape is

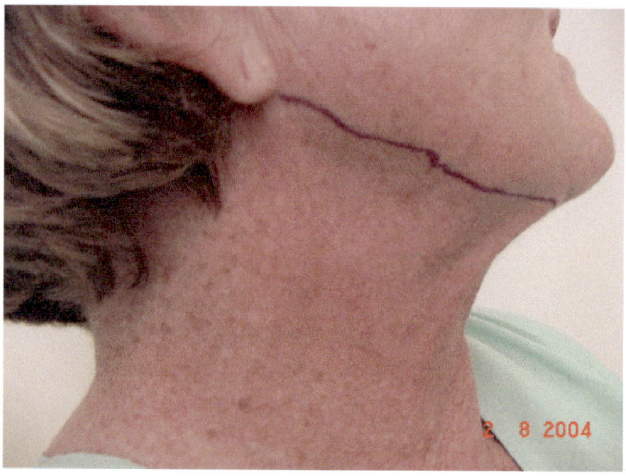

Fig. 6.7 Marking of the lower margin of the treatment area in sitting position is important to avoid demarcation lines

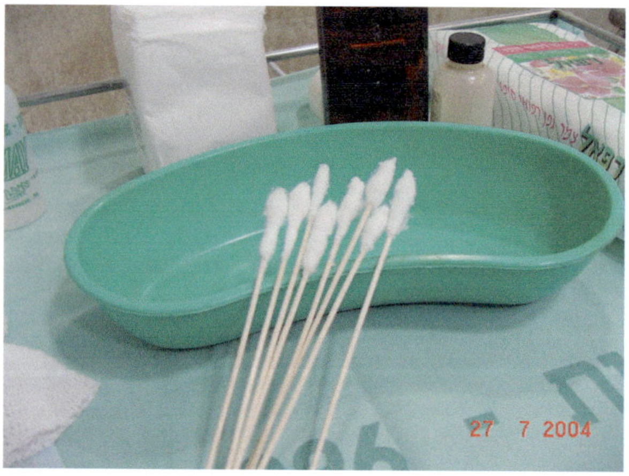

Fig. 6.8 Cotton tips are used to apply peeling solution

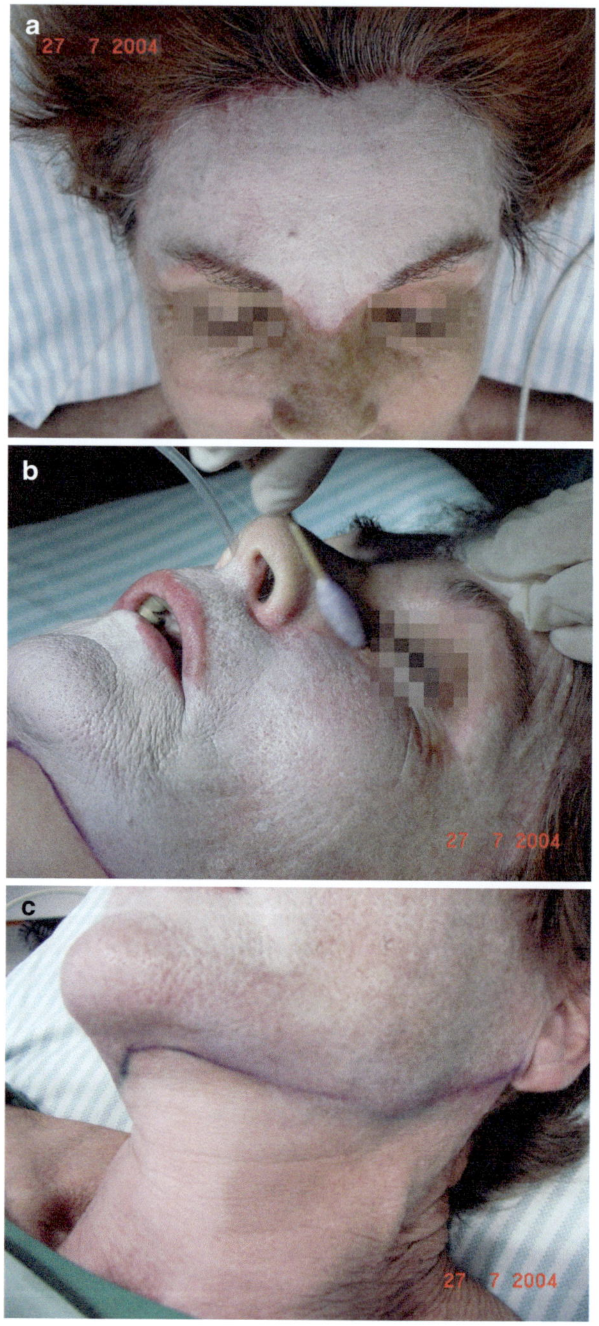

Fig. 6.9 (**a–c**) Application of the peeling solution. Ivory-white color of the skin is the end point of the application

applied to the skin anchoring it to the hairline. Taping is made using short strips of 3.0 cm in the overlapping fashion. Overlapping allows slight motion and flexibility between the strips; therefore, swelling of the face does not cause separation of the tape from the skin surface. All the face is covered except for the upper eyelids and neck. At the end of the procedure, we cover the face with elastic orthopedic grip which keeps the mask adhered tightly to the face (Fig. 6.10).

6.11 Aftercare

After 24 h, the grid is removed. Following removal of the grid, the mask gets off the face almost with no effort, since the skin exudate lifts the tapes. Analgesia is not required, since the procedure is almost painless. Occasionally, some physicians remove the mask at 48 h, but we find it unnecessary and more troublesome for the patients, since while the tape mask is on, the eyelids are frequently swollen shut. We feel that this inconvenient period must be shortened to minimum.

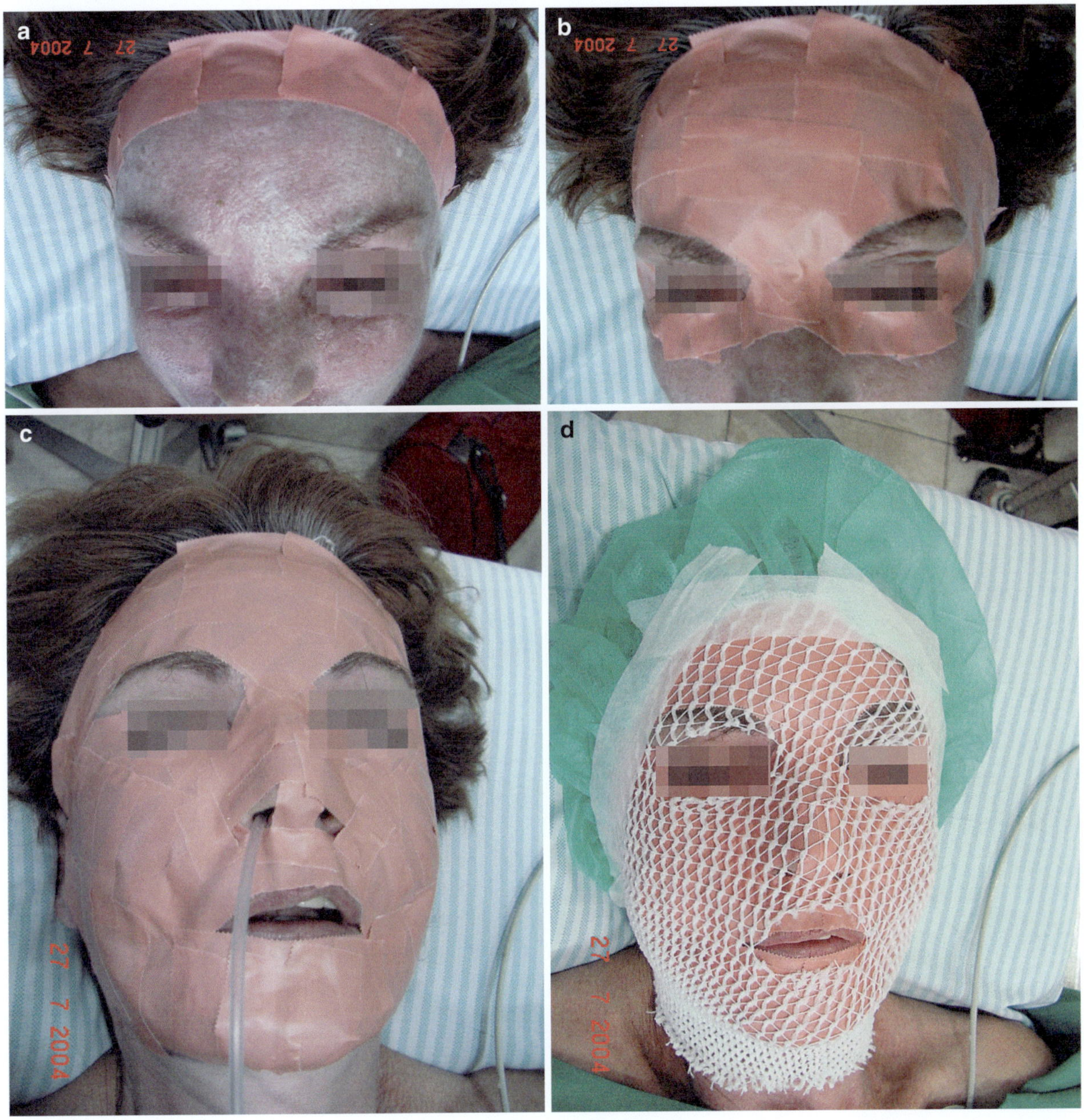

Fig. 6.10 (**a–c**) Waterproof zinc oxide non-permeable tape is applied to the skin in short stripes in overlapping fashion. (**d**) Elastic orthopedic grip keeps the tape mask adhered to the face while skin liquefaction occurs

After the tape mask removal, the exudate is cleaned by sterile saline. Spot peeling and retaping may be done if the skin looks underpeeled particularly in areas with severe wrinkling. It is usually accompanied by short duration burning sensation. The tape is left for an additional 4–6 h and then removed by a patient. We cover the face with bismuth subgalate antiseptic powder for 7 days (Fig. 6.11). Other options include occlusive moisturizers, antibiotic ointments, and biosynthetic occlusive dressings, such as Meshed Omiderm.

At this stage, we recommend to use regular painkillers every 4 h for the first 2 days. Some physicians administer systemic corticoids to reduce the swelling and inflammation after the peel. Neck swelling is expected after deep peel. It disappears during 4–6 days.

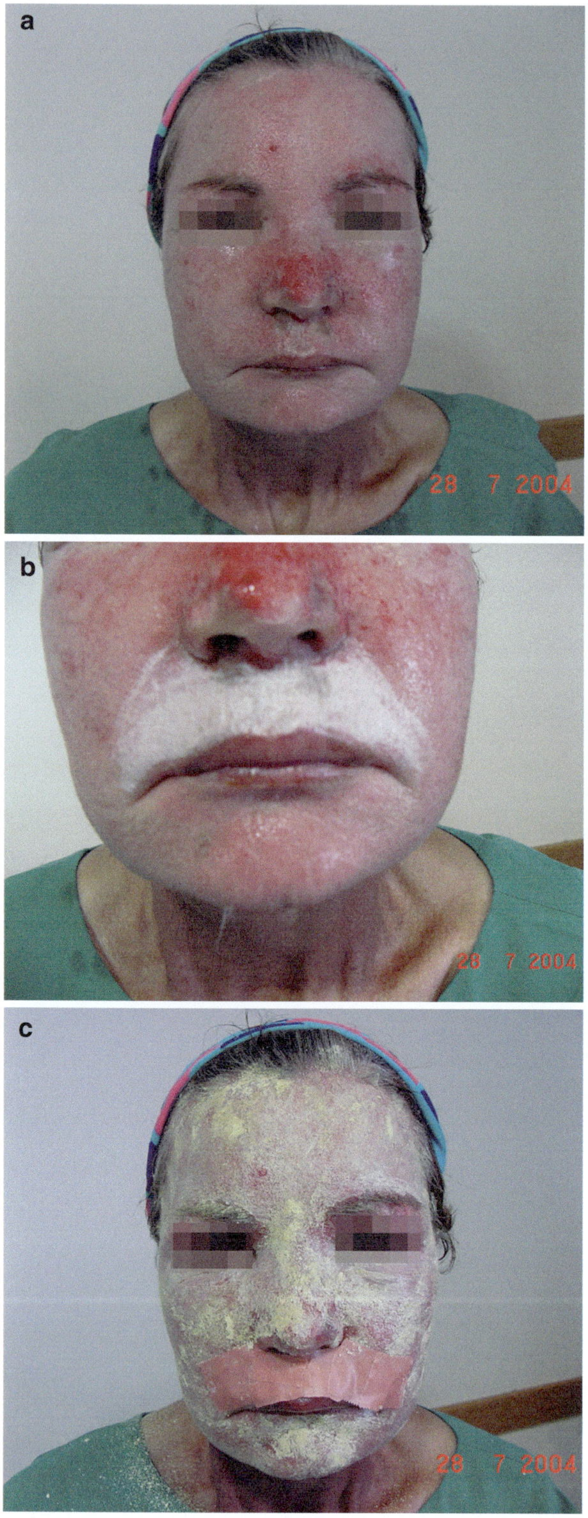

Fig. 6.11 (**a**) Tape mask removal after 24 h; (**b**) Spot re-peeling and re-taping is performed of needed; (**c**) Face is covered by bismuth subgalate antiseptic powder

Bismuth subgalate powder acts as regenerative mask and absorbs skin exudate and gradually creates a firm and rigid mask. It may crack in some areas, usually around the mouth and eyes. Some patients experience itching and can be helped by oral antihistamines. On the eighth day, wet soaking with tap water while standing in the shower is used to soften the powder mask. Repeated applications of vaseline enhance the detachment of the "second mask" from a newly formed skin (Fig. 6.12).

After the procedure, the patient is advised to use water-based lotion creams and potent sunscreens. The erythema is extremely intense in the first 2 weeks, and gradually resolves over about 2-month period. During this time, makeup with a green foundation is encouraged to use to assist the patient to resume all the daily activities. In cases of olive skin patients (Fitzpatrick skin type 3 or 4), the application of Kligman preparation is recommended to prevent reactive hyperpigmentation.

Results of phenol-based peels for various indications are shown below (Figs. 6.12–6.16).

6.12 Complications

6.12.1 Cardiac Arrhythmias

The most important potential complication of phenol-based peels is cardiotoxicity. Phenol is directly toxic to myocardium. Studies in rats showed decrease in myocardial contraction and in electrical activity following systemic exposure to phenol [19]. Since fatal doses ranged widely in these studies, it seems that individual sensitivity of myocardium to this chemical exists. In humans neither sex, age, nor previous cardiac history or blood phenol levels are accurate predictors for cardiac arrhythmia susceptibility [20].

After application of peeling solution, there is a quick absorption of phenol from the skin surface to the circulation [21]. Seventy-five percent of phenol is excreted directly through kidney or detoxified by liver. The other 25% is metabolized to CO_2 and water.

Phenol blood level measured after application of 3 mL of 50% solution of phenol is 0.68 mg/dL, while in patients who survived, accidental oral ingestion of phenol level of 23 mg/dL was found. Application of phenol to one cosmetic unit is equivalent to the application of phenol into a nail matrix for matrixectomy.

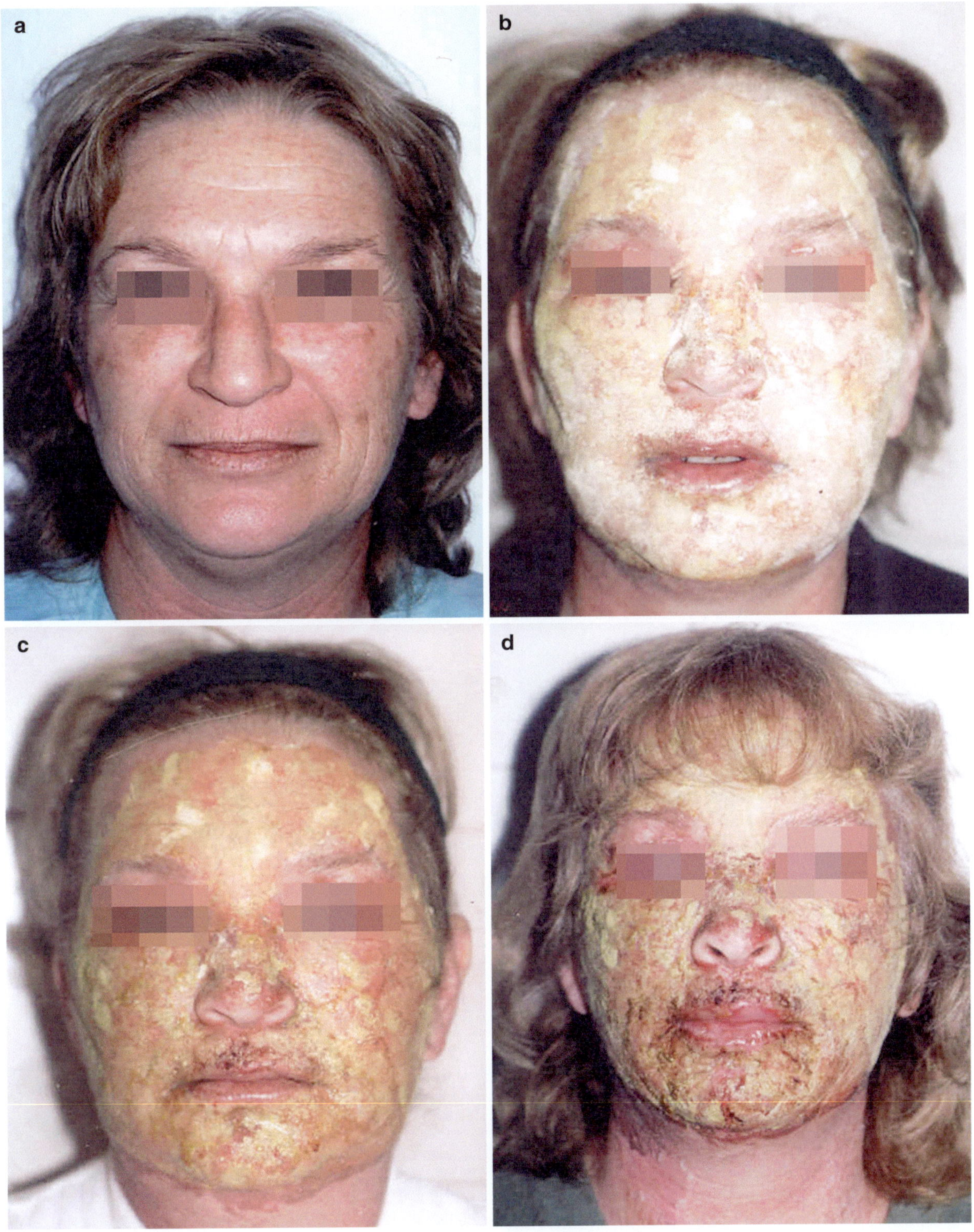

Fig. 6.12 (**a**) A 52-year-old patient with wrinkles and solar lentigines before the peel; (**b**) First day after the peel. The face is covered by powdery bismuth subgalate powder; (**c, d**) Days 3–8. The powder hardens on the face, and creates rigid crust which cracks in the mimetic areas; (**e**) one week after the procedure, a patient with makeup to conceal erythema

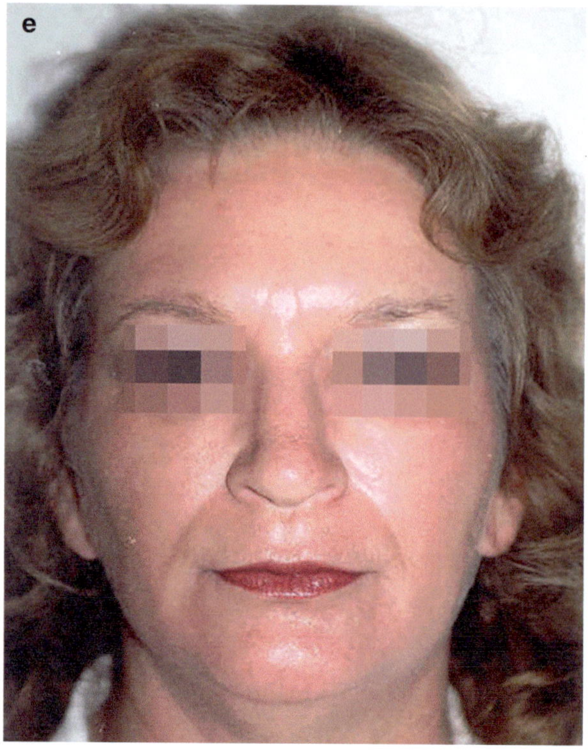

Fig. 6.12 (continued)

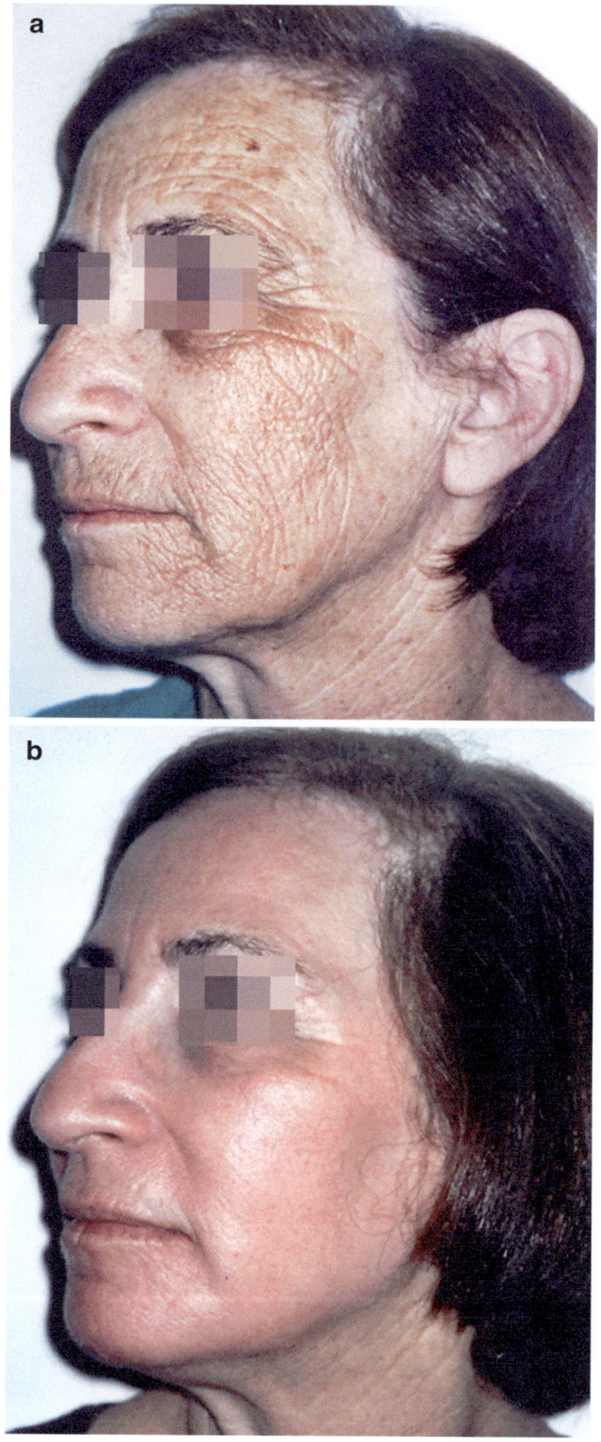

Fig. 6.13 (a, b) A 58-year-old woman with premature skin aging before and 2 weeks after deep peeling

In previous studies in humans, cardiac arrhythmias have been recorded in 23% of patients when full-face peel was performed in less than 30 min. These arrhythmias included tachycardia, premature ventricular beats, bigeminy, and atrial and ventricular tachycardia [22].

In a recent study, cardiac arrhythmia has been recorded in 6.6% of the patients during the procedure and not afterward. Cardiac arrhythmia was more common in patients with diabetes, hypertension, and depression [23].

Full-face phenol-based peel should be always performed under full cardiopulmonary monitoring. The average lag time for the onset of the arrhythmias was 17.5 min from the beginning of the peel, and they are usually not delayed for more than 30 min after the peel. Cardiac arrhythmias are more common while applying the solution on the thin skin of eyelids. In this area, skin absorption is maximal; therefore, application should be performed extremely cautiously. If arrhythmia occurs, the application of phenol should be stopped until normal sinus rhythm returns. To reduce the incidence of arrhythmia, minimal amounts of phenol should be used during the peel. Hydration and diuresis promote metabolism and excretion of phenol and, thus, reduce arrhythmias. Proper pre-peel hydration (oral or intravenous) is imperative while working with phenol. Antiarrhythmia medications are needed if any arrhythmia occurs.

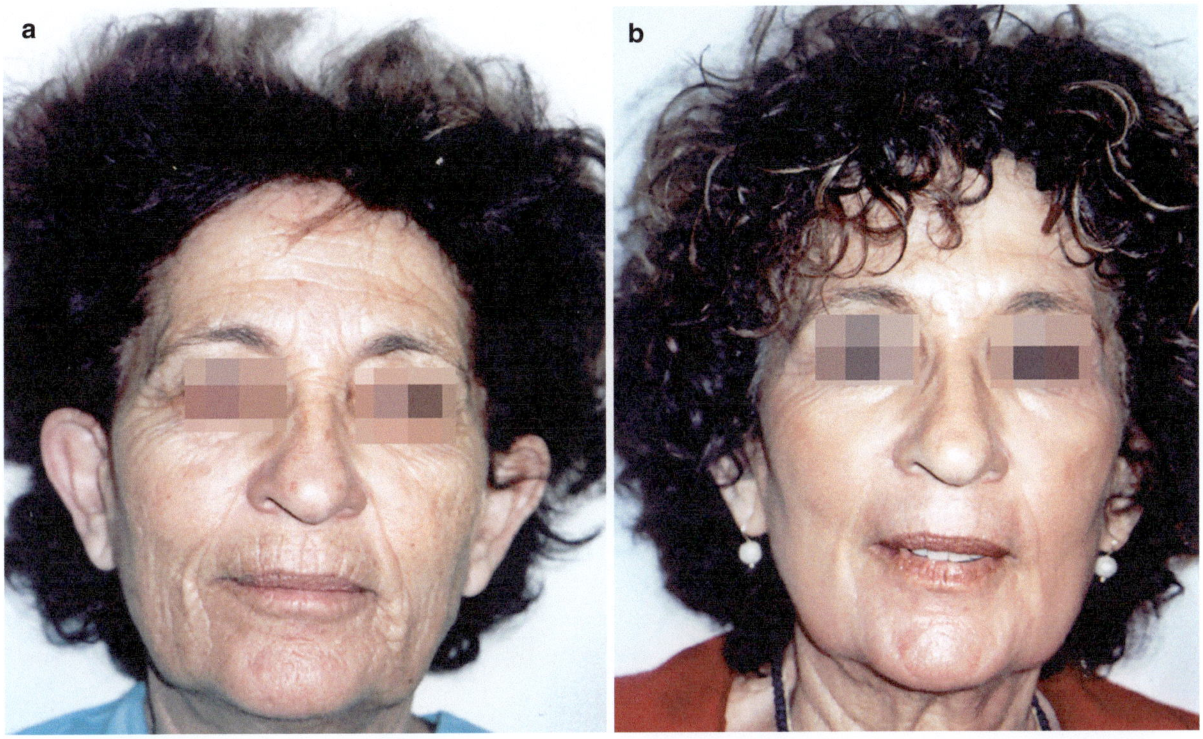

Fig. 6.14 (**a**, **b**) A 63-year-old dark skin woman before and 2 months after deep peeling. Note the effect on the upper eyelid retraction and dramatic improvement of upper lip wrinkles

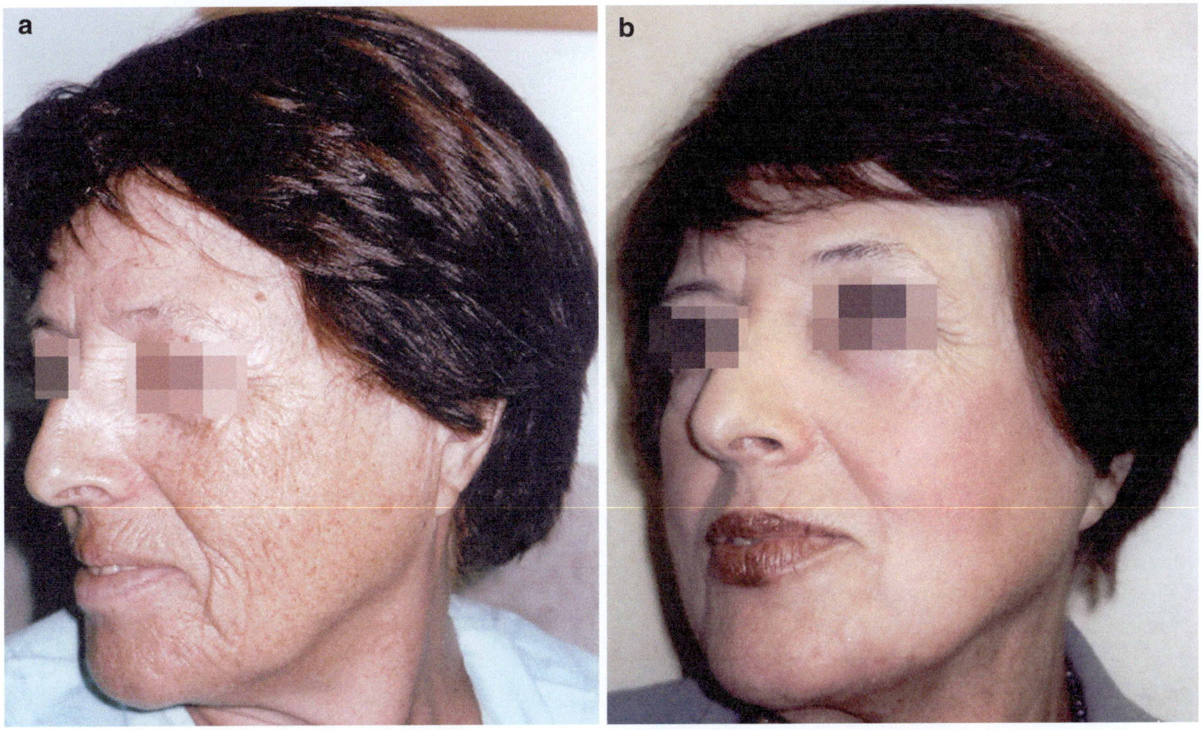

Fig. 6.15 (**a**, **b**) A 68-year-old woman with idiopathic thrombocytopenia, which prevented any cosmetic surgical intervention. One year after the performance of deep chemical peeling

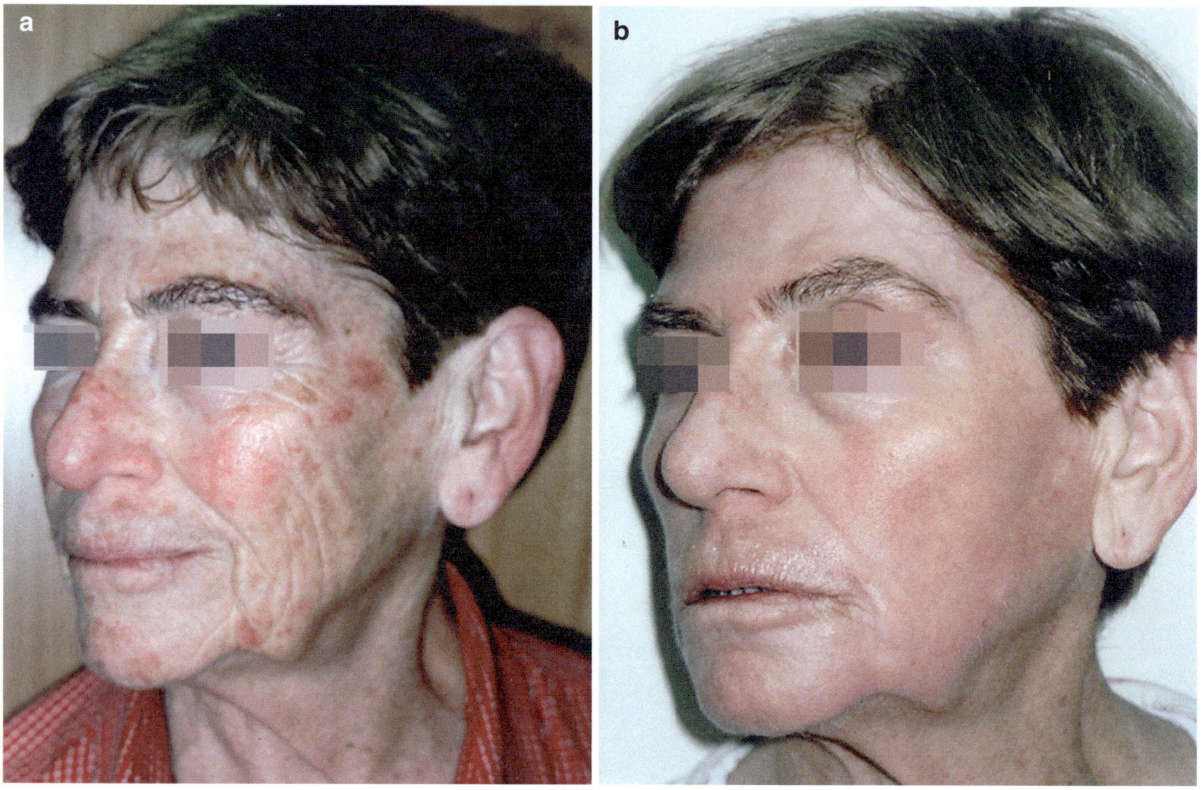

Fig. 6.16 (**a**, **b**) A 72-year-old fair skin woman with farmer skin and multiple solar keratosis. The results 3 months after deep peeling

Oral poisoning after accidental phenol ingestion has caused fulminant central nervous system depression, hepatorenal and cardiopulmonary failure [24]. No hepatorenal or central nervous system toxicities have been reported in the literature with properly performed chemical peels [25].

6.12.2 Pigmentary Changes

Delayed hypopigmentation is a reason why some doctors dislike the long-term results of deep peels. Hypopigmentation after phenol peels is proportional to the depth of the peel, amount of the solution used, inherent skin color, and post-peel sun-related behavior. Complete avoidance of any sun exposure years after the peel creates ivory skin color.

Reactive hyperpigmentation can occur after any depth of chemical peels. Usually lighter complexion has lower risk for hyperpigmentation, but genetic factors play an important role, and sometimes light patients with "dark genes" will hyperpigment unexpectedly. Therefore, we recommend to introduce bleaching preparation 2–3 weeks after the peel in all the patients and keep on them until erythema fades. Demarcation lines can be avoided if the boundaries of the peeling area are hidden under the mandibular line and feathered gradually to the normal skin (Fig. 6.17).

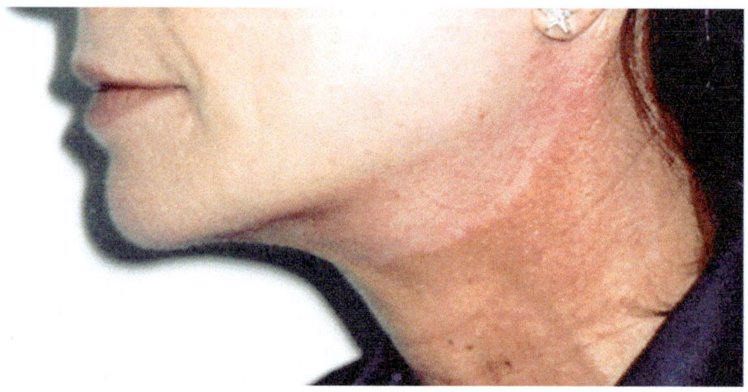

Fig. 6.17 Demarcation line due to wrong positioning of the lower margin of the treatment area

Medium depth neck peel is required in patients with blotchy pigmentation of the neck and in those with no clear mandibular line. Accentuation of the pigment in previously existing intradermal nevi is common and should be recognized when it occurs to avoid any unnecessary alarm of "changing mole" (Fig. 6.5d).

6.12.3 Scarring

Scarring remains to be the most dreadful complication of chemical peels. The contributing factors are not well defined yet. Incidence of scarring with traditional Baker's formula is less than 1% [26], while with less aggressive phenol peels, the incidence is lower. The most common location of the scars is in the lower part of the face, probably due to more aggressive treatment in this area or due to the greater tissue movement, because of eating and speaking, during the healing process. Previous surgical lift elevates the neck skin to the higher position "imitating" normal facial skin appearance. Thus, special precautions should be taken while peeling lower lateral portions of the face in postsurgical face-lift patients even years later. We recommend to keep away from a combination of deep chemical peels with any other surgical facial procedure, since skin undermining compromises severely the after-peel healing process and increases the risk of scarring. Isotretinoin therapy interferes with normal tissue healing; therefore, deep peels should be postponed 6–12 months after completing acne therapy. Delayed healing and persistent redness are important alarming signs for forthcoming scarring. Topical antibiotics and potent steroid preparations should be introduced as soon as this diagnosis is made.

6.12.4 Infection

Bacterial and fungal complications in chemical peels are rare, since phenol is bactericidal and fungicidal. Patients with positive history of herpes simplex infection can be treated prophylactically with acyclovir or valacyclovir during healing phase for 10 days.

6.12.5 Milia

Milia can appear in up to 20% of patients after deep peels 6–8 weeks after the procedure. Electrosurgery is a simple and effective method to treat this post-peel complication.

6.12.6 Acneiform Dermatitis

Acneiform eruption after deep chemical peel is a common phenomenon appearing immediately after reepithelialization. Its etiology is multifactorial and is related to either exacerbation of previously existing acne or is due to over-greasing of newly formed skin. Short-term systemic antibiotics together with discontinuation of any oily preparations will usually provide satisfactory solution.

6.12.7 Skin Atrophy

Clinical loss of normal skin markings without scarring is reported after multiple sessions of traditional Baker's peels.

6.13 Advantages

The main advantage of deep chemical peel is in treating of photodamaged skin with wrinkles, dyschromia, and precancerous lesions. Perioral wrinkling is a condition in which deep peel has an obvious advantage over other medical and surgical methods. Facial scars, such as acne scars, especially if of atrophic character, may be significantly improved by deep chemical peel. In general, deep chemical peel is the most powerful and legitimate tool in the hands of practicing dermatologist for facial skin rejuvenation.

6.14 Disadvantages

The main disadvantage of deep peel is a special setup needed for the procedure, due to potential cardiotoxicity of phenol. In addition, special training is needed for the doctor and the office staff before the implementation of this technique to the daily practice.

Patient's Informed Consent

1. I hereby request and authorize Dr. ____________________, M.D., to treat me for the purpose of attempting to improve my appearance.
2. The effect and nature of the treatment to be given, as well as possible alternative methods of treatment, have been fully explained to me.
3. It has been explained that well-qualified and trained personnel will assist with certain portions of the treatment under his supervision.
4. I hereby authorize Dr. _____________, M.D to administer such treatment to me, and agree to hold him/her free and harmless for any claims or suits for damages or injury or complications whatever for any result from conditions beyond the Doctor's control.
5. I know that the practice of medicine and surgery is not an exact science and that, therefore, reputable practitioners cannot properly guarantee results.
6. I acknowledge that no guarantee or assurance has been made to me by anyone regarding the treatment which I have herein requested and authorized.
7. I am advised that though good results are expected, they cannot be and are not guaranteed, nor can there be any guarantee against untoward results.
8. I acknowledge that no guarantee has been given to me as to the number of years I may appear younger following treatment.
9. I acknowledge that no guarantee has been given to me as to the condition of the complexion or size of the skin pores following treatment.

11. I acknowledge that during the procedure my face will be covered by masks during the 8 days.
12. I acknowledge that no guarantee has been given to me as to the painlessness of the procedure. Some individuals, because of emotional makeup or low pain threshold, may experience severe pain. Heavy premedication is given to make the procedure as comfortable for the patient as possible.
13. I have been advised that the following conditions may arise after treatment. These conditions are uncommon and usually not serious, but may appear at any time because of circumstances beyond the Doctor's control:
    a. A darkening of the skin or blotchiness may occur at any time up to 3 months following treatment. This is usually due to excess sun or heat exposure. Special medication may be prescribed for this and will usually clear the condition completely. Occasionally, further treatment may be required, consisting of a second procedure. Persons with dark complexions undergoing treatment are advised that a blotchy complexion may arise which will usually even out over a period of 3–6 months.
    b. The skin may be red for a 6–8 week period or possibly redness is due to increased blood supply to the new skin. Usually it disappears over the 3–6-month period and the final complexion is somewhat lighter than the original complexion.
    c. On occasion, small areas of the neck and chin may show thickening for a variable period of time following treatment. These areas are buildups of underlying collagen and scar tissue and are usually easily controlled by periodic injections of medication.
    d. Every Facial Rejuvenation procedure is accompanied by swelling of the tissue of the face and neck. This is usually only temporary and disappears within a short period of time. On occasion, the swelling may be persistent and will require further medication.
14. I have been advised that exposure to sun must be avoided at all costs for a period of 6 months. No sunbathing is permitted for 6 months. To do so would encourage blotchy skin pigmentation requiring further treatment.

15. I give my permission that my before and after pictures will be used for:
   - □ Educational purposes only
   - □ Patient's demonstration
   - □ Medical congresses and medical articles

   The operation has been explained to me and I fully understand the nature of the procedure and the risks involved. I acknowledge and understand that no expressed or implied warranty has been given to me.

Date__________ Signature ________________

Results

References

1. Mackee GM, Karp FL (1952) The treatment of post acne scars with phenol. Br J Dermatol 64:456–459
2. Bames HO (1927) Truth and fallacies of face peeling and face lifting. Med J Rec 126:86–87
3. Urkov JC (1946) Surface defects of the skin: treatment by controlled exfoliation. Ill Med J 89:75
4. Combes FC, Sperber PA, Reisch M (1960) Dermal defects: treatment by a chemical agent. NY Physician Am Med 56:36
5. Brown AM, Kaplan LM, Brown ME (1960) Phenol induced histological skin changes: hazards, techniques and users. Br J Plast Surg 13:158
6. Litton C (1962) Chemical face lifting. Plast Reconstr Surg 29:371
7. Baker TJ (1962) Chemical face peeling and rhytidectomy. Plast Reconstr Surg 29:199
8. Baker TJ, Gordon HL (1961) The ablation of rhytids by chemical means: a preliminary report. J Fla Med Assoc 48:541
9. Stone PA, Lefer LG (2001) Modified phenol chemical face peels: recognizing the role of application technique. Clin Plast Surg 9:351–376
10. Spira M, Dahl C, Freeman R et al (1970) Chemosurgery: a histological study. Plast Reconstr Surg 45:247
11. Hetter G (2000) An examination of the phenol-croton oil peel: part I. Dissecting the formula. Plast Reconstr Surg 105:239–248
12. Fintsi Y (1997) Exoderm- a novel phenol-based peeling method resulting in improved safety. Am J Cosmet Surg 14:49–54
13. Larson DL, Karmo F, Hetter GP (2009) Phenol-croton oil peel: establishing an animal model for scientific investigation. Aesthet Surg J 29:47–53
14. Baker TJ, Gordon HL, Seckinger DL (1966) A second look at chemical face peeling. Plast Reconstr Surg 37:487
15. Baker TJ, Gordon HL, Mosienko P et al (1974) Long-term histological study of skin after chemical face peeling. Plast Reconstr Surg 53:522
16. Fintsi Y, Landau M (2001) Exoderm: phenol-based peeling in olive and dark skinned patients. Int J Cosmet Surg Aesthet Dermatol 3:173–178
17. Park JH, Choi YD, Kim SW, Kim YC, Park SW (2007) Effectiveness of modified phenol peel (Exoderm) on facial wrinkles, acne scars and other skin problems of Asian patients. J Dermatol 34:17–24
18. Gatti JE (2008) Eyelid phenol peel: an important adjunct to blepharoplasty. Ann Plast Surg 60:14–18
19. Stagnone GJ, Orgel MB, Stagnone JJ (1987) Cardiovascular effects of topical 50% trichloroacetic acid and Baker's phenol solution. J Dermatol Surg Oncol 13:999–1002
20. Litton C, Trinidad G (1981) Complications of chemical face peeling as evaluated by a questionnaire. Plast Reconstr Surg 67:738–744
21. Wexler MR, Halon DA, Teitelbaum A et al (1984) The prevention of cardiac arrhythmias produced in an animal model by topical application of a phenol preparation in common use for face peeling. Plast Reconstr Surg 73:595–598
22. Truppman F, Ellenbery J (1979) The major electrocardiographic changes changes during chemical face peeling. Plast Reconstr Surg 63:44
23. Landau M (2007) Cardiac complications in deep chemical peels. Dermatol Surg 33:190–193
24. Gleason MD, Gosselin RF, Hodge HC et al (1969) Clinical toxicology of commercial products. Williams & Williams, Baltimore, pp 189–192
25. Brody HJ (1997) Chemical peeling and resurfacing, 2nd edn. Mosby, pp 188–189
26. Brody HJ (1997) Chemical peeling and resurfacing, 2nd edn. Mosby, pp 168–178

7 Jessner's Solution

Pearl E. Grimes

7.1 History

Jessner's solution has been used for over 100 years as a therapeutic agent to treat hyperkeratotic epidermal lesions [1]. This superficial peeling agent constitutes a mixture of salicylic acid, resorcinol, and lactic acid in 95% ethanol. Jessner's solution causes loss of corneocyte cohesion and induces intercellular and intracellular edema. Jessner's solution typically induces wounding to the level of the papillary dermis. In the early twentieth century, resorcinol (a key component of Jessner's peels) was used in concentrations of 10–50%; however, such high concentrations of resorcinol were associated with side effects such as allergic contact dermatitis, irritant contact dermatitis, and skin discoloration. Subsequently, Jessner's solution was formulated by Dr. Max Jessner to lower the concentrations of any one agent contained in the mixture and to enhance its overall effects as a keratolytic agent.

7.2 Chemical Background

Each component of Jessner's solution has specific effects (Fig. 7.1). Salicylic acid (ortho-hydroxy-benzoic acid) is a beta-hydroxy acid [2]. It is a lipophilic compound that removes intercellular lipids which are covalently linked to the cornified envelope surrounding epithelial cells [3]. It also enhances penetration of other agents. Resorcinol (*m*-dihydroxy benzene) is structurally and chemically similar to phenol. It disrupts the weak hydrogen bonds of keratin [4]. Lactic acid is an alpha-hydroxy acid which causes corneocyte detachment and subsequent desquamation of the stratum corneum [5].

P.E. Grimes
Division of Dermatology, Department of Medicine, David Geffen School of Medicine, University of California—Los Angeles, Vitiligo and Pigmentation Institute of Southern California, 5670 Wilshire Blvd., Suite 650, Los Angeles, CA 90036, USA
e-mail: pegrimesmd@earthlink.net

7.3 Formulations

The standard formulation of Jessner's solution is listed in Table 7.1. Modified Jessner's solutions are also available which do not contain resorcinol (Delasco, Council Bluffs, IA) (Table 7.2). Like Jessner's solution itself, this modified solution can enhance the effect of trichloroacetic acid (TCA) when the two are applied together [6].

7.4 Indications

Jessner's peels have been used to treat acne, melasma, postinflammatory hyperpigmentation, lentigines, freckles, and photodamage (Figs. 7.2a, b–7.4a, b). For example, modified Jessner's solution in combination with trichloroacetic acid has achieved greater than 70% reductions in Melasma Area Severity Index (MASI) scores in women with Fitzpatrick phototypes III and IV with minimal post-peel postinflammatory hyperpigmentation [6]. And Jessner's solution combined with 5% 5-fluorouracil solution achieved at least 80% clearing of AK lesions and an overall improvement of

A. Tosti et al. (eds.), *Color Atlas of Chemical Peels*,
DOI 10.1007/978-3-642-20270-4_7, © Springer-Verlag Berlin Heidelberg 2012

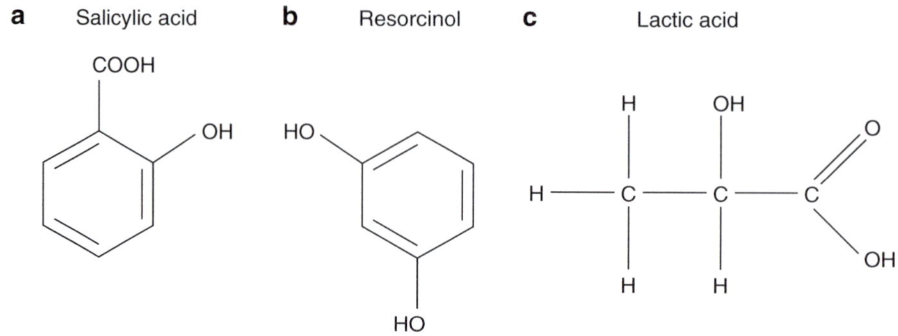

Fig. 7.1 (**a-c**) Chemical structures of Jessner's peel components (salicylic acid, resorcinol, and lactic acid)

Table 7.1 Preparation of Jessner's solution with resorcinol

• Resorcinol 14 g
• Salicylic acid 14 g
• Lactic acid (85%) 14 g
• Ethanol – sufficient quantity to make 100 mL

Table 7.2 Modified Jessner's solution

• 17% lactic acid
• 17% salicylic acid
• 8% citric acid
• Ethanol – sufficient quantity to make 100 mL

photodamaged skin [7]. The authors consider this superficial 5-FU pulse peel to be a safe, well-tolerated, very effective, and inexpensive option for the treatment of multiple, diffuse AKs.

7.5 Contraindications

As with other superficial peeling agents, Jessner's peels are well tolerated with few contraindications. However, there is scant published information on the use of Jessner's peels in Fitzpatrick's skin types V and VI. One study by Ejaz et al. has reported comparable

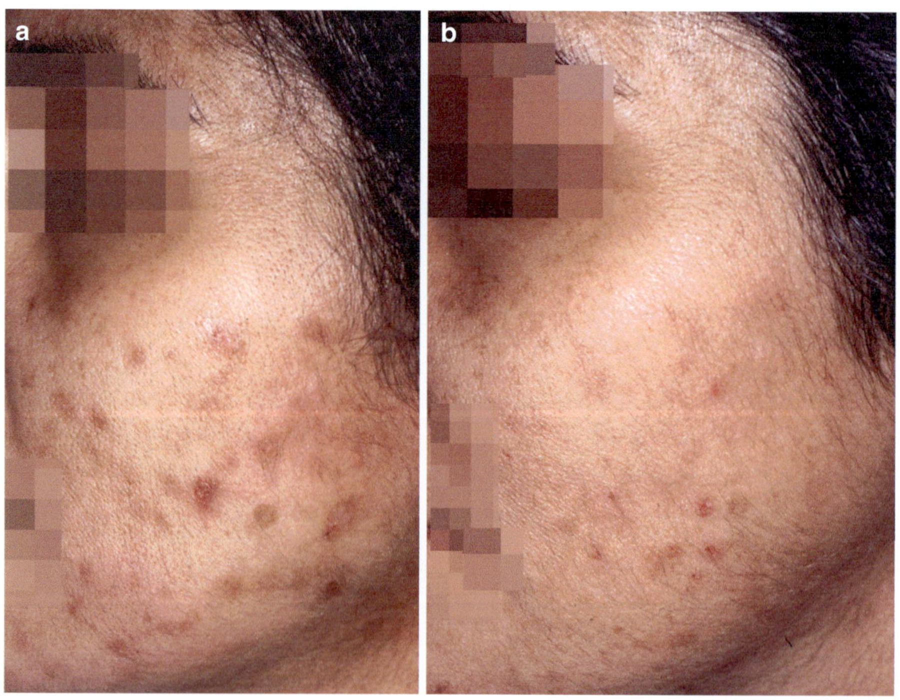

Fig. 7.2 (**a**) Patient with acne with excoriation. (**b**) Patient after treatment with Jessner's peel

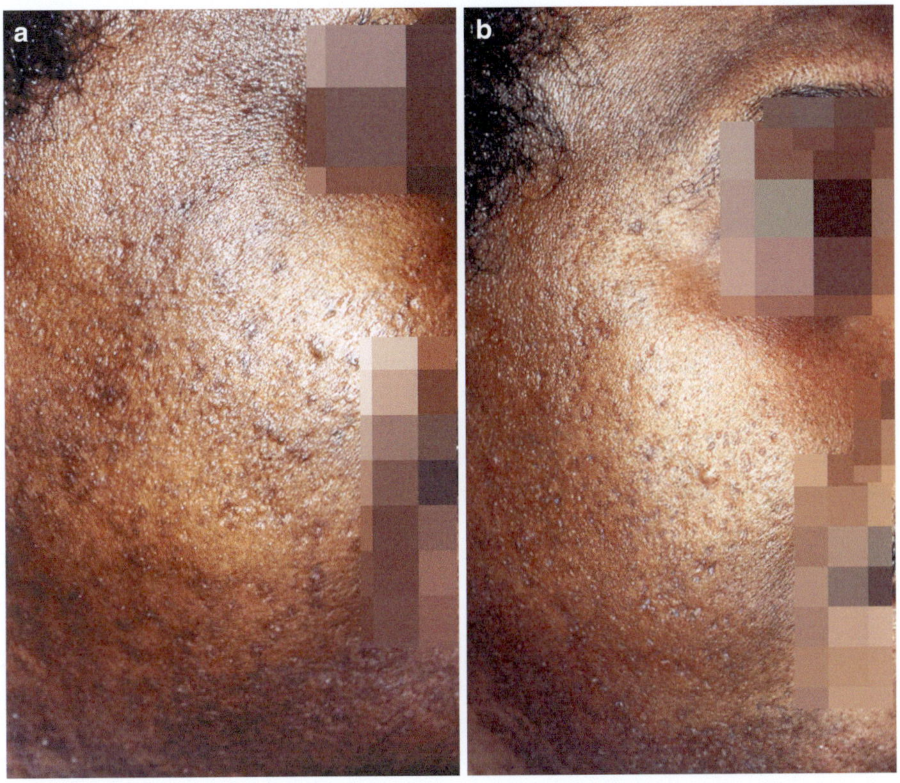

Fig. 7.3 (**a**) Patient with postinflammatory hyperpigmentation. (**b**) Patient after treatment with a series of two Jessner's peels

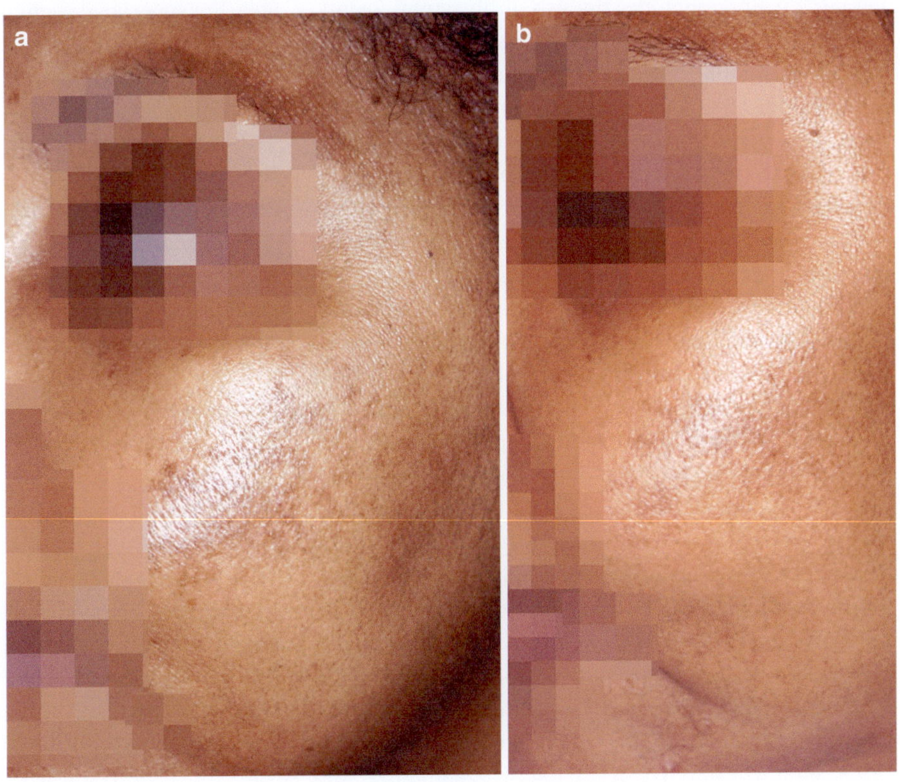

Fig. 7.4 (**a**) Patient with melasma. (**b**) Patient after treatment with Jessner's peeling

tolerability to salicylic acid peeling in a group of Asian patients with melasma and predominantly type V skin tone [8]. Another study, in which repeated applications of Jessner's solution and TCA were used to treat periorbital wrinkles in dark-skinned patients, found that patients experienced only mild adverse events [9]. In the author's experience, Jessner's peels are also well tolerated in these groups. General contraindications include active inflammation, dermatitis, or infection of the area to be treated; isotretinoin therapy within 6 months of peeling; and delayed or abnormal wound healing. Jessner's peels are also contraindicated during pregnancy. Allergies to resorcinol, salicylic acid, or lactic acid are absolute contraindications. Patients should not have unrealistic expectations regarding peel outcomes.

7.6 Skin Preparation

The general goals of preparing the skin for peeling are to maximize peel outcomes while minimizing the potential to develop post-peel complications. A detailed history and cutaneous examination should be performed prior to chemical peeling. Baseline full-face frontal and lateral photos are recommended. Skin preparation for Jessner's peeling includes the use of bleaching agents, topical retinoids, alpha-hydroxy acids, and/or other topical exfoliating agents. However, as with other superficial peeling agents, the patient's diagnosis influences how the skin should be prepared for the peeling procedure. Skin preparation can impact penetration of the peeling agent and the overall efficacy of the peel. In addition, peel preparation can increase or decrease the potential to develop post-peel complications.

Use of topical retinoids (tretinoin, tazarotene, retinol formulations) for 2–6 weeks prior to peeling thins the stratum corneum, and enhances epidermal turnover [10]. Such agents also reduce the content of epidermal melanin and expedite epidermal healing. Retinoids also enhance the penetration of the peeling agent. They should be discontinued several days prior to the peeling procedure. Retinoids can be resumed postoperatively after all evidence of peeling and irritation subsides. When treating conditions such as melasma, acne, and postinflammatory hyperpigmentation, as well as darker skin types, retinoids should be discontinued 1 or 2 weeks before peeling or even eliminated from the prep to avoid post-peel complications, such as excessive erythema, desquamation, and postinflammatory hyperpigmentation. Topical alpha-hydroxy acid or polyhydroxy acid formulations can also be used to prep the skin. In general, they are less aggressive agents in impacting peel outcomes. The skin is usually prepped for 2–4 weeks with a formulation of hydroquinone 4% or higher compounded formulations (5–10%) to reduce epidermal melanin. This is extremely important when treating the aforementioned dyschromias. Although less effective, other topical bleaching agents include azelaic acid, kojic acid, arbutin, and licorice (see Chapter 14). Patients can also resume use of topical bleaching agents postoperatively after peeling and irritation subsides [11, 12]. Broad-spectrum sunscreens (UVA and UVB) should be worn daily (see Chapter 14).

7.7 Peeling Technique

The skin is usually degreased with alcohol followed by a mild acetone scrub. After cleaning, Jessner's solution is applied to the face with a sable brush, cotton-tipped applicators, cotton balls, or 2×2 gauze sponges. The author prefers the use of cotton-tipped applicators. Typically, the cheeks are treated first, working from medial to lateral areas followed by application to the chin and forehead area. For superficial peeling, two coats are usually applied. Additional coats increase the depth of peeling.

Neutralization or dilution with Jessner's solution is not indicated. After application of the product, some visible precipitate may appear on the skin surface. This should be distinguished from true frosting which correlates with the depth of peeling. Extent of erythema and desquamation following a Jessner's peel correlates with extent of and type of pre-peel prepping, number of coats of product applied, and level or degree of frosting during the procedure [11].

7.8 Post-Peel Care

Use of bland cleansers and moisturizers is essential. Recommended moisturizing agents include Cetaphil, SBR-Lipocream, or Aquaphor. Peeling related to Jessner's usually resolves in 2–7 days. Patients can resume the use of general skin care products after peeling subsides. Makeup can be worn to camouflage peeling. Excessive peeling, erythema, or irritation post-peel can be treated with low- or mid- to high-potency steroids for 5–7 days. Use of such agents should be based on the extent of irritation and inflammation.

7.9 Advantages of Jessner's Peeling

- Excellent safety profile
- Can be used in all skin types
- Substantial efficacy with minimal "down time"
- Enhances the penetration of TCA

7.10 Disadvantages of Jessner's Peeling

- Concerns regarding resorcinol toxicity, including thyroid dysfunction
- Manufacturing variations
- Instability with exposure to light and air
- Increased exfoliation in some patients

7.11 Side Effects

Despite concerns regarding resorcinol and salicylate toxicity, Jessner's solution has been extremely well tolerated with minimal side effects. Allergic reactions to resorcinol are reported to be rare [13, 14], but lymph node assay tests have identified resorcinol as a skin sensitizer [15]. Although the potential to induce thyroid disease has been reported, a recent toxicological review on the risk of resorcinol in inducing thyroid abnormalities did not support an association. Resorcinol administered at high doses to rodents can disrupt thyroid hormone synthesis and can produce goitrogenic effects. Clinical case reports from patients undergoing resorcinol therapy for dermatological indications reveal thyroid side effects in instances where copious amounts of resorcinol-containing ointments are applied to integrity-compromised skin for months to years. However, a risk assessment comparing potential worst-case exposures to resorcinol through its use in dermatological preparations supports the conclusion that under real-life conditions, human exposures to resorcinol are not expected to cause adverse effects on thyroid function. In addition, we are aware of no case reports of salicylism from Jessner's formulation. Resorcinol has also been implicated in the induction of exogenous ochronosis in Africa. However, resorcinol has not been implicated in the rare cases of ochronosis in the United States [16].

Patient's Informed Consent

I, ________________, hereby consent to having my ____________ (site) treated with CHEMICAL PEELING USING JESSNER'S SOLUTION. Jessner's peeling is often used to treat sun-damaged skin, dark spots, texturally rough skin, acne, and scarring. It is a peeling agent which causes shedding of the outermost layer of the skin, "the stratum corneum."

The procedure involves first having the peel site prepped with alcohol, acetone, or other pre-peel cleansing agents. The peel is then applied. In general, Jessner's peels are extremely well tolerated. However, the procedure can cause redness, flaking, dryness, or irritation in the area to be treated. The effects could last for 1–2 weeks.

I understand that there is a small risk of developing permanent darkening or undesirable pigment loss at the treated site. There is a rare chance that a scar could develop. There is also a small risk that a bacterial infection could develop or there could be a flare of a pre-existing Herpes infection at the treated site. There is a small chance that the condition being treated could worsen after the peeling procedure. The benefits and side effects of the procedure have been explained to me in detail. All of my questions have been answered.

- I am in stable health.
- I have not used isotretinoin in the past 6 months.
- I have no allergies to resorcinol, salicylic acid, or lactic acid.
- I am not pregnant.

Outcomes are not guaranteed.

______________________________ ____________

Signature of Patient Date

____

Patient Name (Please Print)

______________________________ ____________

Witness Date

Disclaimer The author has no financial interest in any of the products or equipment mentioned in this chapter.

References

1. Monheit GD (1989) Jessner's + TCA peel: a medium depth chemical peel. J Dermatol Surg Oncol 15:945–950
2. Huber C, Christophers E (1977) Keratolytic effect of salicylic acid. Arch Dermatol Res 257:293–297
3. Lazo ND, Meine JG, Downing DT (1995) Lipids are covalently attached to rigid corneocyte protein envelope existing predominantly as beta-sheets: a solid state nuclear magnetic resonance study. J Invest Dermatol 105: 296–300
4. Rook A, Wilkinson DS, Ebling FJG (1972) Textbook of dermatology. Blackwell Scientific, Oxford, pp 2072–2075
5. Van Scott EJ, Yu RJ (1984) Hyperkeratinization, corneocyte cohesion, and alpha hydroxy acids. J Am Acad Dermatol 11(5 Pt 1):867–879
6. Safoury OS, Zaki NM, El Nabarawy EA, Farag EA (2009) A study comparing chemical peeling using modified Jessner's solution and 15% trichloroacetic acid versus 15% trichloroacetic acid in the treatment of melasma. Indian J Dermatol 54(1):41–45
7. Bagatin E, Teixeira SP, Hassun KM, Pereira T, Michalany NS, Talarico S (2009) 5-Fluorouracil superficial peel for multiple actinic keratoses. Int J Dermatol 48(8):902–907
8. Ejaz A et al (2008) Comparison of 30% salicylic acid with Jessner's solution for superficial chemical peeling in epidermal melasma. J Coll Physicians Surg Pak 18:205–208
9. Kadhim KA, Al-Waiz M (2005) Treatment of periorbital wrinkles by repeated medium-depth chemical peels in dark-skinned individuals. J Cosmet Dermatol 4(1):18–22
10. Matarasso SL, Glogau RG (1991) Chemical face peels. Dermatol Clin 9:131–150
11. Rubin MG (1995) Manual of chemical peels: superficial and medium depth. J.B. Lippincott Company, Philadelphia, pp 79–88
12. Brody HJ (1997) Chemical peeling and resurfacing, 2nd edn. Mosby, St. Louis
13. Lynch BS, Delzell ES, Bechtel DH (2002) Toxicology review and risk assessment of resorcinol: thyroid effects. Regul Toxicol Pharmacol 36:198–210
14. Barbaud A, Modiano P, Cocciale M et al (1996) The topical application of resorcinol can provoke a systemic allergic reaction. Br J Dermatol 135:1014–1015
15. Baskettter DA, Sanders D, Jowsey IR (2007) The skin sensitization potential of resorcinol: experience with the local lymph node assay. Contact Dermatitis 56(4):196–200
16. Thomas AE, Gisburn MA (1961) Exogenous ochronosis and myxoedema from resorcinol. Br J Dermatol 73:378–381

8 Combination Salicylic Acid/TCA Chemical Peeling

Pearl E. Grimes

8.1 History

The author has extensive experience using the combination of salicylic acid and TCA 10–15% for facial peeling [1]. She has treated innumerable patients with moderate to severe melasma with this combination regimen. In the initial series of 27 patients, 9 were classified as Fitzpatrick skin type IV, 11 were skin type V, and 7 were skin type VI. Many of the subjects included in the pilot group of patients had not responded to salicylic acid or glycolic acid peels. The concentration of salicylic acid was 20% and 30%, and the TCA concentration was 10%. A series of four peels were performed at 2-week intervals. Thirty percent of the patients experienced moderate improvement, and 70% experienced significant improvement in hyperpigmentation. Sixteen percent had minimal to mild side effects, which cleared within 1 week. The results of the study suggested that the combination peel is safe and efficacious for treatment of moderate and severe melasma. The peel has since been used successfully in all skin types. Swinehart pretreated a series of patients with lentigines, pigmented keratoses, and actinic damage of the dorsal hands with TCA 20% prior to application of a 50% salicylic acid paste [2]. He reported excellent results.

P.E. Grimes
Division of Dermatology, Department of Medicine, David Geffen School of Medicine, University of California—Los Angeles, Vitiligo and Pigmentation Institute of Southern California, 5670 Wilshire Blvd., Suite 650, Los Angeles, CA 90036, USA
e-mail: pegrimesmd@earthlink.net

8.2 Chemical Background/Properties

Salicylic acid (ortho-hydroxybenzoic acid) is a beta-hydroxy acid agent. It is a lipophilic compound which produces desquamation of the stratum corneum via removal of intercellular lipids [3] (see section 7). Given its keratolytic effects, it has become an increasingly popular superficial peeling agent. Salicylic acid peels induce injury via thinning or removal of the stratum corneum [4].

Trichloroacetic acid (TCA) causes precipitation of proteins and coagulative necrosis of epidermal cells [5, 6]. The extent of damage is indeed concentration dependent. Concentrations range from 10% to 50%. Superficial TCA peeling is induced by concentrations of 10–30% whereas higher concentrations cause medium-depth or deep peeling. The combination of salicylic acid followed by TCA 10–15% induces superficial wounding.

8.3 Formulations

Ethanol formulations of salicylic acid (20% and 30%) are used for combination peeling (see salicylic acid section). Trichloroacetic acid is prepared as an aqueous solution, since ethanol solutions do not penetrate the skin. It is prepared by mixing the appropriate concentration of crystals with up to 100 cc of distilled water. Ten percent and 15% TCA is prepared by mixing 10 or 15 g of crystals in up to 100 cc of total volume respectively. Aqueous solutions of TCA remain stable for up to 6 months unless contaminated. Other methods have been used to formulate TCA peeling

A. Tosti et al. (eds.), *Color Atlas of Chemical Peels*,
DOI 10.1007/978-3-642-20270-4_8, © Springer-Verlag Berlin Heidelberg 2012

solutions; however, the weight/volume methods appear to be the most reliable formulation [7]. Premixed TCA solutions are available from a variety of medical suppliers (Delasco – Council Bluffs, Iowa; Moore Medical – New Britain, Connecticut).

8.4 Indications

Despite the benefits of superficial peeling agents such as glycolic acid or salicylic acid, it is not uncommon to observe treatment failures. Some patients may require a more aggressive peeling regimen while minimizing the risk of side effects such as hyperpigmentation or hypopigmentation (Table 8.1). While TCA remains the gold standard of peeling agents, it is maximally efficacious in Fitzpatrick's skin types I through III [8–10]. In darker skin types, even TCA 15% or 20% can be fraught with post-peel complications. The combination of salicylic acid 20%/30% and low-strength TCA peeling produces additional efficacy compared to salicylic acid peels or TCA 10% peels while minimizing complications reported with higher concentrations of TCA or glycolic acid, particularly in darker racial ethnic groups (Figs. 8.1a, b and 8.2a, b).

Table 8.1 Indications for salicylic acid/TCA peeling

Hyperpigmentation
Melasma
Post-inflammatory hyperpigmentation
Solar lentigines
Photodamage
Acne
Texturally rough skin

The combination of salicylic acid and TCA 15% is also an effective treatment for mild to moderate photodamage, acne, and melasma in types I through III. Moderate to excellent improvement has been observed (Figs. 8.3a, b, 8.4a, b and 8.5a, b). Hence, the combination salicylic acid/TCA peeling protocol can be used in all skin types.

8.5 Contraindications

There are few contraindications to combination salicylic acid/TCA peeling. The combination regimen is tolerated in all skin types and all racial/ethnic groups.

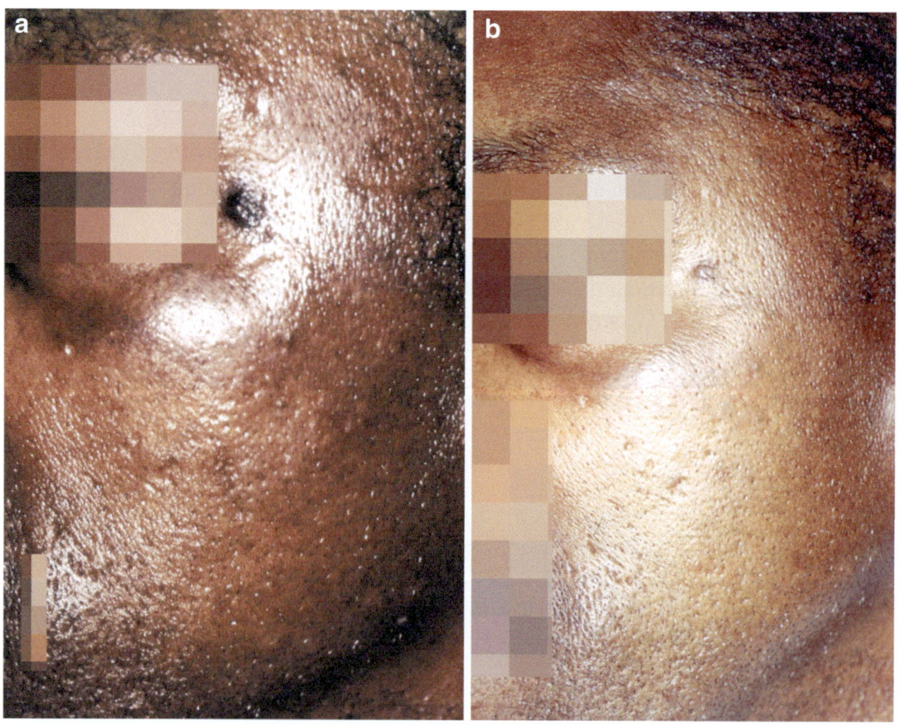

Fig. 8.1 (**a**) African American male with severe post-inflammatory hyperpigmentation. (**b**) Note significant improvement after combination salicylic acid/TCA peeling

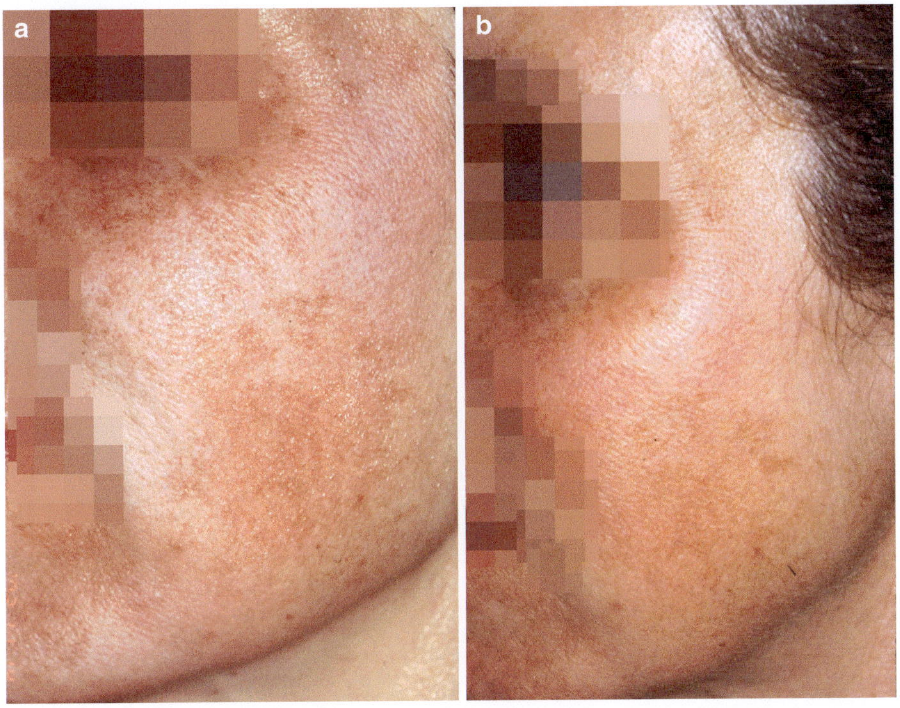

Fig. 8.2 (**a**) Patient with recalcitrant melasma unresponsive to glycolic acid or salicylic acid peels. (**b**) Responded to combination salicylic acid/TCA peeling

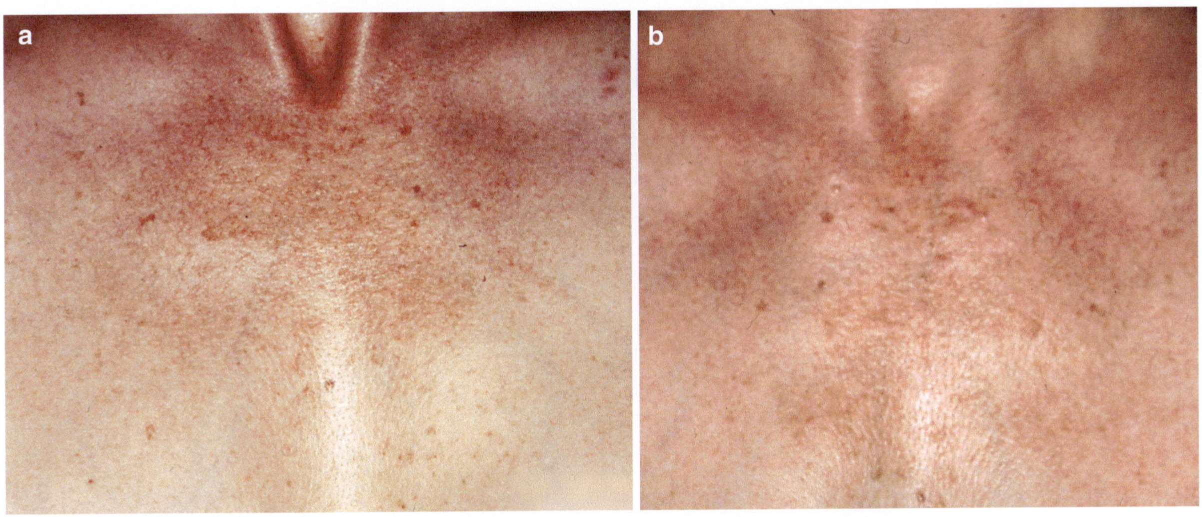

Fig. 8.3 (**a**) Patient with photodamage of the chest. (**b**) Note significant improvement after combination salicylic acid/TCA peel

General contraindications include salicylate hypersensitivity; unrealistic patient expectations; active inflammation/dermatitis of the site to be peeled; acute viral infection; pregnancy; isotretinoin therapy within 6 months of peeling; or history of poor or delayed wound healing. Having peeled more than 1,000 patients with salicylic acid, the author has observed no cases of salicylate hypersensitivity from topical peeling.

8.6 Peeling Preparations

A detailed history and cutaneous examination is performed in all patients prior to chemical peeling. The peeling procedure should be explained in depth to the patient including a discussion of the benefits, as well as the risks of the procedure. In addition, standardized

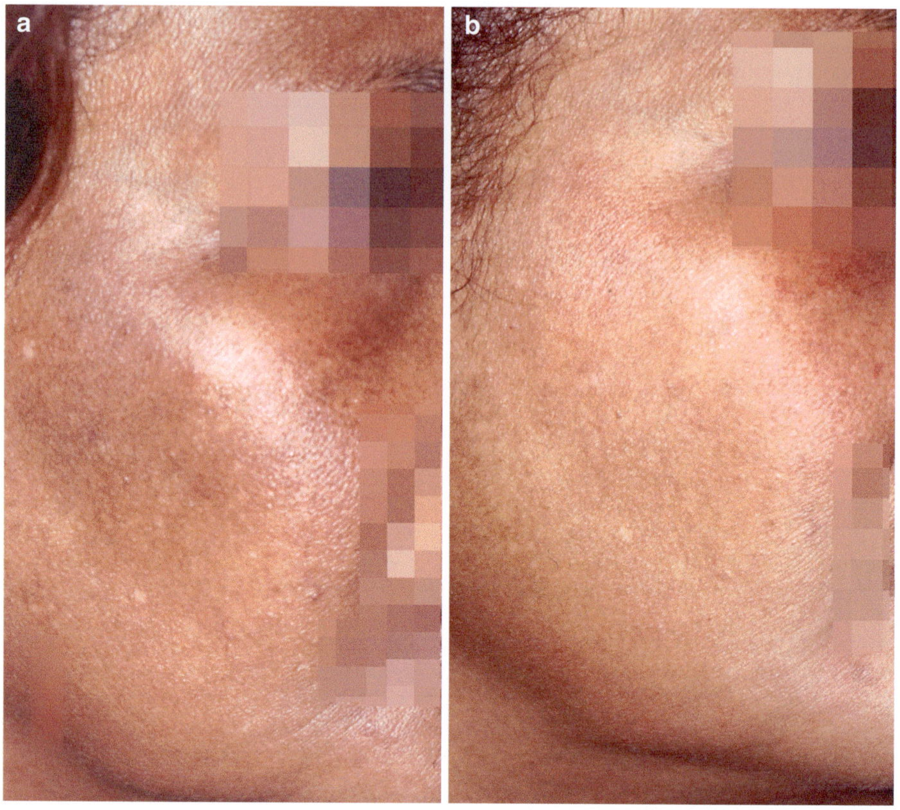

Fig. 8.4 (**a**) Facial melasma in skin type III. (**b**) Note significant improvement after combination salicylic acid/TCA peel

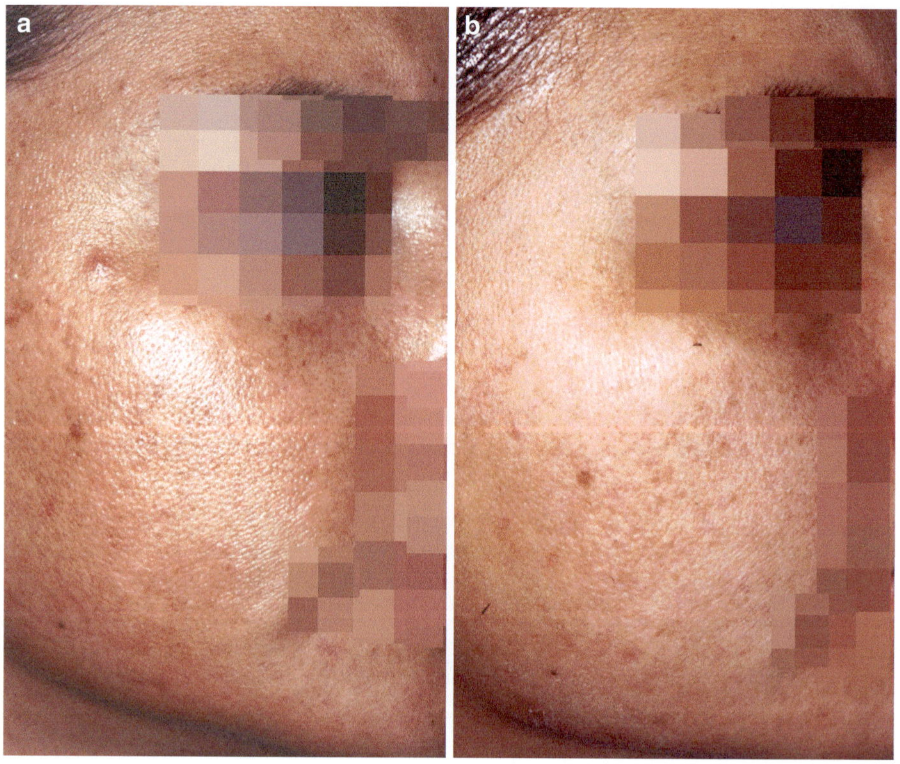

Fig. 8.5 (**a**) Patient with facial melasma. (**b**) Note improvement after combination salicylic acid/TCA peel

photographs are taken of the areas to be peeled including full frontal and lateral views.

The author has never observed a flare of Herpes following a superficial chemical peel. Hence, pretreatment with antiviral therapy is usually not indicated. However, one can prophylactically treat with antiviral therapies including valacyclovir 500 mg bid, famciclovir 500 mg bid, or Acyclovir 400 mg bid for 7–10 days beginning 1 or 2 days prior to the procedure.

Use of topical retinoids (tretinoin, tazarotene, retinol formulations) for 2–6 weeks prior to peeling thins the stratum corneum, and enhances epidermal turnover [8]. Such agents also reduce the content of epidermal melanin and expedite epidermal healing. Retinoids also enhance the penetration of the peeling agent. They should be discontinued several days prior to the peeling procedure. Retinoids can be resumed postoperatively after all evidence of peeling and irritation subsides. When treating conditions such as melasma, acne, and post-inflammatory hyperpigmentation, as well as darker skin types, retinoids should be discontinued 1 or 2 weeks before peeling or even eliminated from the prep to avoid post-peel complications, such as excessive erythema, desquamation, and post-inflammatory hyperpigmentation. Topical alpha-hydroxy acid or polyhydroxy acid formulations can also be used to prep the skin. In general, they are less aggressive agents in impacting peel outcomes. The skin is usually prepped for 2–4 weeks with a formulation of hydroquinone 4% or higher compounded formulations (5–10%) to reduce epidermal melanin. This is extremely important when treating the aforementioned dyschromias. Although less effective, other topical bleaching agents include azelaic acid, kojic acid, arbutin, and licorice (see photoaging section). Patients can also resume use of topical bleaching agents postoperatively after peeling and irritation subsides [9].

8.7 Peeling Technique

After thorough cleansing of the face with alcohol and acetone, two or three coats of salicylic acid (20% or 30%) are applied to the entire face with a 2 × 2 wedge sponge, 2 × 2 gauze sponges, or cotton-tipped applicators for 3–5 min. Typically, the cheeks are treated first, applying the peel from medial-to-lateral areas, followed by application to the chin and forehead. Most patients experience some mild burning and stinging during the procedure. Some patients experience a sensation of peel-related facial anesthesia. Portable handheld fanning during the procedure substantially mitigates the sensation of burning and stinging.

A white precipitate which represents crystallization of the salicylic acid begins to form at 30 s to 1 min following peel application. This should not be confused with frosting or whitening of the skin, which represents protein agglutination. After 3–5 min, the face is thoroughly rinsed with tap water to remove salicylic acid crystals. The face is gently blotted to remove excess water. When treating hyperpigmentation, TCA 10% or 15% is then applied to the areas of hyperpigmentation with a cotton-tipped swab for 2–3 min, producing minimal (Level 1) or no (Level 0) frosting. The face is again rinsed with tap water. If treating photodamage, acne, or texturally rough skin, TCA is applied to the entire face. This protocol usually involves a regimen of two or three combination peels performed at 2–4 week intervals.

8.8 Post-peeling Care and Complications

Bland, non-irritating moisturizers and cleansers are used after peeling until all desquamation and/or erythema subsides. Crusting, desquamation, or erythema can be treated with low- to high-potency steroids for 7–10 days. Given the depth of peeling, the author has observed no cases of scarring or persistent post-peel hyperpigmentation. Any residual post-inflammatory hyperpigmentation has responded to treatment with either hydroquinone 4% or higher strength formulations (5–10%).

8.9 Advantages

The advantages of combination salicylic acid/TCA peeling include:

- Efficacy in all skin types
- Well tolerated in darker racial/ethnic groups

- Most beneficial in treating recalcitrant melasma and post-inflammatory hyperpigmentation

8.10 Disadvantages

- Increased depth of superficial peeling
- Increased desquamation in some patients lasting up to 7–10 days
- Post-inflammatory hyperpigmentation more common than with salicylic acid peeling

8.11 Side Effects

As with salicylic acid peeling, the incidence of side effects is usually low. However, given the combination effects, erythema and desquamation can last longer than the usual changes observed with salicylic acid peels or TCA 10%. In a larger series of 50 patients treated by the author with combination peeling, 6 patients exhibited mild post-inflammatory hyperpigmentation which resolved within 1–2 weeks after the use of mid- to high-potency topical steroids.

Patient's Informed Consent

I, _______________, hereby consent to having my _____________ (site) treated with CHEMICAL PEELING USING A COMBINATION SALICYLIC ACID 20% AND 30% AND TRICHLOROACETIC ACID 10% OR 15%. The peeling procedure can improve dark spots (hyperpigmentation), photodamage (sun damage), textural roughness, acne, tone, and the overall appearance of the treated area. This combination peeling agent will cause shedding of the outermost layers of the skin. There may or may not be visible peeling. The procedure involves first having the peel site prepped with alcohol, acetone, or other pre-peel cleansing agents. The salicylic acid peeling agent is applied first, followed by application of the trichloroacetic acid. The area is rinsed and blotted dry.

You may experience redness, crusting, and flaking of the skin. The effects could possibly last for 1–2 weeks. In general, the combination salicylic acid/Trichloroacetic acid peel is extremely well tolerated.

I understand that there is a small risk of developing permanent darkening or undesirable pigment loss at the treated site. There is a rare chance that a scar could develop. There is a small risk that a bacterial infection could develop. There is a small chance the peel could also trigger a flare of a pre-existing Herpetic infection at the treated site. There is a small chance that the condition being treated could worsen after the peeling procedure. The benefits and side effects of the procedure have been explained to me in detail. All of my questions have been answered.

- I am in stable health.
- I have not used isotretinoin in the past 6 months.
- I have no allergies to salicylic acid, or trichloroacetic acid.
- I am not pregnant.

Outcomes are not guaranteed.

___________________________________ ______________

Signature of Patient Date

____

Patient Name (Please Print)

___________________________________ ______________

Witness Date

Disclaimer The author has no financial interest in any of the products or equipment mentioned in this chapter.

References

1. Grimes PE, Rendon M, Pallerano J (2008) Superficial chemical peels in aesthetics & cosmetic surgery in darker skin types. Lippincott Williams & Wilkins, Philadelphia, pp 155–169
2. Swinehart JM (1992) Salicylic acid ointment peeling of the hands and forearms. Effective nonsurgical removal of pigmented lesions and actinic damage. J Dermatol Surg Oncol 18(6):495–498
3. Lazo ND, Meine JG, Downing DT (1995) Lipids are covalently attached to rigid corneocyte protein envelope existing predominantly as beta-sheets: a solid state nuclear magnetic resonance study. J Invest Dermatol 105: 296–300
4. Imayama S, Ueda S, Isoda M (2000) Histologic changes in the skin of hairless mice following peeling with salicylic acid. Arch Dermatol 136:1390–1395
5. Matarasso SL, Glogau RG (1991) Chemical face peels. Dermatol Clin 9:131–150
6. Rajalingam D, Loftis C, Xu JJ, Kumar TK (2009) Trichloroacetic acid induced protein precipitation involves the reversible association of a stable partially structured intermediate. Protein Sci 18:980–993
7. Bridenstine JB, Dolezal JF (1994) Standardizing chemical peel solution formulations to avoid mishaps. Great fluctuations in actual concentrations of trichloroacetic acid. J Dermatol Surg Oncol 20(12):813–816
8. Nguyen TH, Rooney JA (2000) Trichloroacetic acid peels. Dermatol Ther 13:173–192
9. Rubin MG (1995) Manual of chemical peels: superficial and medium depth. J.B. Lippincott Company, Philadelphia, pp 79–88
10. Brody HJ (1997) Chemical peeling and resurfacing, 2nd edn. Mosby, St. Louis

Home Peeling: A Combined Technique

9

Brigitta Maria Cavegn

9.1 From a Dermatological Clinical Treatment to a New Kind of Home Peel

The spectacular results achieved with chemical peels containing all kinds of substances are well documented, since for decades, they have been carried out in a proper, controlled manner, and empirically for much longer.

Although a peel in a clinic may be an excellent treatment option, not everyone is interested in undergoing one.

However, most people are interested in having the most beautiful skin possible, judging by the immense offer of beauty-care products in the market, including a number of home peels. Every cosmetic brand has its own version: from Elizabeth Arden, Lancôme, and La Prairie to REN, Pevonia, and Neutrogena, and several doctors even have their own lines, such as SBT, Dr. Patricia Wexler, and Dr. Sebag, to name but a few. Although in the past, most home peels were mechanical exfoliators (scrubs), there is today a clear tendency toward chemical or enzymatic peels. Rarely are peels combined with a mechanical and chemical component such as DERMAdoctor Physical Chemistry. They are always integrated in their product line.

Over the years, I have seen so many patients in my dermatological clinic who have, to a certain extent, been confused by the enormous offer of skin-care products. Again and again I am asked for simple, fast home solutions to improve people's skin, not least as the result of today's lifestyle, but also for simple and fast solutions for maintaining or priming the skin after or before procedures performed in the clinic.

The challenge was to satisfy the many and diverse requirements of my patients in one unique basic product. The Peeling B SAND was created and produced in cooperation with the reputable pharmaceutical and cosmetics company Louis Widmer SA of Zurich, Switzerland, and shortly afterward received the international "Annabelle Prix de Beauté 2009" award for the best new face-care product.

9.1.1 What is the Peeling B SAND?

It is a skin-care product based on the concept of "fast, easy, effective." To satisfy this concept, the product had to be in the form of a peel, but to satisfy all my patients' requirements, it had to be much more than that.

It is the most compact, and perhaps the only doctor's brand to consist of just one product. It is a basic skin-care product in the form of a bi-phase exfoliant that was inspired by techniques of esthetic dermatology (microdermabrasion and chemical peel) with integrated preliminary hydration.

Thanks to the combination of mechanical exfoliation, the chemical effects of AHAs, and the integrated care provided by biostimulators (amino acids), B SAND improves the structure of skin of all ages and slows down the aging process in just one single, fast step.

B.M. Cavegn
Private Dermatologic Clinic, Via Praella 11,
6850 Mendrisio, Switzerland
e-mail: info@bsand.ch

A. Tosti et al. (eds.), *Color Atlas of Chemical Peels*,
DOI 10.1007/978-3-642-20270-4_9, © Springer-Verlag Berlin Heidelberg 2012

Table 9.1 Ingredients and effects

Active ingredients	Effects
Polyethylene beads	Mechanical exfoliation
Fruit acid complex	Chemical exfoliation
Biostimulators	Hydrate the skin
D-panthenol, polidocanol	Reduce skin irritations
Undecylenic acid	Mildly antibacterial

9.1.2 Characteristics

B SAND has three fundamental functions:

- Ultra deep cleansing
- Preliminary hydration
- Antiaging qualities

In particular, thanks to the unique blend of various ingredients (Table 9.1) and the synergetic mode of action (Table 9.2) B SAND is

- A primary cure:
  It is intended for the treatment of various skin problems such as restricting sebum production in oily skin, moisturizing dry skin, disinfecting acne lesions, reducing pores, diminishing blackheads, lightening marks and blemishes, reducing fine lines, and leaving the complexion bright and radiant.
- A complementary cure:
  It can be combined with any other skin-care and antiaging product.
- A prerequisite for subsequent treatments:
  It is a booster, and increases the effectiveness of other products/treatments.

The skin is made over in just 3 min. Unlike earlier peels, which only exfoliated, this peel delivers amino acids and AHAs to the skin as it is being exfoliated. The peel resurfaces and replenishes the skin simultaneously, which is a new approach to skin rejuvenation. Amino acids moisturize the skin while AHAs (especially undecylenic acid) minimize congestion/breakouts.

9.1.3 Mechanisms of Action

The combination of the mechanical and biochemical phases (Table 9.2) has a synergistic effect. Corneocytes are easily dissociated and exfoliated, and the barrier of the skin is thinned so it can better absorb the remaining principal active ingredients. Epidermal growth is stimulated by the partial removal of the stratum corneum. Although the concentration of the AHAs may be minimal, which guarantees the optimum tolerance, there is no loss of performance because it is a combined peel. As a further aid to tolerance, we added amino acids to moisturize the skin, help rebuild its support structure, and improve firmness and elasticity while minimizing the appearance of fine lines and wrinkles. Polidocanol

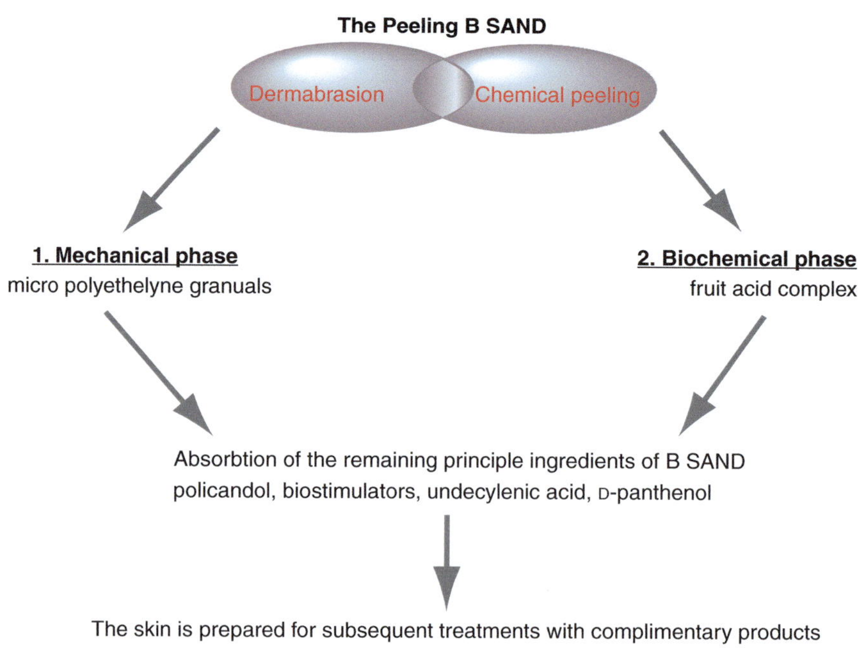

Table 9.2 Combination of mechanisms of actions

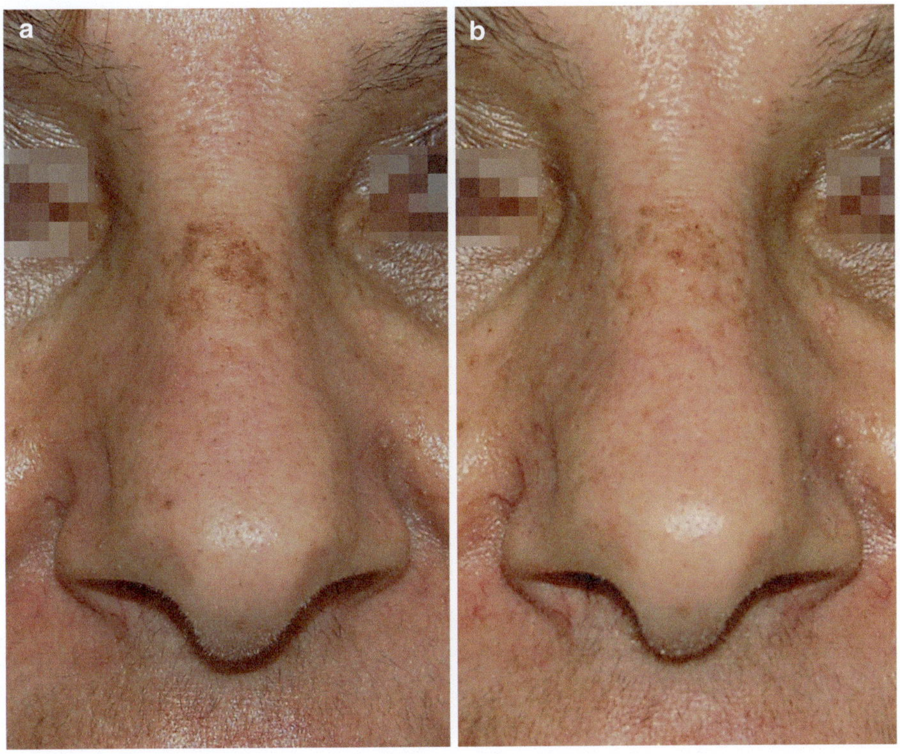

Fig. 9.1 (**a**, **b**) before and after using only The Peeling B SAND, four times a week, during 4 weeks (From www.bsand.ch/products/effect, with permission)

and D-panthenol reduce skin irritations and repair tiny lesions. Massaging with microgranules improves the blood circulation and thus all the natural skin functions (defense, protection, regulation, production of collagen fibers), which slows down the skin's aging process and enhances skin rejuvenation.

9.1.4 Results and Patient Satisfaction

To monitor general satisfaction, we followed 100 patients in the clinic after 2, 4, and 6 weeks using B SAND twice a week (normal or sensitive skin) and four to five times a week (oily and acne skin). The patients continued their usual local skin-care regimen including ongoing local therapies. The only additional skin care was B SAND.

In 30 patients (16 with sensitive skin, 10 with normal skin, 4 with oily skin), we performed an epicutane test with B SAND.

We observed the following:

- No allergic reaction or irritation resulted from the epicutane test.
- Overall patient satisfaction with B SAND is excellent.
- In most cases, the skin structure and pore size were improved, the complexion appeared more uniform, the skin was better hydrated, and acne lesions were reduced (Figs. 9.1–9.5).

9.1.5 Indications and Application

Thanks to the original blend of components, the optimum tolerance and safety profile of B SAND is indicated for all skin types after puberty (Table 9.3).

Use once or twice a week on sensitive and dry skin, 2–3 times a week on greasy skin and skin that is prone to breakouts.

Massage gently onto wet skin. Leave to work for 3–4 min, then rinse off with plenty of water.

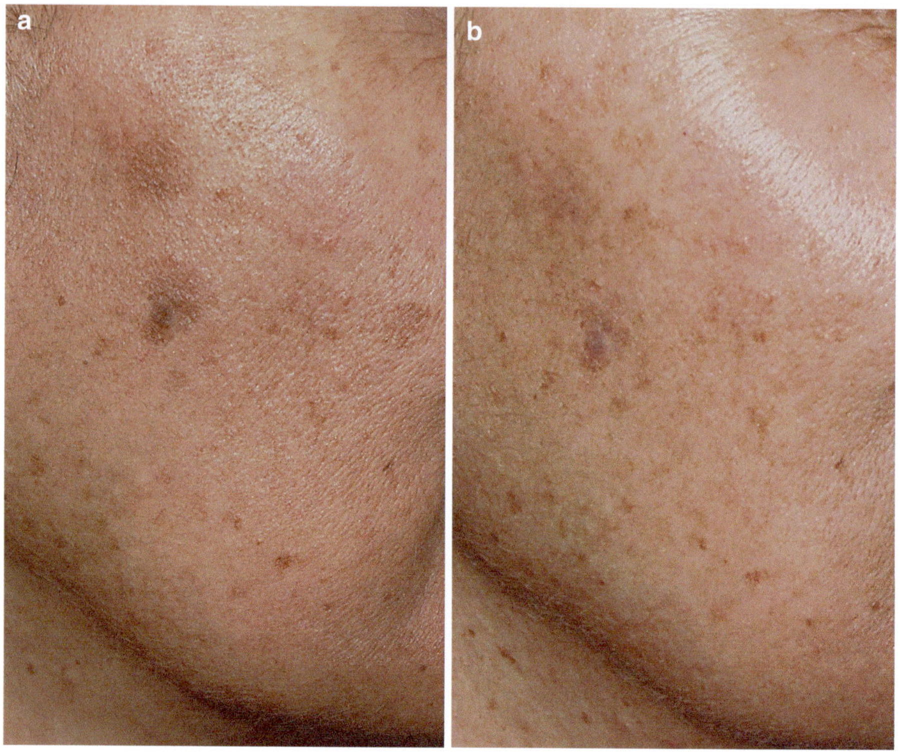

Fig. 9.2 (**a**, **b**) Before and after using only The Peeling B SAND, four times a week, during 4 weeks

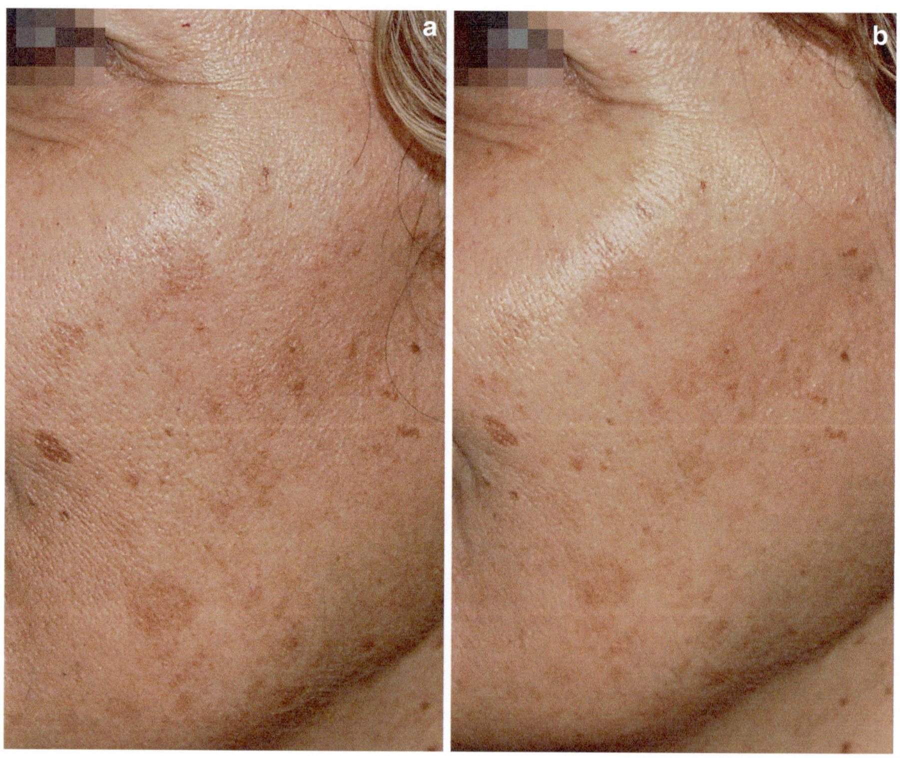

Fig. 9.3 (**a**, **b**) Before and after using only The Peeling B SAND, four times a week, during 4 weeks

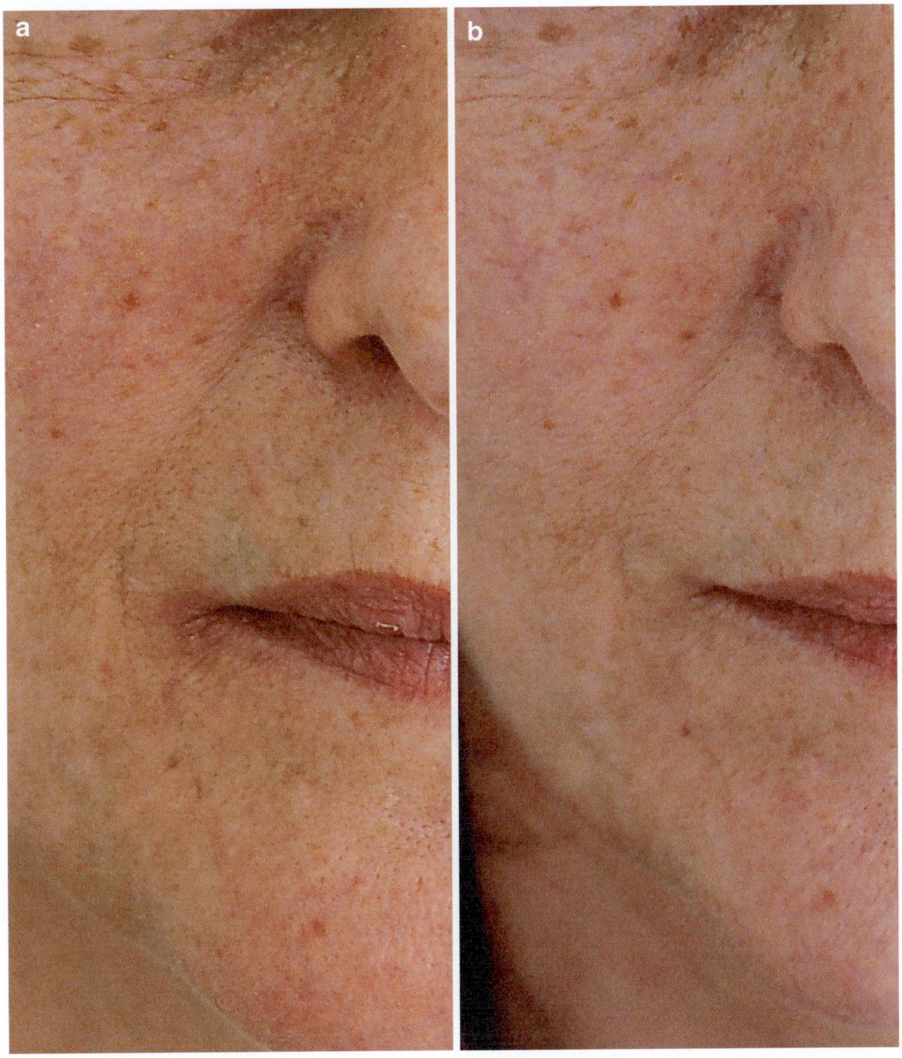

Fig. 9.4 (**a**, **b**) Before and after using only The Peeling B SAND, three times a week, during 4 weeks besides a mild soap and hydration

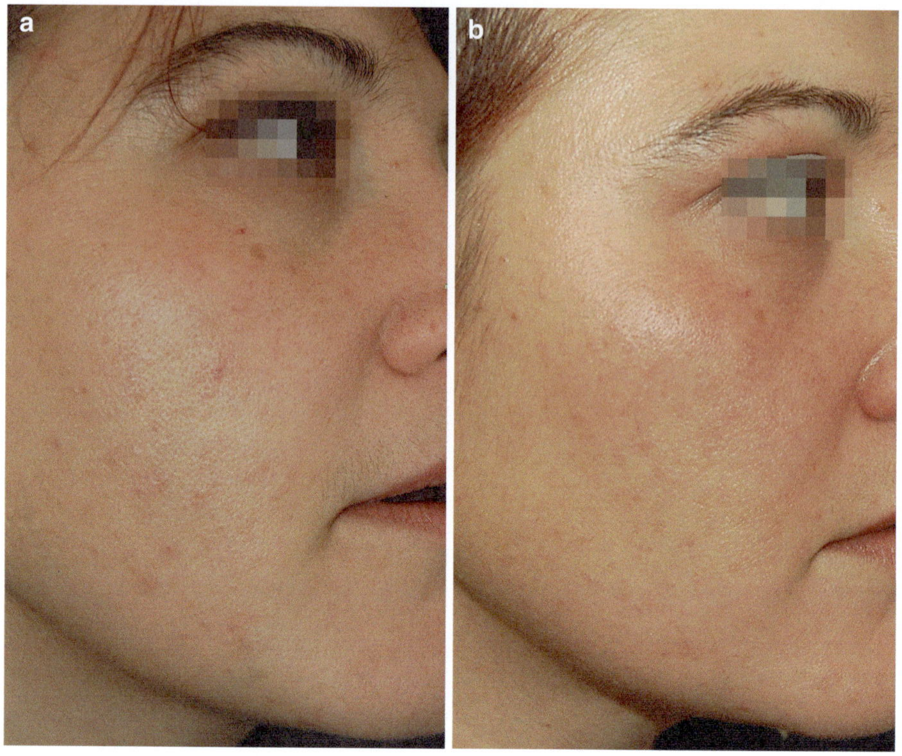

Fig. 9.5 (**a**, **b**) Before and after using The Peeling B SAND, daily, during 4 weeks (From www.bsand.ch/products/indications, with permission)

Table 9.3 Indications

Age	15	25	35	50
Indications	• Acne • Oily skin • Imperfections	• Dishydrated skin • Stressed skin • Fine lines	• Aging signs • Wrinkles • First spots • Open pores	• Wrinkles • Spots
		Booster for secondary anti-aging treatments (25–50)		

Combination of Peelings and Bio-rejuvenation

10

Maria Pia De Padova and Antonella Tosti

Bio-rejuvenation or bio-revitalization (mesolift) is a technique that utilizes the injection of absorbable and biocompatible substances into the superficial dermis in order to increase skin firmness, brightness, and moisturization. Most utilized agents include nonreticular hyaluronic acid 0.2–3% alone or associated with vitamins, amino acids, minerals, coenzymes, nucleic acids, antioxidants and beta-glucan, polynucleotidic macromolecules, organic silicium, autologous cultured fibroblasts, growth factors, and homeopathic products.

We usually utilize bio-revitalization before combined peeling with 25% salicylic acid followed by 25% TCA in patients with photoaging of the face, hands, neck, or decoltè who complain of skin dryness and hyperpigmentation. Combining the two procedures enhances results of treatments as bio-revitalization improves skin brightness and moisturization and chemical peeling improves skin texture and color (Fig. 10.1a, b, c).

After cleaning the skin with antiseptic solution (without alcohol), we microinject 1–2 mL of the active solution using a 2.5-mL Luer-lock syringe with 30½G or 32G 4-mm needle or a syringe with a 2.5-mm S.I.T. needle (needle for Skin Injection Therapy) (Fig. 10.2).

M.P. De Padova
Ospedale Privato Nigrisoli,
Bologna, Italy
e-mail: mdepadova@gmail.com

A. Tosti (✉)
Department of Dermatology and Cutaneous Surgery,
Miller School of Medicine, University of Miami, US
e-mail: atosti@med.miami.edu

Injection should be performed in the superficial dermis either as single punctures (Picotage) or serial threading (Cross-linking).

- Picotage (Fig. 10.3)

  Inject one drop of the product into the superficial dermis (the needle needs to penetrate 2–2.5 mm). The injections are placed at a distance of 2 mm.
- Serial threading
- Insert the needle for all its length and inject during the extraction phase (Fig. 10.4)

  Injections are placed at a distance of 1 cm (Fig. 10.5). This method is useful for the cheeks and low neckline (Fig. 10.6).

A gentle massage improves uniform distribution of the treatment. The procedure usually requires 20–30 min, depending on the treated area and does not produce any visible side effect except for small short-lasting bruises. Mild stinging during injection occurs with products containing vitamin C. The combination peeling can be performed immediately after bio-rejuvenation. We first apply the 25% salicylic acid solution on the whole area to be treated, and after precipitation of the salicylic acid, we then apply the 25% TCA gel, which should be applied with pressure on hyperpigmented spots.

Treatments should be repeated every 2 weeks for 3–4 weeks, then once a month for 3–4 months, and then once or twice a year.

This protocol may vary according to the patient's age, clinical presentation, and response to initial treatments.

Improvement of skin brightness is usually visible after the first treatment due to the vascular stimulus induced by the microinjections.

A. Tosti et al. (eds.), *Color Atlas of Chemical Peels*,
DOI 10.1007/978-3-642-20270-4_10, © Springer-Verlag Berlin Heidelberg 2012

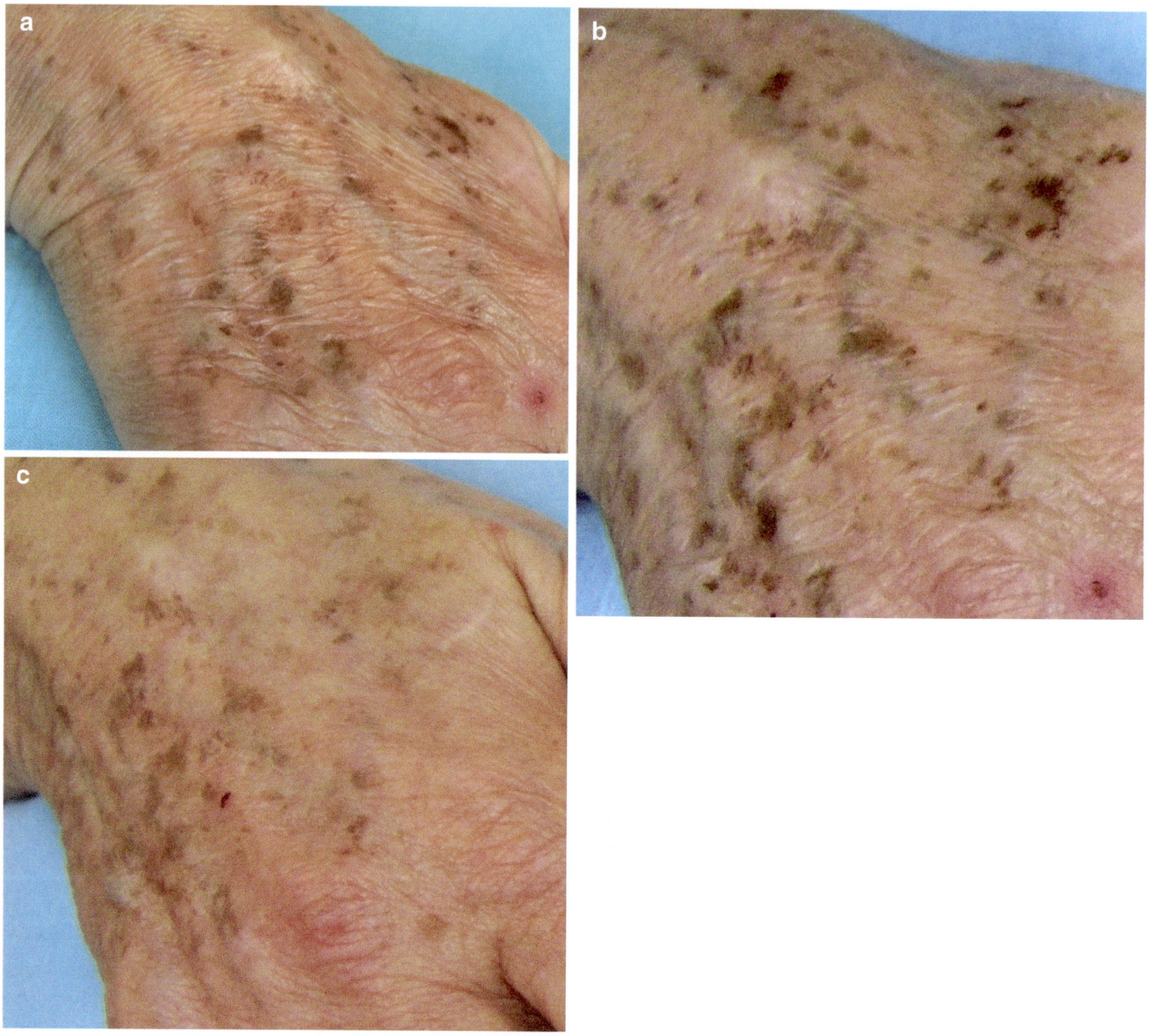

Fig. 10.1 Severe hand photoaging before (**a**), after 1 week (**b**), and after four sessions (**c**) of bio-rejuvenation followed by combination 25% salicylic acid and 25% TCA. Note crusting (**b**) on the hyperpigmented lesions treated with spot TCA

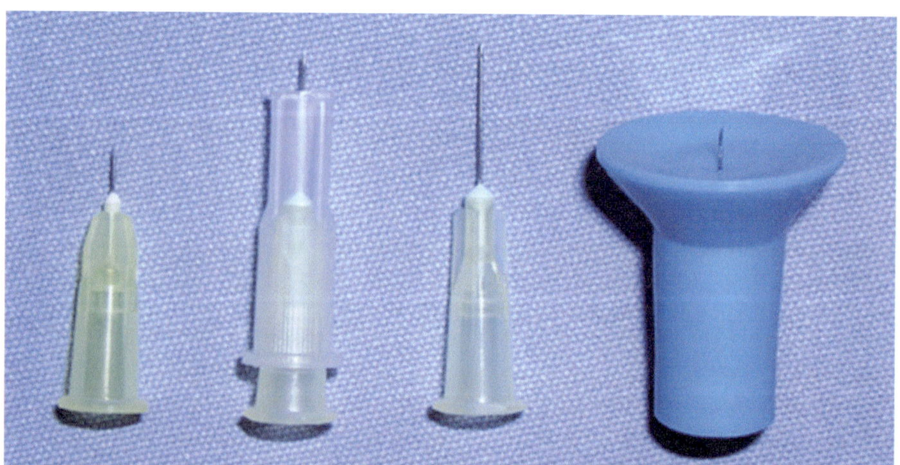

Fig. 10.2 Needles utilized for bio-rejuvenation. *From left*: 32G 4-mm long needle; 30½G needle: we cut the needle cover in order to obtain a 3–4-mm long needle; 30½G needle to be utilized for serial threading injections; 2.5-mm S.I.T. needle

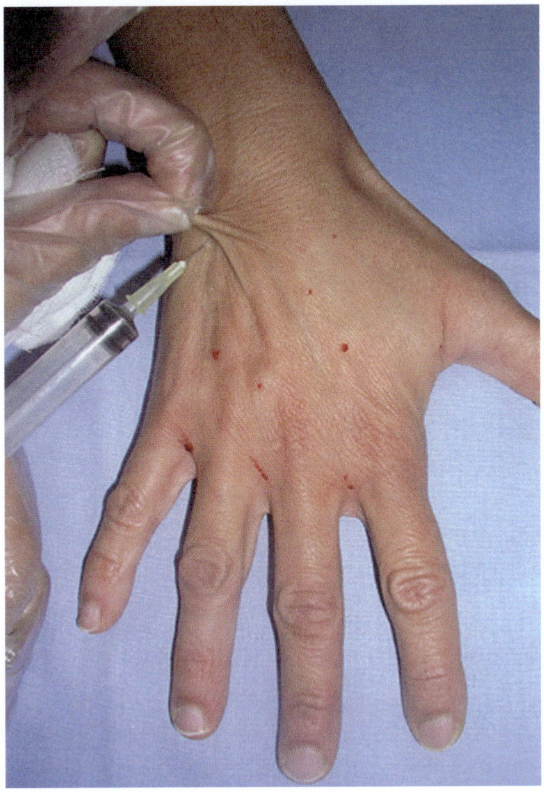

Fig. 10.3 Picotage

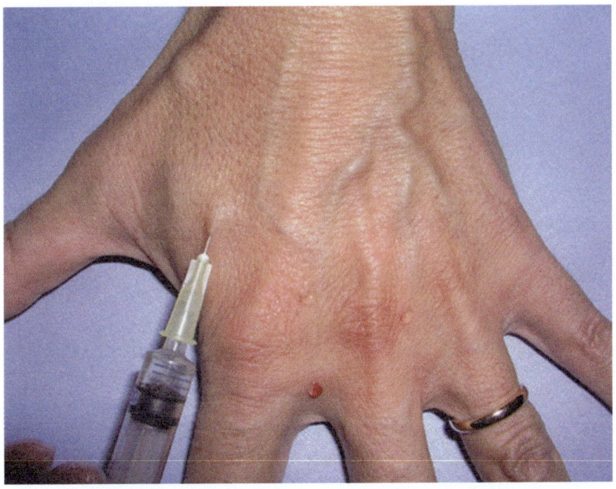

Fig. 10.4 Serial threading technique: insert the needle superficially under the skin surface

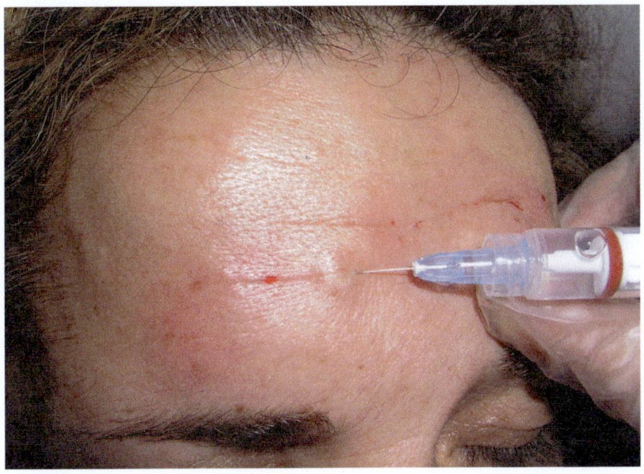

Fig. 10.5 The solution is injected during the extraction phase (retrograde technique)

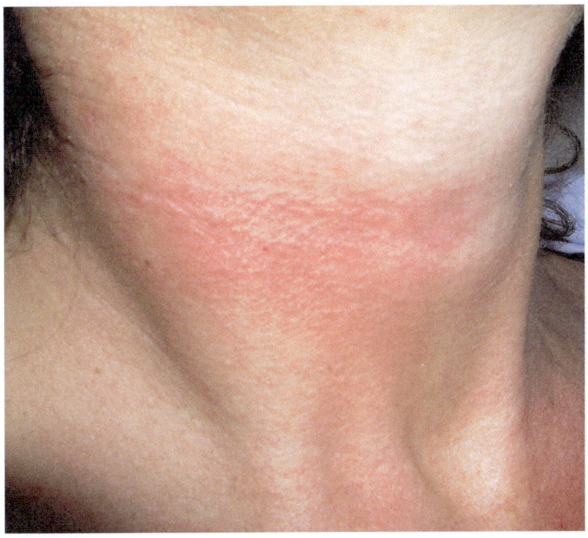

Fig. 10.6 Erythema after bio-rejuvenation with serial threading technique on the neck

10.1 Advantages of Bio-rejuvenation

- Easy to perform
- Almost painless
- No necessity of skin test
- No recovery or down time
- Limited side effects (mild erythema and bruising)

11 Combination of Microdermabrasion and Chemical Peels

Pearl E. Grimes

11.1 Introduction

Microdermabrasion is a popular technique for superficial resurfacing of the skin [1]. It involves the propulsion of abrasive microcrystals on to the treatment area in short strokes using a special handpiece. The handset simultaneously vacuums away the used abrasive particles and skin debris. The speed of the particles (and the vacuum suction) can be adjusted by the operator to control the volume of particles bombarding the skin. Other factors influencing the intensity of the treatment are the speed of movement of the handpiece and the number of times it is passed over the skin. An increased depth of microdermabrasion is achieved when the handpiece is moved slowly and repeatedly over a specific site [2]. Overall, the technique is considered to be minimally invasive with few complications [2]. Particle-free microdermabrasion units have become extremely popular. Such units utilize a disposable or reusable diamond wand to induce abrasion. Numerous microdermabrasion units are available globally.

Clinically, microdermabrasion results in a visible brightening of the skin and improvement of surface texture as the superficial skin cells are removed. The appearance of fine wrinkles, shallow acne scars, and hyperpigmentation may also be ameliorated. Although the histopathological effects of microdermabrasion have not been fully elucidated, research shows that a single treatment triggers a chain of molecular events that may ultimately result in dermal remodeling [3]. These events included the induction of matrix-degrading enzymes and of primary cytokines including interleukin 1b (IL-1b) and tumor necrosis factor alpha (TNF-α). Significant effects on collagen synthesis were not, however, demonstrated [3]. Rajan and Grimes have demonstrated that dermabrasion with aluminum oxide or sodium chloride is associated with significant improvements in epidermal barrier function [4]. They speculated that this might contribute to observed improvements in skin tone and texture. Other studies have shown that microdermabrasion can increase epidermal thickness, decrease melanization of the epidermis, increase dermal thickness as well as increase elastin and collagen production [1].

Chemical peels are treatments that involve the application of caustic chemicals to the skin to induce controlled destruction and shedding of components of the epidermis and dermis [5]. Chemical peels are classified according to the depth of peeling and include superficial, medium-depth, and deep peels. Superficial peeling agents target the stratum corneum to the papillary dermis. They include glycolic acid, salicylic acid, Jessner's solution, tretinoin, and tricholoracetic acid (TCA) in concentrations of 10–30%. Medium-depth peels penetrate to the upper reticular dermis and include TCA (35–50%), combination glycolic acid 70%/TCA 35%, Jessner's/TCA 35%, and phenol 88%. Deep chemical peels utilize the Baker-Gordon formulas and penetrate to the midreticular dermis. Peeling triggers repair and regeneration processes in the epidermis and the dermis, resulting in the remodeling of the skin surface. Chemical peels are often used to improve the appearance of scars,

P.E. Grimes
Division of Dermatology, Department of Medicine, David Geffen School of Medicine, University of California—Los Angeles, Vitiligo and Pigmentation Institute of Southern California, 5670 Wilshire Blvd., Suite 650, Los Angeles, CA 90036, USA
e-mail: pegrimesmd@earthlink.net

A. Tosti et al. (eds.), *Color Atlas of Chemical Peels*,
DOI 10.1007/978-3-642-20270-4_11, © Springer-Verlag Berlin Heidelberg 2012

dyschromias such as melasma and postinflammatory hyperpigmentation, and photoaged skin. They are also used in the treatment of acne and actinic keratoses.

Recent years have seen the introduction of new microdermabrasion units that release chemicals onto the skin following microdermabrasion so that a chemical microdermabrasion process is achieved. The superficial physical abrasion of the stratum corneum and epidermis achieved by microdermabrasion has been shown to increase the uptake of hydrophilic agents across the lipophilic epidermal barrier. For example, absorption of 5-aminolevulinic acid prior to photodynamic therapy is increased and accelerated by microdermabrasion [6]. In the same way, microdermabrasion has the potential to boost the penetration and activity of chemical peeling agents. This may result in a more pronounced overall effect, compared with either process used alone [7–10]. For example, in a small pilot study, patients who underwent microdermabrasion with aluminum oxide particles prior to a superficial chemical peel with 5% retinoic acid reported greater satisfaction (in terms of the texture, pigmentation, and general appearance of the treated skin) than those who received the retinoic acid peel only [9]. Similar results were obtained when microdermabrasion plus 15% TCA was compared with microdermabrasion alone for the treatment of hyperpigmentation [10]. In his histological study comparing the effects of microdermabrasion alone and in combination with a chemical peel, Kisner found that there was a complete removal of the epidermis following the combined treatment, producing a medium-depth wound [8]. In contrast, the effects of light microdermabrasion were confined to the stratum corneum, while more intensive microdermabrasion caused pinpoint bleeding and resulted in uneven epidermal stripping. Combined microdermabrasion and chemical peeling has been advocated for treatment of more severe acne scarring, moderately deep rhytides, and photodamaged skin, and for patients with a history of procedures [8, 9]. Briden et al. have also concluded that combined procedures – when used every other month, or seasonally, depending on the patient – can be effectively used as maintenance therapy [9].

11.1.1 Indications

Combined microdermabrasion and superficial chemical peeling is indicated for skin conditions which do not respond adequately to microdermabrasion or peeling alone. These include: photodamage (roughness, sallowness, solar lentigines, rhytides, and keratosis); hyperpigmentation; pronounced acne scars; and moderately deep wrinkles (Figs. 11.1–11.3). Although rosacea is considered an indication for superficial chemical peeling, it is regarded as a relative contraindication for microdermabrasion [1, 11].

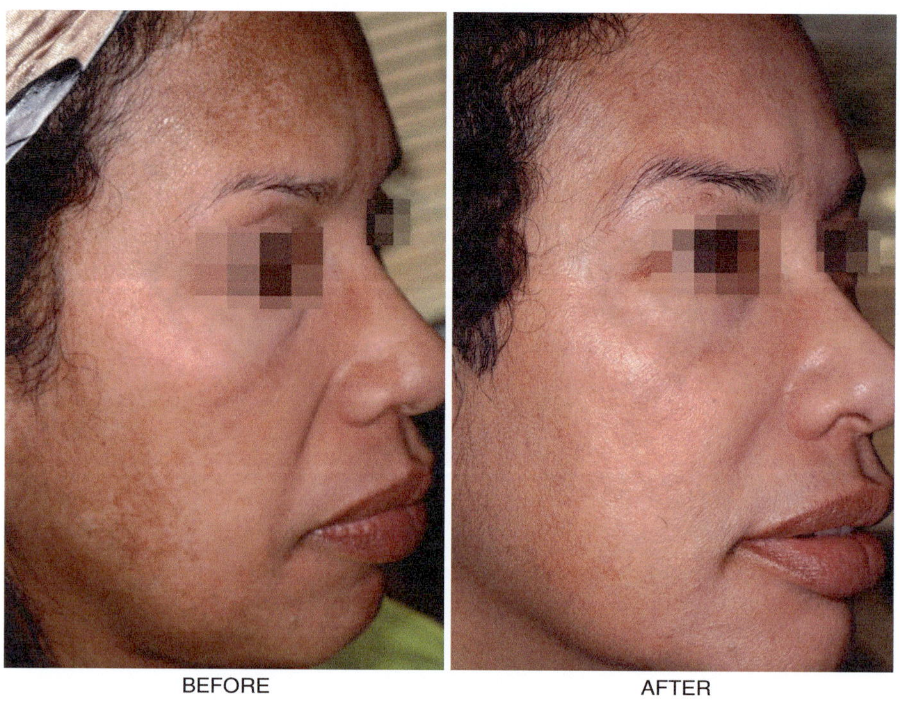

Fig. 11.1 Patient with Melasma before a series of 3 salicylic acid peels and 3 microdermabrasion treatments

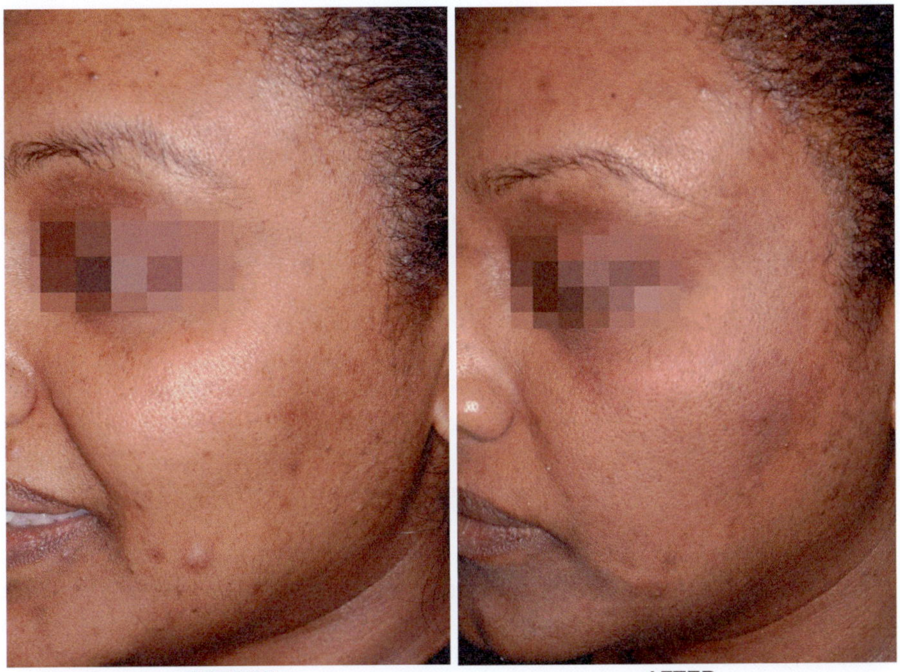

Fig. 11.2 Patient with post inflammatory hyperpigmentation and textural changes after 2 glycolic peels and 2 microdermabrasions

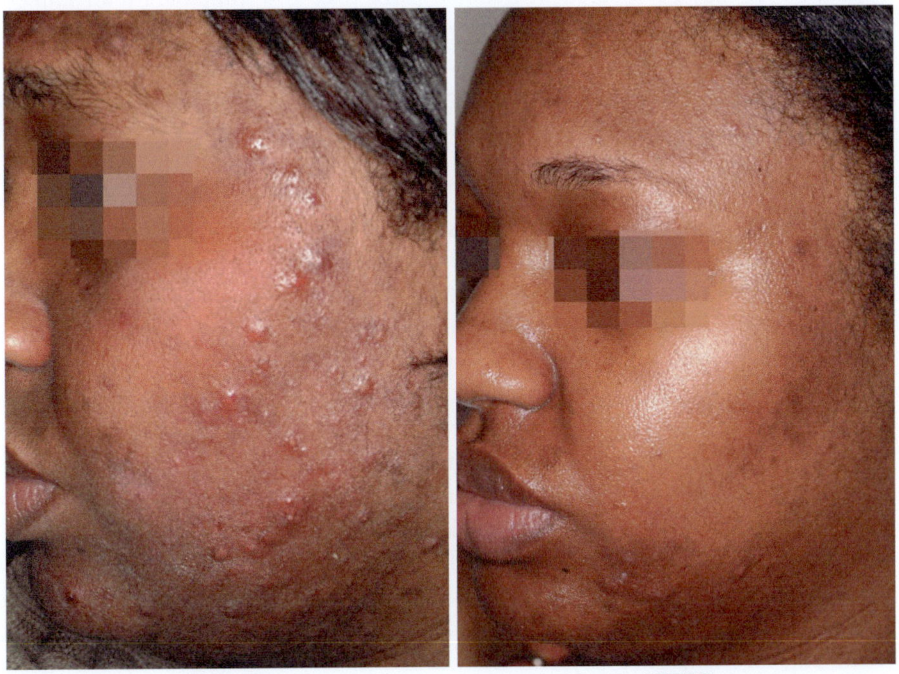

Fig. 11.3 Patient with acne vulgaris after 3 salicylic acid peels and 3 microdermabrasion treatments

11.1.2 Contraindications

Generally speaking, microdermabrasion is regarded as a safe, minimally invasive treatment, with a low potential for side effects. Microdermabrasion is, however, contraindicated in cases of active infection, such as herpes simplex, impetigo and flat warts, and active pustular or cystic acne [12]. Malignant tumors, keratoses, and evolving dermatosis are also contraindications. Relative contraindications include rosacea and telangiectasia [1]. Chemical peels are contraindicated in pregnant and nursing mothers and in cases of active herpes simplex or cold sores [5]. Other contraindications include isotretinoin treatment in the last 6 months and use of drugs that can induce hyperpigmentation (tetracycline, oral contraceptives) [11].

11.1.3 Skin Preparation

A detailed history and cutaneous examination should be performed in all patients prior to combined microdermabrasion and chemical peeling. Standardized photos are taken of the face, including frontal and lateral views. The exact technique used is likely to vary somewhat between physicians. In addition, skin preparation will vary with the condition being treated. For instance, when treating dyschromias such as melasma or postinflammatory hyperpigmentation. The skin can be prepped for 2–4 weeks with hydroquinone 4% or higher concentrations (5–10%) if the patient has stubborn areas of hyperpigmentation. Alternatively, other hypopigmentation formulas can also be used. Topical retinoids should be discontinued several days prior to the procedure. Retinoids will indeed enhance to depth of penetration of the chemicals utilized during the peeling procedure. Immediately before treatment, the patient's facial skin is thoroughly cleansed and degreased with isopropyl alcohol or acetone [11]. The patient's eyes may be covered with moist gauze pads or commercial pads (Sperian Derm-Aid®, Rhode Island, USA) designed to cover the eyes for microdermabrasion to protect them from contact with microdermabrasion crystals.

11.1.4 Techniques for Using Units

After the patient has been made comfortable in a supine or reclining position, the physician holds the skin taut and applies the handpiece of the microdermabrasion unit. This action triggers the flow of abrasive crystals through the handpiece. Typically, three passes in different directions are made over each treatment site, progressing through the various esthetic subunits of the face in a symmetrical fashion. It may be necessary to reduce the suction and crystal flow pressure over sites where the skin is thin and delicate, such as the eyelid. At the end of the microdermabrasion treatment, any remaining crystals are washed away, either with mild cleanser and water. The chemical peel is then applied using an applicator, brush, cotton balls, for a timed period or until the development of white frosting. At the end of the procedure, the peeling agent is removed with either cold water or a neutralizing spray. This combined procedure should be used with extreme care and caution in darker skin types.

11.2 Post-procedure Care

Following a combined microdermabrasion and chemical peeling procedure, Kisner recommends applying antibiotic ointment and cold compresses to the skin. I rarely use antibiotic ointments. Instead, a bland cleanser and moisturizer such as CeraVe or Cetaphil are used for 7 days. If the patient has irritation, hydrocortisone cream 2½% can be applied daily, sunscreens are worn daily. In their pilot study, Hexsel et al. washed the skin with running water 4 h after retinoid acid application and prescribed 1% hydrocortisone cream for the following 3 days [7]. This was combined with thrice daily application of SPF 15 sun cream for 1 week.

11.3 Advantages of Combined Microdermabrasion and Chemical Peeling

- Suitable for all skin types.
- Microdermabrasion enhances the penetration of chemical peeling agents.
- Combined treatment more effective than microdermabrasion alone in treating deeper wrinkles and acne scars.
- Fewer appointments required compared with separately administered treatments.

11.4 Disadvantage

- Minimal documentation available to support efficacy of combined approach

11.5 Side Effects

Common and immediate side effects of microdermabrasion are erythema, which usually subsides within 24 h but may occasionally be prolonged, and a slight burning sensation [13]. Purpura and petechiae may develop, especially on more delicate areas of skin, but these usually resolve spontaneously. Other potential complications are postinflammatory hyperpigmentation and, if excessive pressure is used, streaking marks. One unusual case of a severe urticarial response to microdermabrasion has been reported, which may have been due to latex allergy [14]. There is a risk of ocular complications if aluminum crystals enter the patient's eye; sodium chloride crystals, on the other hand, can be easily dissolved and washed away with prompt rinsing. Such events are easily prevented by the use of adhesive ocular shields. Likewise, practitioners should wear masks to minimize the risk of inhaling aluminum particles [1]. Side effects associated with chemical peeling include erythema, desquamation, and transient mild hyperpigmentation. With darker skin tones and deeper peels, there is also an increased risk of hyperpigmentation and solar lentigines. Careful use of sunscreen post treatment is recommended to reduce this risk.

A further potential side effect of combined microdermabrasion and chemical peeling is herpetic infection, which was reported by Kisner [8]. This can be treated with systemic acyclovir.

11.6 Summary

A number of small studies have indicated that the amelioration of more severe acne scars, moderately deep rhytides, and the effects of photoaging, which are often recalcitrant to standard treatment regimens, can be improved by combining microdermabrasion and superficial chemical peels in one treatment session. While more published data to support the use of this combined technique would be welcome, the data that are available indicate that it is highly effective, well tolerated, and more convenient for patients.

Patient Informed Consent

I______________________ hereby consent to have my ___________(site) treated with a combination procedure utilizing microdermabrasion and chemical peeling (superficial or medium-depth peel). The procedure will be performed to improve the appearance of my skin at the site(s) of treatment. This combination procedure is used to improve acne vulgaris, acne scars, hyperpigmentation (dark spots), sun damage (photodamage), and textural changes including rough texture.

Your face will be photographed prior to the procedure. The procedure first involves having the treatment site (_____) prepped with alcohol, acetone, or other pre-peel cleansing agents. Then the face is treated with a microdermabrasion machine (particle, nonparticle). This involves the propulsion of abrasive microcrystals such as aluminum chloride or sodium bicarbonate onto the treatment area from a wand-like hand piece while simultaneously vacuuming away the used abrasive particles and skin cells. Alternatively, a machine may be used which abrades the skin without the use of particles. The skin is then revised to remove debris and crystals from the face.

The chemical peel (type) is then applied using a brush, cotton balls, or other applications for either a timed period or until frosting or a whitish color appears at the end of the procedure; the peeling agent is either removed with either cold water or a neutralizing mist or spray.

In general, this combination procedure is well tolerated. However, it can cause irritation, redness, crusting, swelling, dryness, and obvious swelling of the face which could last 7–10 days.

I understand that there is a small risk of developing permanent darkening after the procedure. There is a rare chance that the peel could cause: undesirable pigment loss at the treated site, or the condition being treated could worsen after the peeling procedure; or a scar could develop. In addition, there is a small chance that a bacterial infection could develop, or the peel could also trigger a flare of a pre-existing herpetic infection at the treated site. In addition, there have been uncommon cases of allergic reactions to salicylates (the active peel ingredient). The benefits and side effects of the procedure have been explained to me in detail. All of my questions have been answered.

- I am in stable health.
- I have not used isotretinoin in the past 6 months.
- I have no allergies to aluminum chloride, sodium bicarbonate (peeling agent used for procedure).
- I am not pregnant.

Outcomes are not guaranteed.

__________________________ _____________________

Signature of Patient Date

____

Patient Name (Please Print)

__________________________ _____________________

Witness Date

References

1. Grimes PE (2005) Microdermabrasion. Dermatol Surg 31:1160–1165
2. Grimes PE. (2010) Microdermabrasion. In: Cosmetic dermatology. Wiley-Blackwell, Oxford, pp 418–425
3. Karimipour DJ, Kang S, Johnson TM et al (2005) A molecular analysis following a single treatment. J Am Acad Dermatol 52:215–223
4. Rajan P, Grimes PE (2002) Skin barrier changes induced by aluminum oxide and sodium chloride microdermabrasion. Dermatol Surg 28:390–393
5. Fischer TC, Perosino E, Poli F et al (2010) Chemical peels in aesthetic dermatology: an update 2009. J Eur Acad Dermatol Venereol 24:281–292
6. Karimipour DJ, Karimipour G, Orringer JS (2010) Microdermabrasion: an evidence-based review. Plast Reconstr Surg 125:372–377
7. Hexsel D, Mazzuco R, Dal'Forno T, Zechmeister D (2005) Microdermabrasion followed by a 5% retinoid acid peel vs. a 5% retinoid acid peel for the treatment of photoaging – a pilot study. J Cosmet Dermatol 4:111–116
8. Kisner AM (2001) Microdermabrasion with chemical peel. Aesthet Surg J 21(2):191–193
9. Briden E, Jacobsen E, Johnson C (2007) Combining superficial glycolic acid (alpha-hydroxy acid) peels with microdermabrasion to maximize treatment results and patient satisfaction. Cutis 79(1 Suppl Combining):13–16
10. Cotellessa C, Peris K, Fargnoli MC, Mordenti C, Giacomello RS, Chimenti S (2003) Microabrasion versus microabrasion followed by 15% trichloroacetic acid for treatment of cutaneous hyperpigmentations in adult females. Dermatol Surg 29(4):352–356
11. Zakopoulou N, Kontochristopoulos G (2006) Superficial chemical peels. J Cosmet Dermatol 5:246–253
12. AlKhawam L, Alam M (2009) Dermabrasion and microdermabrasion. Facial Plast Surg 25(5):301–310
13. Song JY, Kang HA, Kim M-Y et al (2004) Damage and recovery of skin barrier function after glycolic acid chemical peeling and crystal microdermabrasion. Dermatol Surg 30:390–394
14. Farris P, Rietschel R (2002) An unusual acute urticarial response following microdermabrasion. Dermatol Surg 28:606–608

Combination of Chemical Peels and Needling for Acne Scars

12

Gabriella Fabbrocini and Maria Pia De Padova

12.1 Definition

Skin needling, percutaneous collagen induction (PCI), collagen induction therapy (CIT), dry tattooing, needle dermabrasion, intradermabrasion, dermal remodeling, multitrepannic collagen actuation, intradermabrasion (MCA), these are all names for the same treatment. Skin needling is a procedure that involves using a sterile roller comprised of a series of fine, sharp needles to puncture the skin. Performed under local anesthetic with sedation, the device is "rolled" over the surface affected by acne scars to create many microscopic channels deep into the dermis of the skin, which is stimulated to produce new collagen. Skin needling is a procedure that ensures better results if it is associated with alpha-hydroxy acids (AHAs) treatment.

AHAs are organic carboxylic acids that are characterized by the presence of an –OH group and a –COOH group to the alpha position of the carboxylic carbon atom All the acids of the AHA family are different in the length of their atomic chains. They could be soluble in water or in biological lipids. They can cause loss of corneocyte cohesion. Among AHA family, glycolic acid is the acid more useful for an association therapy with skin needling.

G. Fabbrocini
Section of Dermatology, Department of Systematic Pathology, University of Naples Federico II, Via Sergio Pansini 5, 80133, Napoli, Italy
e-mail: gafabbro@unina.it

M.P. De Padova (✉)
Ospedale Privato Nigrisoli, Bologna, Italy
e-mail: mdepadova@gmail.com

12.2 Epidemiology

Although severe scarring is also secondary to chickenpox or other infectious diseases such as leishmaniasis, variola major, and variola minor, acne is the most common cause of scarring. Acne is a common condition seen in up to 80% of people between 11 and 30 years of age and by up to 5% of older adults. In some patients, the severe inflammatory response results in permanent scars. Scars can involve textural change in the superficial and deep dermis, and they can be associated with erythema, and less often, may also present pigmentary change.

12.3 Pathophysiology

PCI results from the natural response to wounding of the skin, even though the wound is minute and mainly subcutaneous. When a needle penetrates into the skin, it causes some localized damage and bleeding by rupturing fine blood vessels. A completely different picture emerges when thousands of fine pricks are placed close to each other. This promotes the normal wound healing that develops in three phases (Fig. 12.1). The inflammation (Phase 1) starts soon after the injury. Platelets are important in causing clotting and releasing chemotactic factors, which cause an invasion of other platelets, leucocytes, and fibroblasts. After the platelets have been activated by exposure to thrombin and collagen, they release numerous cytokines.

After 5 days, (Phase 2) neutrophils are replaced by monocytes. They remove cellular debris and release several growth factors including platelet-derived

A. Tosti et al. (eds.), *Color Atlas of Chemical Peels*,
DOI 10.1007/978-3-642-20270-4_12, © Springer-Verlag Berlin Heidelberg 2012

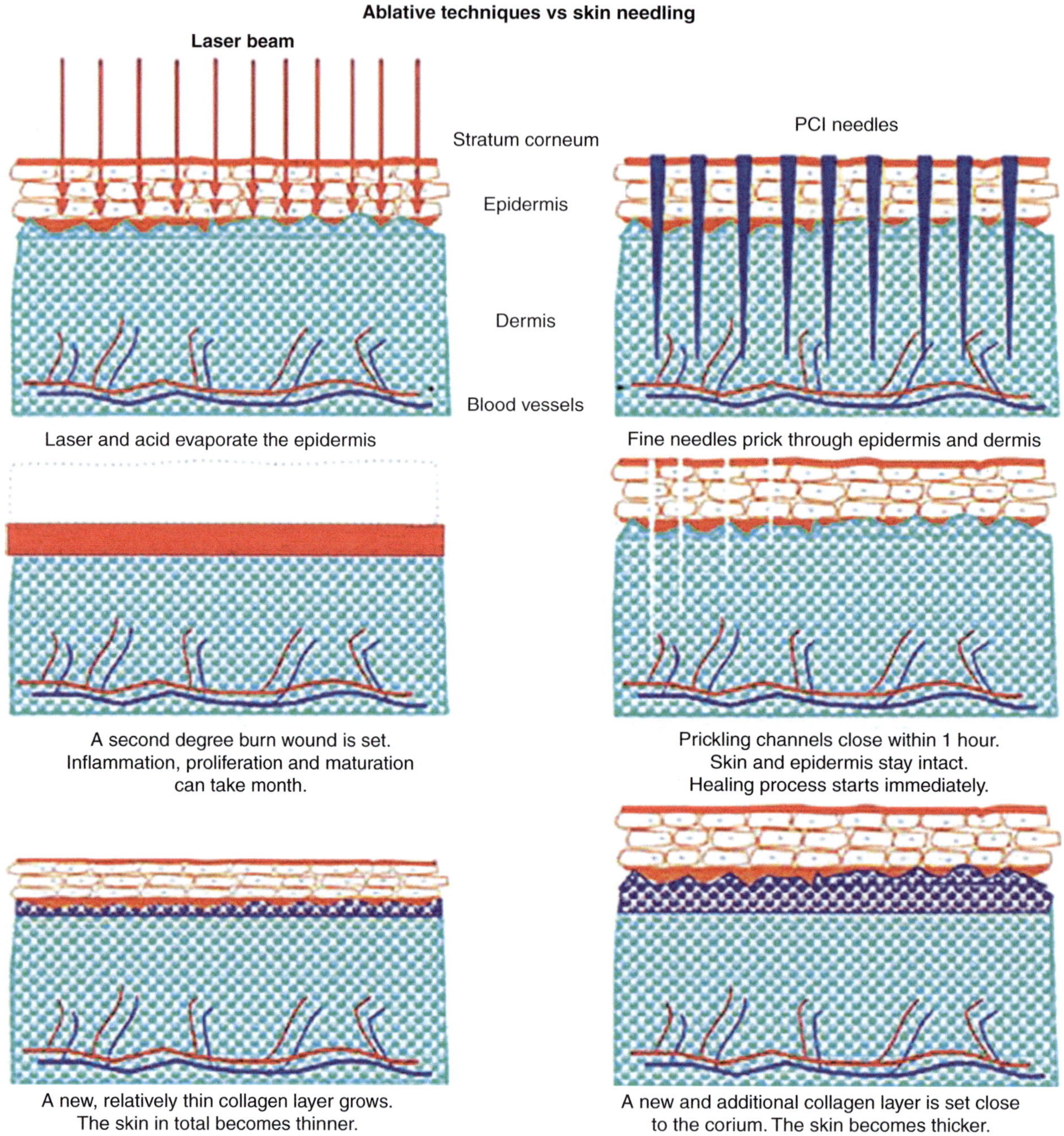

Fig. 12.1 Ablative techniques vs. Derma Roller (From www.dermaroller.de, with permission)

growth factor, fibroblast growth factor, TGF-b, and TGF-a, which stimulate the migration and proliferation of fibroblasts and the production and modulation of extracellular matrix. Tissue remodeling (Phase 3) continues for months after the injury and is mainly done by the fibroblasts. By the fifth day after injury, the fibronectin matrix is laid down along the axis in which fibroblasts are aligned and in which collagen will be laid down. TGF-b and other growth factors play an important part in the formation of this matrix. Recently a new theory has been proposed to explain the PCI mechanism of action [1]. The formation of new tissue (wound healing: inflammation–proliferation–maturation) is a complex series of reactions and interactions among cells and mediators. But it seems that these processes are somewhat cut short, when the skin is treated with needles. As a series of needles – not longer than 1.5 mm – do not set a wound in the classical sense, according to this theory, bioelectricity – also called demarcation current – triggers the cascade of growth factors immediately to the maturation phase. When stainless steel microneedles penetrate the skin, they set fine wounds. Cells react to this intrusion with a "demarcation current." This demarcation current is additionally increased by the needles' own electrical potential. The electrical potential difference is typical in the wound-healing process. The materials that penetrate the membrane are ionic and cells change the membrane potential by losing or gaining ions. Relative to its size, the cell membrane potential is enormous. On an average, its thickness is 70–100 nm. This would be equivalent to a 10-million-volt potential difference over 1 m. It can be further hypothesized that microneedles do not cause overt injury in the classical sense. The body is only somehow "fooled" into believing that an injury has occurred! Cell membranes react to the local change in electrical potential with increased cell activity and with the release of potassium ion, proteins, and growth factors.

This peel, as other AHA do, is able to produce these effects on the epidermis:

- Increase of epidermal thickness (increased turn over)
- Increase of glycosaminoglycans physiological production
- Less cellular alteration
- Less melanin "compact areas"

All these effects, in addition to needling effect on the collagen and other structural matrix components, can play a synergic role, very useful for acne scars.

12.4 Clinical Types

Acne scars have been subclassified into ice pick, boxcar, and rolling scars [2]. Over the past several decades, numerous descriptive terms and classifications have been suggested for acne scars. We used the classification recently proposed by Goodman et al. [3]. This classification defines as Grade 1 macular scarring or flat scarring characterized by flat areas of increased or decreased pigmentation visible from greater than 50 cm. Grade 2 includes mild disease visible at distances of less than 50 cm and that can be covered by makeup (e.g., mild rolling acne scars). Moderate disease that is visible at 50 cm or greater and is not easily covered with makeup or the normal shadow of a shaved beard is classified as Grade 3. In this type of acne scar stretching, the skin can flatten the scar. Examples include more significant rolling scars, shallow boxcar scars, and mild-to-moderate hypertrophic scars. Grade 4 includes severe disease as in grade 3 but scarring is not flattened by stretching the skin. Examples include severe boxcar scars, deep divots, ice pick scars, and hypertrophic keloid scarring (very raised/pigmented scars).

12.5 Therapy

12.5.1 Patient Preparation

The first step toward skin health is to topically replace photosensitive vitamin A and the other antioxidants, vitamins C and E, and carotenoids, which are normally lost on photoexposed skin. Vitamin A is utterly essential for the normal physiology of skin, and yet, it is destroyed by exposure to light so that it is prevented from exerting its important influence on skin and preserving collagen. Vitamin A in physiologic doses will stimulate cell growth, the release of growth factors, angiogenesis, and the production of healthy new collagen. The DNA effects of vitamin A interact in parallel with the growth factors released by PCI. Adequate nourishment of the skin with vitamin A will ensure that the metabolic processes for collagen production will be maximized and the skin will heal as rapidly as possible. Vitamin C is similarly important for collagen formation but is destroyed by exposure to blue light. Both of these vitamins need to be replaced every day so that the natural protection and repair of DNA can be maintained. As a result, the skin will take on a more youthful appearance. The skin is routinely prepared by using topical vitamins A and C and antioxidants for at least 3 weeks, but preferably for 3 months if the skin is very much damaged by the Sun. It can be used also as a topical product containing alpha-omega HA, omega-hydroxy acids, enoxolone, and zinc. If the stratum corneum is thickened and rough, a series of mild TCA peels (2.5–5% TCA) will get the surface of the skin prepared for needling and maximize the result. At first,

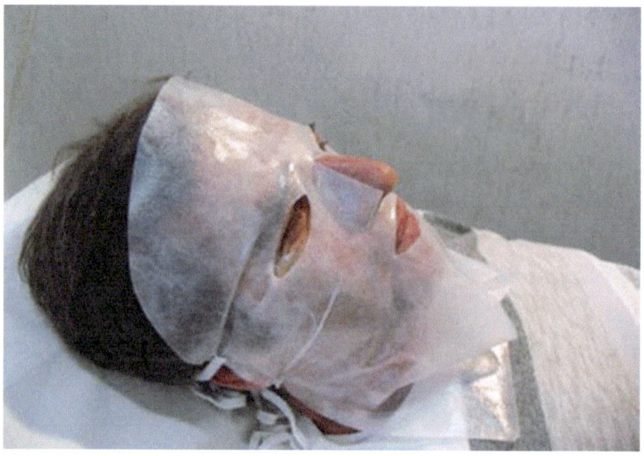

Fig. 12.2 Occlusion application of local anesthetic before the needling treatment

facial skin must be disinfected, then a topical anesthetic (EMLA) is applied leaving for 60 min (Fig. 12.2).

The skin-needling procedure is realized by rolling a performed tool on the skin areas affected by acne scars. Actually, there is a number of skin rollers available for professional and home use that come in many different needle lengths, diameters, and numbers, which can make it very confusing for their users. In an attempt to determine the best combination for treating scars and rejuvenating the skin, the number of needles on a roller is the least important feature, as repeated rolling causes numerous dermal injuries. Needle diameter is very important, as we are seeking to maximize the dermal injury without creating a new scar. In our experience, 0.25-mm needle diameter is the maximum size that can be used without causing a new scar in the skin. Smaller diameter needle-skin rollers can be used but do not maximize the dermal injury and, therefore, will be slower to produce results. Needle length is also a critical issue. The target of the needle action is a layer in the upper dermis called the intermediate reticular dermis. This dermal layer contains the highest number of stem cells that are able to produce new collagen. The epidermis (the outer layer of the skin) varies in depth from 0.05 mm on the eyelids to 1.5 mm on the soles of the feet. The epidermis of the face (other than the eyelids) varies from 0.3 to 1 mm in depth and, therefore, a 0.75-mm to 2-mm long needle is more than adequate to reach the intermediate reticular dermis. To treat acne scars, it is recommended that the professional device be used that is equipped with a rolling barrel 10-mm wide and 96 needles in four rows (Dermaroller model MS4). The needles used should have a length of 1.5 mm and a diameter of 0.25 mm. Depending on the applied pressure (pressing too hard is not necessary for excellent results and if you are needling the face, do not use the rolling barrel on the eyelids or lips), they penetrate the scar tissue between 0.1 and 1.3 mm. Rolling consists in moving, with some pressure, four times in four directions: horizontally, vertically, and diagonally right and left. This ensures an even pricking pattern resulting in about 250–300 pricks per square centimeter. The microneedles penetrate through the epidermis but do not remove it; thus, the epidermis is only punctured and will rapidly heal. The needle seems to divide cells from each other rather than cutting through the cells so that many cells are spared. Because the needles are set in a roller, every needle initially penetrates at an angle and then goes deeper as the roller turns. Finally, the needle is extracted at the converse angle; therefore, the tracts are curved, reflecting the path of the needle as it rolls into and then out of the skin, for about 1.3 mm into the dermis.

The epidermis and particularly the stratum corneum remain "intact," except for these tiny holes, which are about four cells in diameter. The treatment times can range from 10 to 60 min, depending on the size of the area being treated. Naturally, the skin bleeds for a short time, but that soon stops. The skin develops multiple microbruises in the dermis that initiate the complex cascade of growth factors that eventually results in collagen production.

It can be useful to perform some AHA clinical peeling sessions 2 weeks before and 2 weeks after the needling session. Our experience is very positive with 70% glycolic acid and 30% salicylic acid. The choice of the peeling to perform in combination with skin needling depends on the skin type and scar type. For the treatment of deeper skin-scars, it is preferable to use salicylic or TCA 10% acid compared to glycolic acid. For photosensitive skin type, it is preferable to use glycolic acid.

12.6 Posttreatment Care

Postprocedure appearance [4] includes the following:

Day 1 and 2: Depending on how deeply the technician inserts the needle into the epidermis, the tissue may have slight to moderate swelling and may be tender, red, and bruised, with a slight lymph discharge from the treated areas. Minor itching may occur and the "needled" tissue may exhibit the appearance of "cat scratches."

Day 3: The treated areas slightly crust and remain faintly pink to red.

Day 4–5: The redness has diminished.

Day 5–7: There is barely any evidence of a procedure.

Healing time is 4–7 days and makeup can be worn after 2–3 days. Immediately after the treatment, the skin looks bruised, but bleeding is minimal, and there is only a small ooze of serum that soon stops. It is a good practice to apply cold compresses (no ice!) and vitamin-C mask. Some practitioners recommend soaking the skin with saline swabs for an hour or two and then cleaning the skin thoroughly with an oil-based cleanser. A thin layer of Vaseline or equivalent may be applied to reduce skin humidity loss. The patient is encouraged to use topical vitamin A and vitamin C as a cream or an oil to promote better healing and greater production of collagen. No products have to be applied on the treatment areas for 36 h after treatment. Makeup and sunblock can be applied on Day 2 post treatment, if the treatment area is dry and unbroken. Normal skincare can be recommended once the treatment area is completely healed. It is very important to continue using the topical vitamin cream for at least 6 months post procedure to ensure the production of healthy collagen and elastin. The addition of peptides, like palmitoyl pentapeptide, could possibly ensure even better results. At home, the patient should stand under a shower for a long time, allowing the water to soak into the surface of the skin. Bathing is discouraged because of potential contamination from drains and plugs. Patients should be reminded to use only tepid water because the skin will be more sensitive to heat. While the water is running over the face or body, the patient should gently massage the treated skin until all serum, blood, or oil is removed. The importance of a thorough but gentle washing of the skin, a few hours after the procedure, cannot be stressed enough. The following day, the skin looks less dramatic and by day 4 or 5, the skin has returned to a moderate pink flush, which can easily be concealed with makeup. The patient should avoid direct sun exposure for at least 10 days, if possible, and use a broad-brimmed hat or scarf to protect the facial skin. To obtain best results, it is recommended to repeat skin-needling treatments over a period of 1–2 years. The outcome of collagen induction therapy combined with a prescribed posttreatment skin care routine can produce dramatic results that will last for years. So it is recommended that patients continue home needling to ensure the longevity of their scar improvement. The home needling can be safely combined with the use of peptide serum and/or tretinoin to maximize improvements in depressed scarring.

Among peeling session and needling session, some patients can be treated with nourishing creams and AHA creams that can enhance the efficacy of the treatment.

References

1. Liebl H (2009) Abstract reflections about Collagen-Induction- Therapy (CIT). A hypothesis for the mechanism of action of collagen induction therapy (cit) using micro-needles. January 2–7. http://www.dermaroller.de/us/science/abstractreflections- 26.html. Feb Accessed 15 Apr 2009
2. Jacob CI, Dover JS, Kaminer MS (2001) Acne scarring: a classification system and review of treatment options. J Am Acad Dermatol 45:105–117
3. Goodman GJ, Baron JA (2006) Postacne scarring: a qualitative global scarring grading system. Dermatol Surg 32: 1458–1466
4. Church S. Skin Needling – Natural Collagen Renewal. International Institute of Permanent Cosmetics. Internet paper. http://www.spmuc.com.au/downloads/Skin-Needling-What.pdf

Part III

How to Choose the Best Peeling for the Patient

13 Acne

Gabriella Fabbrocini, Maria Pia De Padova,
S. Cacciapuoti, and Antonella Tosti

13.1 Definition

Acne vulgaris is one of the most common dermatologic diseases, and it is the skin disease most commonly treated by physicians. It is a disease of the pilosebaceous units, clinically characterized by seborrhea, comedones, papules, pustules, nodules, and, in some cases, scarring. Acne vulgaris affects more than 80% of people at some point in their life [1]. Acne cannot be regarded as a serious disease or measured in terms of life and death, but it has a nuisance value out of all proportion to its seriousness, affecting, as it does, young people at an age when they are most sensitive to any disfigurement. For these reasons, morbidity can be high and associated with loss of confidence, and impairment of normal social and workplace function, with documented effects on quality of life including depression, dysmorphobia, and even suicide [2].

G. Fabbrocini • S. Cacciapuoti
Section of Dermatology, Department of Systematic Pathology, University of Naples Federico II, Via Sergio Pansini 5, 80133, Napoli, Italy
e-mail: gafabbro@unina.it; sara.cacciapuoti@libero.it

M.P. De Padova (✉)
Ospedale Privato Nigrisoli, Bologna, Italy
e-mail: mdepadova@gmail.com

A. Tosti
Department of Dermatology and Cutaneous Surgery, Miller School of Medicine, University of Miami, US
e-mail: atosti@med.miami.edu

13.2 Epidemiology

Acne is a most common disease affecting all ages and ethnic groups and is the leading dermatologic diagnosis with 10.2 million diagnoses (25.4% of the 10 most common dermatologic diagnoses) according to a National Ambulatory Medical Care Survey conducted in 1995 in the USA. Acne vulgaris develops earlier in females than in males, which may reflect the earlier onset of puberty in females. The most severe forms of acne vulgaris occur more frequently in males, but the disease tends to be more persistent in females [3]. The hormonal changes of puberty are almost always related to the beginning of typical acne vulgaris. Adrenal maturation and gonad development lead to the production of androgens and subsequent increase in sebaceous glands, with the eventual eruption of acne at this age group. In fact, acne affects 95% and 83% of 16-year-old boys and girls respectively, but it is clearly no longer a problem confined to teenagers: Recently, attendance at general practitioner surgeries for this condition and referral for specialist opinion has significantly increased among people aged over 20 [4]. The prevalence of adult acne is 3% in men and between 11% and 12% in women [5, 6] with a significant decline from 45 years of age. Moreover, at 40 years of age, 1% of men and 5% of women exhibit acne lesions.

13.3 Pathophysiology

The pathogenesis of acne is thought to be an interplay between a number of factors including:

- Hyperkeratinization with occlusion of the follicular unit
- Colonization by pathogenic *Propionibacterium acnes*

A. Tosti et al. (eds.), *Color Atlas of Chemical Peels*,
DOI 10.1007/978-3-642-20270-4_13, © Springer-Verlag Berlin Heidelberg 2012

- Inflammation
- Sebum hypersecretion

Blockage of the follicular opening due to hyperkeratosis of epithelium in the follicular canal is the basis for microcomedones formation. Microcomedones are the first acne lesions and can be found in normal-looking skin. The distended follicular may rupture, causing further inflammatory reaction, leading to the formation of papules, pustules, cystis, and nodules.

However, ongoing research is modifying the classical view of acne pathogenesis through identification of upstream mechanisms.

The very early stage of acne lesion development, namely the beginning of microcomedones, is associated with vascular endothelial-cell activation and involvement of inflammatory events [7] which corroborates the suggestion that acne may represent a genuine inflammatory disorder without involvement of bacteria in its initiation. In fact, hyperkeratinization, obstruction of sebaceous follicles resulting from abnormal keratinization of the infundibular epithelium, stimulation of sebaceous gland secretion by androgens, and microbial colonization of pilosebaceous units by *P. acnes* promote perifollicular inflammation. For these reasons, it has been hypothesized that *P. acnes* could act in acne pathogenesis not as pathogen by itself, but by triggering inflammation indirectly. This confirms the essential role played by inflammation in acne pathogenesis. Acne vulgaris is likely to be a genuine inflammatory disease with androgens and environmental factors being agents able to interrupt the natural cycling of the sebaceous follicles and lead microcomedones to form comedones and inflammatory lesion.

13.4 Clinical Patterns

Acne is a polymorphic disease with a wide spectrum of severity. Severity of the disease varies markedly from one individual to the other depending upon the interplay of various factors involved in the development of acne vulgaris. Several methods have been proposed in order to standardize clinical evaluation of acne severity. Grading systems based on the clinical appearance of lesions as well as "lesion counting" are useful in assessing the severity of acne vulgaris.

Methods of measuring the severity of acne vulgaris include simple grading based on clinical examination, lesion counting, and those that require complicated instruments such as photography and fluorescent photography. The two commonly used measures are grading and lesion counting.

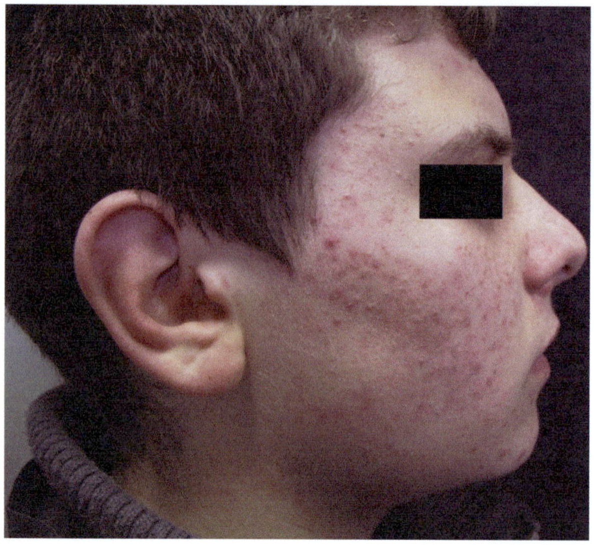

Fig. 13.1 Patient with pores, blackheads and open comedones

Although no grading system has been accepted universally, one of the most frequently used is a system of points, the Global Acne Grading System [8]. This system considers six locations on the face, chest, and upper back, with a grading factor for each location based roughly on the affected surface area, distribution and density of pilosebaceous units. A global score is obtained by summing up the individual local scores. The individual lesions of acne vulgaris are divisible into three types: non-inflamed lesions, inflamed lesions, and scars.

The first pattern is that of essentially *noninflammatory disease*, which tends to be an early phase often seen in the peri-pubertal age group. There is increased sebum production on the face, chest, back, and shoulders. This may be accompanied by an increase in pores, blackheads, or open comedones (Fig. 13.1).

The second clinical pattern is that of *inflammatory disease*, which is the pattern that tends to lead to more scarring. This may span the full gamut from papules, pustules, nodules, and cysts and any combination of these (Fig. 13.2). Postinflammatory macular disease may follow resolution and these may be red or hyperpigmented, representing a component of postinflammatory change. Most patients have a mixture of non-inflamed and inflamed lesions (Fig. 13.3).

In some patients, the severe inflammatory lesions result in permanent, disfiguring *scars* (Fig. 13.4). Scars can involve textural change in the superficial and deep dermis, and can also be associated with erythema, and less often,

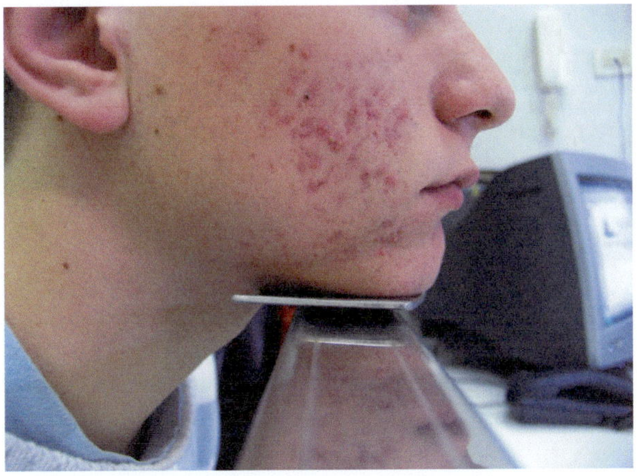

Fig. 13.2 Patient with papulopustolar acne

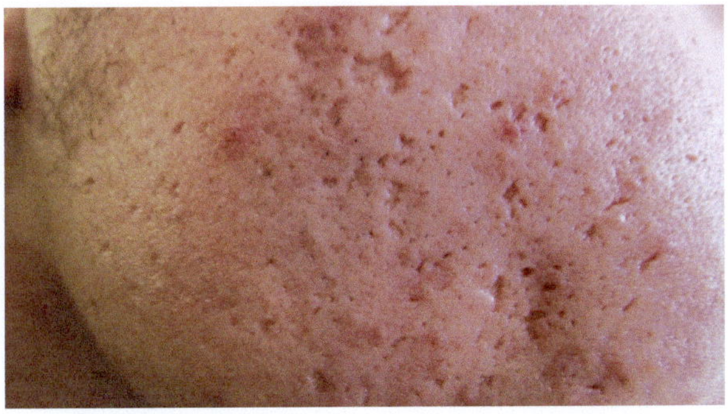

Fig. 13.4 Acne scars

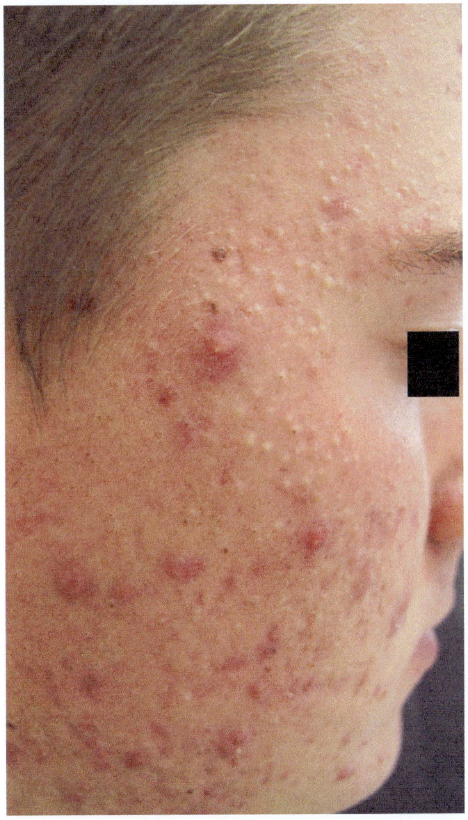

Fig. 13.3 Mixture of noninflamed and inflamed lesions

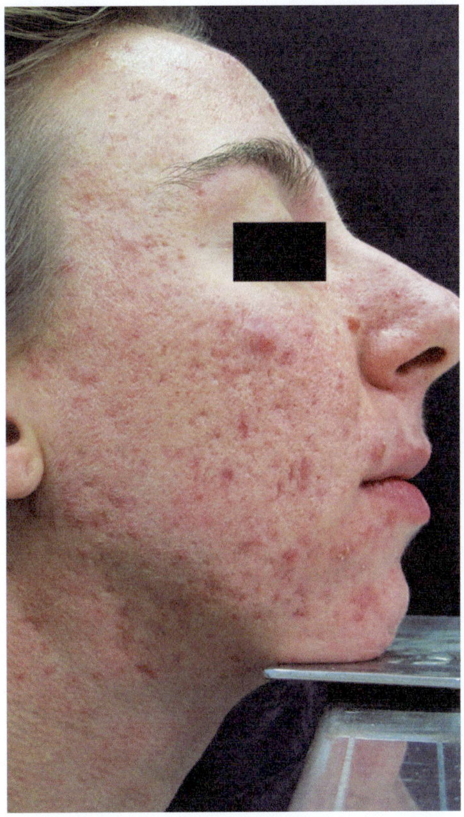

Fig. 13.5 Patients with acne scars and pigment changes

with pigment change (Fig. 13.5). Acne scars have been subclassified into ice pick, boxcar, and rolling scars. [9] suggested a comprehensive and functional scheme of classification based on the severity of acne scars (Table 13.1).

Unfortunately, scarring may affect up to 95% of patients and is maximally related to severity and duration of acne before adequate therapy is instituted [11]. Early and effective treatment of acne is the most appropriate way to prevent scarring and to minimize the psychological effects of acne and its resultant scarring.

13.5 Clinical Types

In Table 13.2, we summarize clinical features characterizing different acne clinical types.

Table 13.1 Classification of acne scars (Goodman and Baron [10])

Grade	Description
Grade 1	Macular scarring or flat scarring characterized by flat areas of increased or decreased pigmentation visible at distances of greater than 50 cm
Grade 2	Mild disease visible at distances of less than 50 cm and that can be covered by makeup. Examples include mild rolling acne scars
Grade 3	Moderate disease that is visible at 50 cm or greater and is not easily covered with makeup or the normal shadow of a shaved beard. Stretching the skin can flatten the scar. Examples include more significant rolling scars, shallow boxcar scars, and mild-to-moderate hypertrophic scars
Grade 4	Severe disease as in grade 3 but scarring is not flattened by stretching the skin. Examples include severe boxcar scars, deep divots, ice pick scars, and hypertrophic keloid scarring (very raised/pigmented scars)

Table 13.2 Acne clinical types

Clinical types	Clinical features
Acne neonatorum	Closed comedones on the forehead, nose, and cheeks
Infantile acne	Comedones/inflammatory papulopustules to cysts
Acne vulgaris	Microcomedones Closed comedones (whiteheads) Open comedones (blackheads) Papules Pustules Nodules Cysts
Adult acne	Papules Pustules Nodules Cysts Seborrhea
Acne conglobata	Cystic abscesses Confluent follicular and perifollicular inflammations Intercommunicating cysts
Acne inversa	Recurrent draining sinuses and abscesses in skin folds that carry terminal hairs and apocrine glands
Acne fulminans	Ulcerative nodules associated with systemic complications: • Hematologic manifestations • Arthritis • Musculoskeletal symptoms
Acne cosmetica and iatrogenic acne	Papules and pustules monomorphous in their appearance often associated with systemic signs of drug toxicity
Acne excoriée	Excoriated areas with inflammation and superficial crusting

Acne neonatorum occurs in up to 20% of newborns [12]. It typically consists of closed comedones on the forehead, nose, and cheeks, although other locations are possible. Open comedones, inflammatory papules, and pustules can also develop. Neonatal acne is thought to result from stimulation of sebaceous glands by maternal or infant androgens. Parents should be counseled that lesions usually resolve spontaneously within 4 months without scarring.

However, severe, unrelenting neonatal acne accompanied by other signs of hyperandrogenism should prompt an investigation for adrenal cortical hyperplasia, virilizing tumors, or underlying endocrinopathies.

Infantile acne is a rare occurrence and has its onset at 3–6 months and is less common than neonatal acne. Clinically, the lesions range from comedones to inflammatory papulopustules to cysts. It is probably associated with a premature secretion of gonad androgens. These patients may develop severe acne as teenagers.

Acne vulgaris is the most frequent form of acne and resolves slowly after the teenage years. Acne vulgaris is more frequent, but less severe in women than men and it involves more frequently face in women, but chest in men. Its evolution is unpredictable with the tendency to complete or incomplete remissions particularly in summer time, and subintrant exacerbations at the time of the menses, with overwork, etc. Lesions of all the various stages can be seen at the same time (Figs. 13.6 and 13.7).

Adult acne can be a continuation of teenage acne or appear *de novo*. It may differ clinically showing fewer comedones and more inflammation, affecting most commonly the perioral, chin, and jawline regions. A typical clinical characteristic of acne in adult women refers to topography of lesions: predominance of lesions in the upper half of the face, in addition to dorsum of younger patients. In the meantime, adults presented more lesions in the neck, in addition to face (Fig. 13.8).

Acne conglobata is a disease characterized by the presence of cystic abscesses, confluent follicular and perifollicular inflammations, and intercommunicating cysts. These lesions affect primarily the face, neck, chest, and shoulders and are the causes of serious and disfiguring scars. This disorder typically begins in adulthood and presents as numerous comedones, papules, pustules, nodules, abscesses, and draining sinus tracts involving the chest, back, and buttocks. Patients with this disease are usually from 15 to 25 years of age

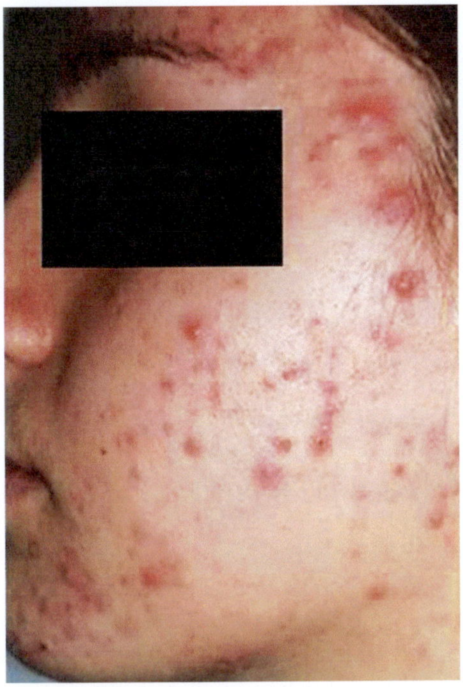

Fig. 13.6 Lesional pleomorphism in acne patient

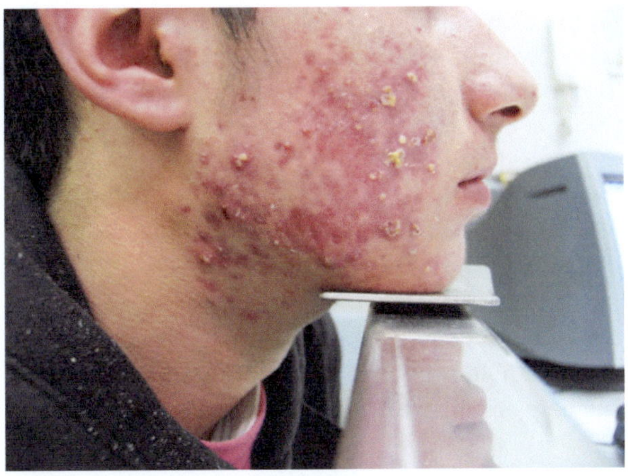

Fig. 13.7 Lesional pleomorphism in acne patient

and have an antecedent history in most cases of acne vulgaris of varying degrees of severity.

Acne inversa (also known as Hidradenitis suppurativa) is a chronically relapsing inflammatory disease that is characterized by recurrent draining sinuses and abscesses occurring predominantly in skin folds that carry terminal hairs and apocrine glands. Healing occurs with substantial scarring.

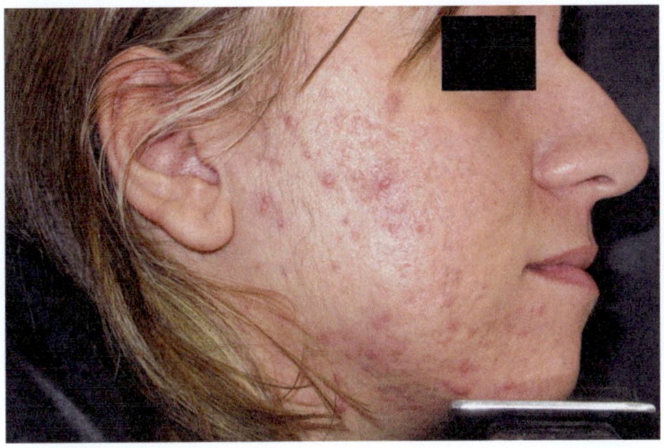

Fig. 13.8 Patient with adult acne

Acne fulminans is a severe form of cystic acne primarily affecting Caucasian adolescent males. It is a rare form of acne characterized by ulcerative nodules and associated with systemic complications. Musculoskeletal symptoms and hematologic manifestations frequently are associated with this disorder. An associated arthralgia or arthritis frequently occurs.

Acne cosmetica and iatrogenic acne result from the use of cosmetic-containing comedogenic substances (such as lanolin, certain vegetable oils, butyl stearate, lauryl alcohol, and oleic acid) and resolve with the cessation of the use of the causative agent. Moreover, there are several drugs that can cause or exacerbate acne, such as corticosteroids, anabolic steroids, antiepileptics, antidepressive, antituberculous, antineoplastic, and antiviral drugs. For these reasons, any medical history excludes the precipitating factors indicated above: medications and comedogenic cosmetics.

Acne excoriée results by picking of the spots that aggravates the appearance of the acne patient. This type of acne excoriated is characterized by areas with inflammation and superficial crusting, and it occurs predominantly in females and often results from personality or psychological problems.

13.6 Differential Diagnosis

Diagnosis is usually easy, but acne may be confused with folliculitis, rosacea, or perioral dermatitis. However, in these skin conditions, there are no comedones. Comedonal acne has to be differentiated from milia and sebaceous hyperplasia. Inflammatory acne could mimic rosacea or perioral dermatitis. Rosacea is characterized by persistent erythema and telangiectasia predominantly of the cheeks, frequently followed by papules and pustules but no comedones, the elementary lesion of acne. Perioral dermatitis affects mostly perioral area and seldom periorbital area. Acne could result in differential diagnosis with a lot of other dermatologic diseases: lupus miliaris disseminatus, pseudofolliculitis of the beard, and syphilide's follicular lesions. However, the sprouting of typical acne lesions (comedones, papules, pustules and nodules) on the face, on the chest, and on the neck is pathognomonic.

13.7 Therapy

The aims of treatment are to prevent scarring, limit the disease duration, and reduce the impact of the psychological stress that may affect over half of sufferers. The four major steps in the pathophysiology of acne govern its therapeutic principles. In fact, the goals of the drugs most commonly used in acne treatment are the following:

- Exert an anti-inflammatory effect.
- Correct the altered pattern of follicular keratinization.
- Decrease sebaceous gland activity.
- Decrease the follicular bacterial population (*P. acnes*).

Some general measures contribute to reach these aims. We summarize them in Table 13.3.

However, specific pharmacological measures are necessary to obtain a significant clinical improvement. We can distinguish local therapy from systemic therapy (see Table 13.4).

Table 13.3 General measures in acne management

Measures	Goals to reach
Perform a successful skin detersion to respect skin's physiological and structural equilibrium	To favor the removal of the excess of sebum and of desquamated corneocytes, helping containing the presence of bacteria on the skin
Use moisturizing emulsions after detersion	To avoid massive skin water loss damaging skin structures and hydrolipidic film
Use sebum regulators such as piroctone olamine, nicotinamide, serenoa repens, zinc, and phytosphingosine	To reduce seborrhea obtaining an opaque effect
Use keratolytics such as alpha-hydroxy acids	To remove follicular obstruction and enhance cells' turnover

Table 13.4 Acne therapy

Local therapy	• Topical retinoids
	• Topical antibiotics
	• Benzoyl peroxide
	• Chemical peels
	• Emergent topical therapy
Systemic therapy	• Oral retinoids
	• Oral antibiotics
	• Hormonal therapy in women

13.7.1 Local Therapy

13.7.1.1 Topical Retinoids

The retinoids [13] are a class of chemical compounds that are related chemically to vitamin A. They are able to bind and activate retinoic acid receptors (RARs) and activate specific gene transcription. Most used topical retinoids are tretinoin, adapalene, tazarotene, and isotretinoin. Tretinoin has a great comedolytic and anticomedogenic action, an indirect antimicrobial action with a weak anti-inflammatory effect. Adapalene is a third-generation retinoid with a better therapeutical profile than tretinoin: It has a huge anti-inflammatory action with less adverse effect (irritative dermatitis). Tazarotene, also a synthetic retinoid, exerts action through its metabolite, tazarotenic acid. It has been introduced as a drug for the treatment of psoriasis but for the high price, the strong cutaneous irritative process, and the potential teratogenicity, it has become a second choice drug in acne. All topical retinoids can be contact-irritants (Fig. 13.9) and cause severe xerosis (Fig. 13.10). Advising patients to apply the product on alternate nights during the first few weeks of treatment can help ensure greater tolerability (Fig. 13.11a, b).

13.7.1.2 Topical Antibiotics

Erythromycin and clindamycin are the most common used topical antibiotics for the treatment of acne [14]. Topical antibiotics have a bacteriostatic and bactericidal effect, reducing *P. acnes* colonization of the sebaceous follicle. However, topical antibiotics have not to be used in monotherapy due to the high risk of increasing *P. acnes* resistance. The development of resistance is less frequent in patients who are treated with combination therapy (benzoyl peroxide/erythromycin; benzoyl peroxide/clindamycin). These associations enhance the bactericidal effect, reducing the risk of drug-resistance.

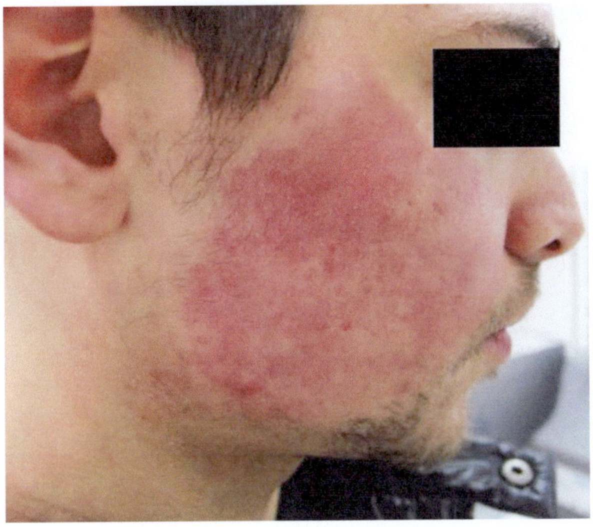

Fig. 13.9 Adverse effect (erithema) of topical retinoids

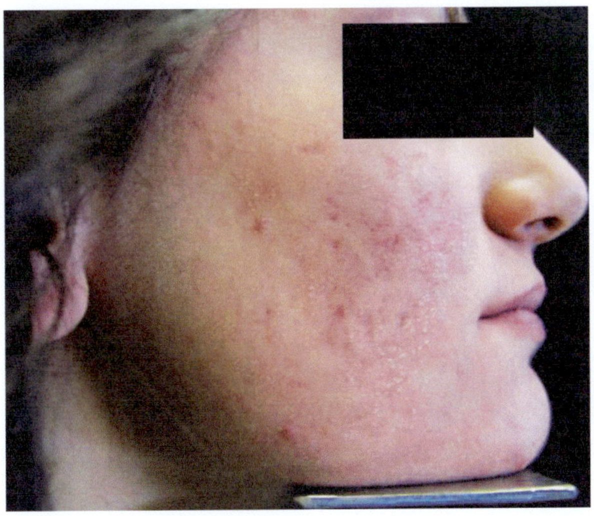

Fig. 13.10 Patient with xerosis retinoids-induced

13.7.1.3 Benzoyl Peroxide

This topical agent exercises a potent antimicrobial activity through the release of free oxygen radicals, resulting in a decrease in bacterial population and an accompanying decrease in the hydrolysis of triglycerides. This action is much faster than antibiotics and avoids the inconvenience of drug-resistance. In fact, benzoyl peroxide maintains its efficacy after years of use, making it the ideal agent for combination therapy. Benzoyl peroxide preparations are available in gels, creams, lotions, and soaps. Gel products are generally considered more effective.

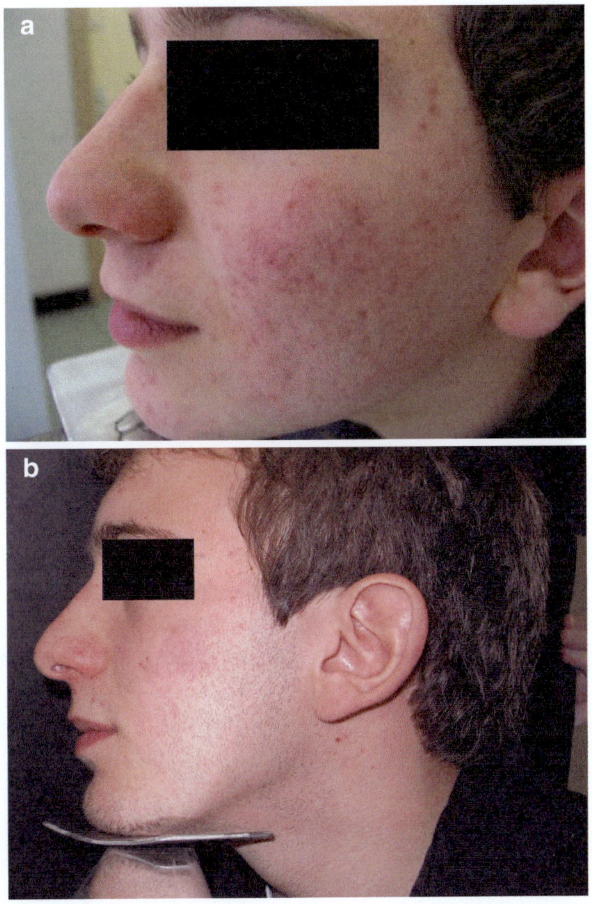

Fig. 13.11 (**a**) Erithema in patient with daily retinoid scheme. (**b**) Good compliance in the same patient treated with alterned retinoid scheme

Dryness and irritation are the most frequent side effects.

13.7.1.4 Chemical Peels

Chemical peel is a dermocosmetic technique that uses one or more exfoliating agents in a well-determined time to interact with epidermis and derma. The aim is to remove corneum stratum, enhancing physiological cell turnover. The acids used are distinguished on superficial, medium, and deep. In the following topics the goal is to explain the real efficacy of some of the caustics used to treat acne vulgaris.

- *Superficial peels:* Various chemicals have been used as peeling agents, out of which the most fruitful one is the alpha-hydroxy acid such as glycolic acid. Alpha-hydroxy acid (AHA) works inducing epidermolysis and subsequent desquamation within few

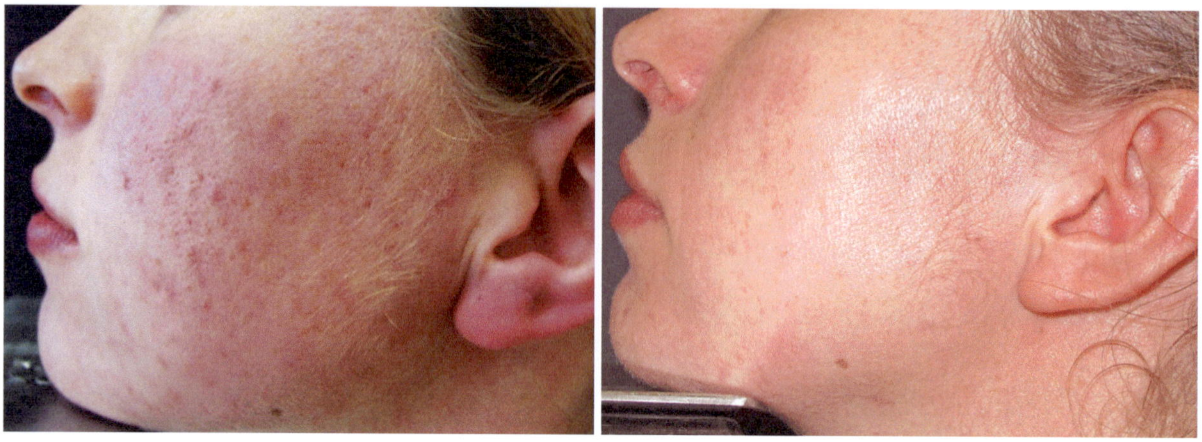

Fig. 13.12 Mild papular acne treated with TCA peel (10%): before and after the treatment

minutes of application. The intensity of the AHA peel is determined by both the concentration of the acid and the chemical vehicle used that the acid is soluted. Among AHA, glycolic acid is the most readily available commercial peeling agent. Chemical peeling by physicians is usually performed with a 30–70% glycolic acid solution. Mandelic acid (30%) is another alpha-hydroxy acid that causes a superficial exfoliation. Another class is beta-hydroxy acids. The most frequently used beta-hydroxy acid is Salicylic acid (ortho-hydroxybenzoic acid). Salicylic acid is a naturally occurring substance found in the bark of the willow tree. In concentrations of 3–5%, it functions as a keratolytic agent and enhances the penetration of other peeling agents and topical preparations. At a concentration of 15%, it can be considered as a superficial peel. Retinoid acid is a chemical derivative of Vitamin A which is able to stimulate the cellular differentiation and to improve the tissue's architecture. It is still used as topical formulation for the treatment of acne in the 0.01, 0.025, and 0.05 concentrations. Trichloroacetic acid (TCA) is an inorganic compound which is present in crystalline form. For the treatment of acne, we used a concentration of 10%. These types of chemical peels are indicated in comedonal acne and mild papular acne (Fig. 13.12a, b).

- *Medium peels:* Glycolic acid (concentration of 70%) combined with other alpha hydroxy acids such as pyruvic acid and malic acid (30%), kojic acid (10%) and azelaic acid (30%), salicylic acid (33%) and TCA (15%). These acid associations could lead to the frosting phenomena (skin whitening due to protein precipitation). These peels are used for papulopustular acne and in case of dyschromia exists.
- *Deep peels:* TCA (30%), salicylic acid (50%). These peels cause a deep frosting phenomena and they require home postpeeling management for the intense erythema. These peels are used in medium and deep acne scars. Ice-pick and boxcar scars can be treated with TCA 30% application all over the face when they are diffuse. When they are isolated, TCA cross 50–90% using cotton tips is the gold standard [15] (Fig. 13.13a. b). In Table 13.5, we summarize the principal chemical peels and their indication in acne.

13.7.1.5 Emergent Topical Therapy

Resveratrol is a phenolic-like molecule naturally contained in red grape with these important properties:

- Antioxidant action
- Pro-apoptotic action
- Anti-cancer action
- Estrogen like properties
- Antiatherogenic

Recent studies [16] show activities that can be used to inhibit the pathogenesis of acne in vitro. At submicromolar concentration too, it can inhibit the proliferation of human keratinocytes, while at higher concentrations (40–100 μmol), it can be toxic. Besides, resveratrol has a bactericidal action on *P. acnes* at a concentration of 200 mg/L and a bacteriostatic activity at lower doses [17]. In spleen mice cells treated with resveratrol for 2–4 weeks, there is a reduction of the TNF alpha production [18].

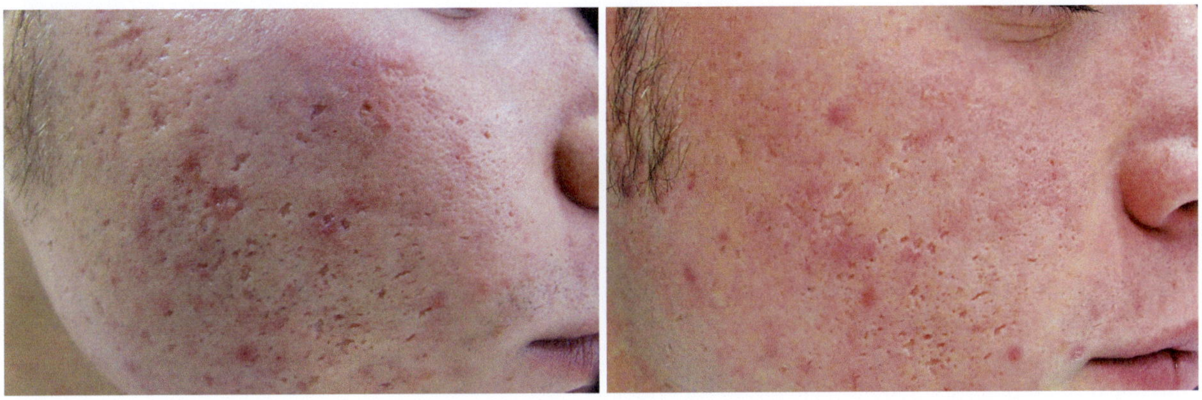

Fig. 13.13 Patient with ice-pick and boxcar scars treated with TCA CROSS 50%: before and after the treatment

Table 13.5 Principal chemical peels and their indication in acne

Type of chemical peel	Acid concentration	Indication in acne
Superficial peels	• Glycolic acid 30–70%	• Comedonal acne
	• Retinoid acid 5–10%	• Mild papular acne
	• Salicylic acid 15%	
	• TCA 10%	
	• Mandelic acid 30%	
Medium peels	• Glycolic acid (70%)	• Papular and pustular acne
	• Pyruvic acid (30%)	
	• Malic acid (30%)	
	• Kojic acid (10%)	
	• Azelaic acid (30%)	
	• Salicylic acid (33%)	
	• TCA (15%)	
Deep peels	• TCA (30%)	• Acne scars (ice pick, boxcar, and rolling scars)
	• Salicylic acid (50%)	

Based on these acquisitions, it has been proposed that the resveratrol could inhibit the production of TNF alpha on the skin too, blocking the inflammatory process at an initial phase or stopping all the inflammatory cascade with the inhibition of NF-Kb. Resveratrol, moreover, through the inhibition of the human keratinocytes differentiation, could limit the hyperproliferation of the keratinocytes that could take to the follicular obstruction and, through the *P. acnes* growth inhibition, minimize the genesis of acne lesions. Experimental studies to confirm this activity in vitro are under processing. To investigate the therapeutic effects of resveratrol on acneic skin, Fabbrocini et al. [19] incorporated it in a carboxymethylcellulose-based gel. The authors compared the Global Score of the beginning with the one obtained at the end of the study. Moreover, with the innovative technique of follicular biopsy, areas of acneic skin were prepared for histopathology. The average area occupied by microcomedones at the baseline was compared with the same average area at the end of the treatment. All patients were satisfied; none of them suffered side effects. Clinical evaluation, calculated with the Global Score, showed a reduction equal to 54.75% in the treated hemiface. These data were supported by histological analysis showing a reduction of density of microcomedones equal to 62.3%.

13.7.2 Systemic Therapy

13.7.2.1 Oral Retinoids

Although isotretinoin is approved for the treatment of severe, recalcitrant, nodular acne, it is commonly used in other acne clinical type such as significant acne unresponsive to other treatments which results in significant physical or emotional scarring. Isotretinoin is effective in a high percentage of patients. Some advantages of this approach are the completeness of the remission in almost all cases and the longevity of remission which lasts for months to years after treatment suspension. The high frequency of side effects limits its use.

For sexually active women, it is necessary to require a pregnancy test before the start of therapy with isotretinoin and at monthly intervals during use of the drug plus use of 2 forms of contraception or sexual abstinence, beginning 1 month before the drug is started, continued during drug use, and for 1 month after stopping the drug. It requires blood tests to check for effect on blood cells, the liver, and fat levels. Systemic adverse effects are headache, and it has been associated with depression, suicidal thoughts, attempted suicide, and (rarely) completed suicide. Some common side effects are: dry eyes, chapped lips, and drying of the mucous membranes.

13.7.2.2 Oral Antibiotics

Oral therapy is indicated for moderate to severe and widespread forms of acne, particularly those patients who are at risk of scarring. Effective systemic therapies for acne include: tetracyclines (including its relatives minocycline and doxycycline), erythromycin and trimethoprim alone or in combination with sulfamethoxazole.

Minocycline is the most widely prescribed systemic antibiotic for acne. Tetracyclines have a bacteriostatic and bactericidal activity, reducing inflammatory and noninflammatory lesions. The most important adverse effects are photosensibility, serious gastric intestinal problems, enterocolitis, headaches, and, above all, a bacterial resistance. Women who are pregnant or breastfeeding should not take tetracyclines as they can stain teeth permanently and inhibit bone growth, leading to skeletal defects in a fetus. They are also contraindicated for children under 12, for the same reasons. Erythromycin is less popular owing to frequent induction of resistance by *P. acnes* and *Staphylococcus epidermidis* [20]. Erythromycin and macrolids in general offer a bacteriostatic effect linked to the action on bacteria ribosomes, blocking protein synthesis. At high doses, they can offer a bactericidal action too. Long-term use of antibiotics may induce hepatotoxicity [21]; therefore, periodic monitoring of blood chemistry is advisable.

13.7.2.3 Hormonal Therapy in Women

The sebaceous gland is an androgen target organ, and moderate acne may respond to antiandrogens. Oral contraceptives have been particularly useful in the treatment of acne since the advent of combination contraception where the progestin is actively antiandrogenic. Cyproterone acetate is the most common agent added to ethinyl estradiol. An alternative drug for treating hormonal acne in women is spironolactone, which can be combined with oral contraceptive therapy. Other antiandrogenic therapies that may prove useful include flutamide, finasteride, and gonadotropin-releasing hormone agonists [22, 23].

References

1. Chu TC (1997) Acne and other facial eruptions. Medicine 25:30–33
2. Niemeier V, Kupfer J, Gieler U (2006) Acne vulgaris – psychosomatic aspects. J Dtsch Dermatol Ges 4(12):1027–1036
3. Simpson NB, Cunliffe WJ (2004) Disorders of sebaceous glands. In: Burns T, Breathnach S, Cox N, Griffiths C (eds) Rook's textbook of dermatology, 7th edn. Blackwell Publishing, Oxford, pp 43.1–43.75
4. Simpson NB (1992) Acne and the mature female. Science Press, London
5. Goulden V, Stables GI, Cunliffe WJ (1999) Prevalence of facial acne in adults. J Am Acad Dermatol 41:577–580
6. White GM (1998) Recent findings in the epidemiologic evidence, classification, and subtypes of acne vulgaris. J Am Acad Dermatol 39:S34–S37
7. Jeremy AHT, Holland DB, Roberts SG, Thomson KF, Cunliffe WJ (2003) Inflammatory events are involved in acne lesion initiation. J Invest Dermatol 121:20–27. (http://www.ncbi.nlm.nih.gov/pubmed/12839559)
8. Doshi A, Zaheer A, Stiller MJ (1997) A comparison of current acne grading systems and proposal of a novel system. Int J Dermatol 38:416–418
9. Jacob CI, Dover JS, Kaminer MS (2001) Acne scarring: a classification system and review of treatment options. J Am Acad Dermatol 45:105–117
10. Goodman GJ, Baron JA (2006) Postacne scarring: a qualitative global scarring grading system. Dermatol Surg 32: 1458–1466
11. Layton AM, Henderson CA, Cunliffe WJ (1994) A clinical evaluation of acne scarring and its incidence. Clin Exp Dermatol 19:303–308
12. Katsambas AD, Katoulis AC, Stavropoulos P (1999) Acne neonatorum: a study of 22 cases. Int J Dermatol 38(2): 128–130
13. Thielitz A, Gollnick H (2008) Topical retinoids in acne vulgaris: update on efficacy and safety. Am J Clin Dermatol 9(6):369–381
14. Adişen E, Kaymak Y, Gurer MA, Durukan E (2008) Topical tetracycline in the treatment of acne vulgaris. J Drugs Dermatol 7(10):953–955
15. Fabbrocini G, Cacciapuoti S, Fardella N, Pastore F, Monfrecola G (2008) Cross technique: chemical reconstruction of skin scars method. Dermatol Ther 21:S29–S32

16. Holian O, Walter RJ (2001) Resveratrol inhibits the proliferation of normal human keratinocytes in vitro. J Cell Biochem Suppl. (Suppl 36):55–62
17. Docherty JJ et al (2007) Resveratrol inhibition of *Propionibacterium acnes*. J Antimicrob Chemother 59(6): 1182–1184, Epub Apr 21, 2007. (http://jac.oxfordjournals.org/content/59/6/1182.full)
18. Gao X et al (2003) Immunomodulatory activity of resveratrol: discrepant in vitro and in vivo immunological effects. Biochem Pharmacol 66(12):2427–2435
19. Fabbrocini G, Staibano S, De Rosa G, Battimiello V, Fardella N, Ilardi G, La Rotonda MI, Longobardi A, Mazzella M, Siano M, Pastore F, De Vita V,Vecchione ML, Ayala F (2011) Resveratrol-Containing Gel for the Treatment of Acne Vulgaris: A Single-Blind, Vehicle-Controlled, Pilot Study. Am J Clin Dermatol 12(2):133–141
20. Eady EA, Jones CE, Tipper JL, Cove JH, Cunliffe WJ, Layton AM (1993) Antibiotic resistant propionibacteria in acne: need for policies to modify antibiotic usage. BMJ 306:555–556
21. Thiim M, Friedman LS (2003) Hepatotoxicity of antibiotics and antifungals. Clin Liver Dis 7:381–399
22. Wang HS, Wang TH, Soong YK (1999) Low dose flutamide in the treatment of acne vulgaris in women with or without oligomenorrhea or amenorrhea. Changgeng Yi Xue Za Zhi 22:423–432
23. Wolff H (1999) Finasteride: also effective in acne vulgaris? Hautarzt 50:815

14 Photoaging

Pearl E. Grimes

14.1 Etiology

All humans experience intrinsic aging. Typically, it is characterized by smooth, relatively atrophic, finely wrinkled, or lax skin. Histologically, the stratum corneum is normal. However, the epidermis is atrophic and there is flattening of the dermo-epidermal junction. Dermal features include decreased thickness, loss of elastic fibers, and a decrease in the biosynthetic capacity of fibroblasts [1, 2] (Table 14.1).

In contrast, photoaging results from the long-term deleterious effects of sun exposure. Sunlight is divided into three components including ultraviolet (UV), visible, and infrared light with UV light representing the most important component. Ultraviolet light is divided into three groups based on the wavelength of light. It includes UVC (100–280 nm) which has minimal effects on the earth's surface because it is blocked by the ozone layer. UVB (290–320 nm) causes erythema, sunburn, DNA damage, solar elastosis, hyperpigmentation, and skin cancer. UVA (320–400 nm) requires a much higher dose to induce erythema; however, because it is more abundant and penetrates deeper, it is thought to play a more substantial role in the induction of photodamage [2].

Clinically, photodamaged skin is characterized by coarse and fine wrinkling, mottled pigmentary changes, sallowness, textural roughness, and telangiectasias. Histological features of photoaged skin include significant epidermal and dermal alterations [3]. The epidermal thickness may be increased or decreased corresponding to areas of hyperplasia or atrophy. There is loss of polarity of epidermal cells and keratinocyte atypia. Dermal features include elastosis, degeneration of collagen, and anchoring fibrils. Blood vessels become dilated and twisted. Ultraviolet light exposure activates matrix-degrading metalloproteinase enzymes including collagenase. Cytokines are released from keratinocytes. The cumulative effect of these changes is chronic dermal inflammation [1, 2, 4].

14.2 Epidemiology

Photoaging affects all races and skin types. Genetics plays an important part in this, with different combinations of genetic mutations determining not only skin and hair color but also the extent to which the skin is able to protect itself from the effects of the sun. These genomic differences may be leveraged when choosing the most appropriate and efficacious form of therapy for the individual patient [5]. Signs of photoaging may begin at an early age as evidenced by freckles following UV light exposure; however, the manifestations of photodamage may differ in lighter compared to darker skin types. In individuals with Fitzpatrick's skin types I to III, or lighter complexioned races, the clinical signs of photoaging (wrinkles, dyschromia, and sallowness) may also be accompanied by an increased occurrence of premalignant and malignant skin lesions including actinic keratoses, basal cell carcinoma, squamous cell carcinoma, and melanoma [6]. In contrast to lighter

P.E. Grimes
Division of Dermatology, Department of Medicine, Vitiligo and Pigmentation Institute of Southern California, David Geffen School of Medicine, University of California—Los Angeles, 5670 Wilshire Blvd., Suite 650, Los Angeles, CA 90036, USA
e-mail: pegrimesmd@earthlink.net

A. Tosti et al. (eds.), *Color Atlas of Chemical Peels*,
DOI 10.1007/978-3-642-20270-4_14, © Springer-Verlag Berlin Heidelberg 2012

Table 14.1 Clinical and histological features of intrinsic and extrinsic aging

Feature	Intrinsic aging (chronological)	Extrinsic aging (photoaging)
Clinical features	Smooth, atrophic Finely wrinkled Laxity, unblemished	Fine and course wrinkles sallowness, laxity, mottled pigmentation, textural roughness, telangiectasias
Epidermis	Stratum corneum normal thickness (basket weave pattern), epidermis thinned, atrophic, flattened rete ridges	Basket weave or compact stratum corneum, Acanthosis and/or atrophy, keratinocyte atypia, flattened rete ridges
Dermis	Absent Grenz zone, loss of elastic fibers, elastogenesis, decreased thickness, microvasculature normal, no evidence of inflammation	Grenz zone prominent, elastogenesis, elastosis, collagen degeneration, loss of anchoring fibrils Microvasculature abnormal: Blood vessels dilated, twisted later stages – sparse, perivenular lymphohistiocytic infiltrates

Modified from Gilchrest [3]

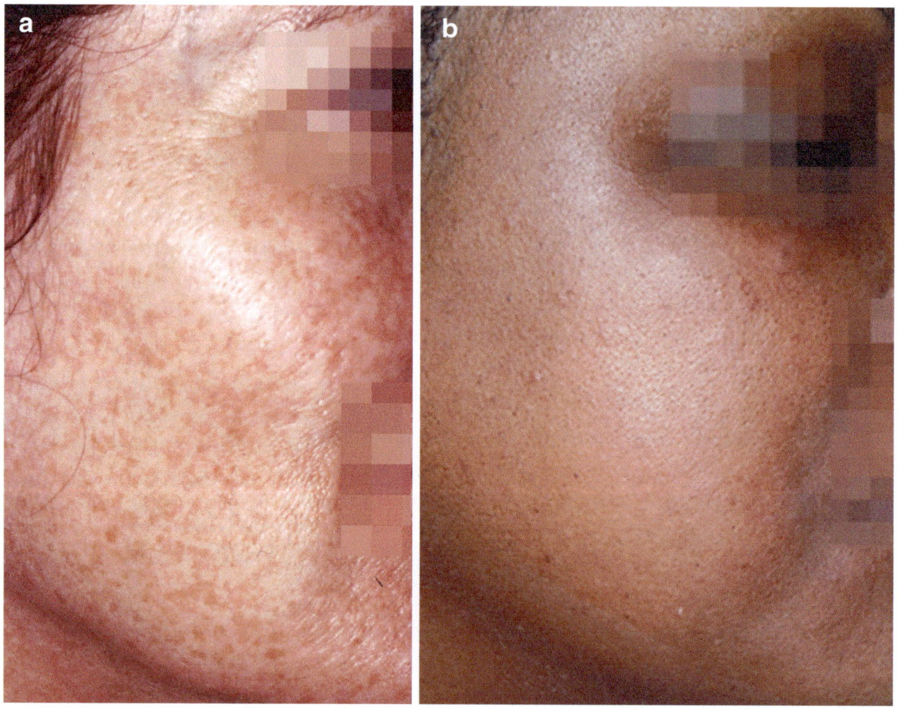

Fig. 14.1 (**a**) A 57-year-old Caucasian woman with fine wrinkling and significant mottled hyperpigmentation. (**b**) A 56-year-old African American woman with some textural irregularities, but no wrinkles

skin types, clinical observations document that people of color (skin types IV through VI) show less wrinkling with age than lighter-skinned individuals [7] (Fig. 14.1a, b). The biological basis for these observations correlates with many of the well-documented morphological and physiological skin differences in dark as opposed to white skin. (See section on dark skin) There appears to be a spectrum of photodamage in individuals with Fitzpatrick's skin types IV through VI with deeply pigmented skin showing minimal histological evidence of solar-induced changes (Fig. 14.2a, b). Clinical photodamage in black skin appears to be a subtle phenomenon, manifesting itself as diffuse or patchy hyperpigmentation and texturally rough skin. In addition, there is a significantly lower incidence of skin cancer in deeply pigmented people [8].

14.3 Clinical Types

Glogau [9] classified the severity of photodamage based on the extent of epidermal and dermal degenerative changes (Table 14.2; Fig. 14.3a–d). Severity of photodamage is categorized from I through IV ranging from mild, moderate, advanced, to severely photodamaged skin. Patients with mild photodamage often respond

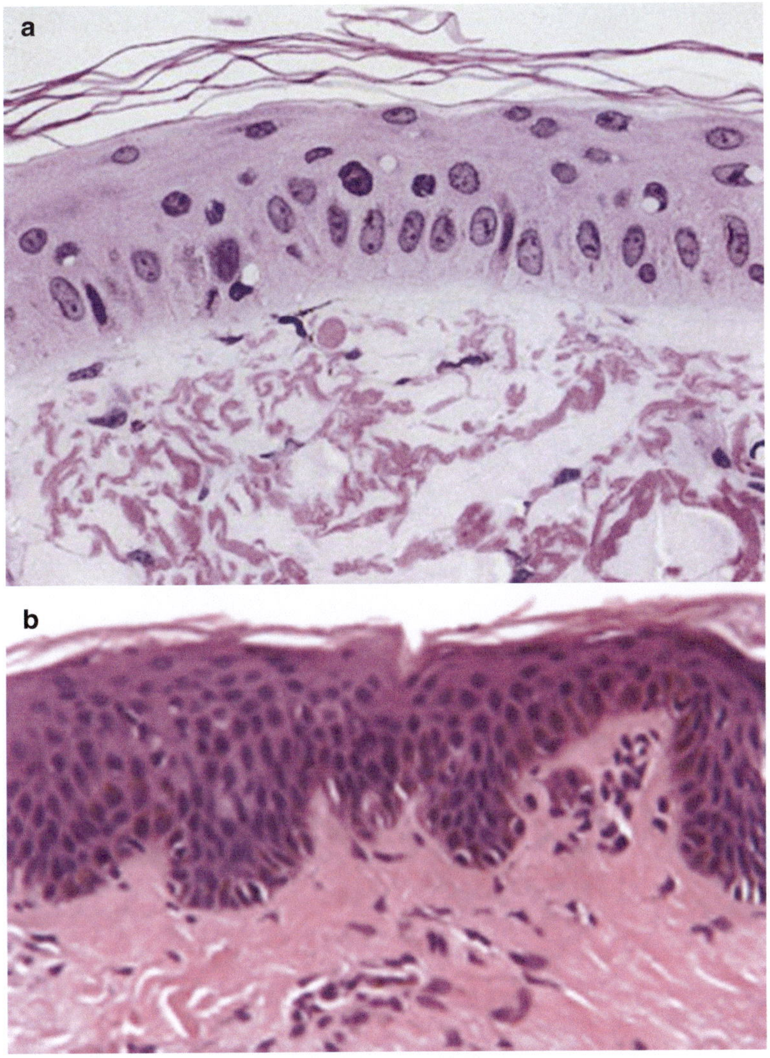

Fig. 14.2 (**a**) Biopsy of a 50-year-old Caucasian (Hispanic) woman showing significant epidermal atrophy and collagen degeneration. (**b**) Biopsy of a 50-year-old African American woman showing minimal to no evidence of photodamage

to topical antiaging regimens and superficial chemical peeling agents, whereas moderate to advanced photodamage often requires a medium-depth peel for substantial improvement (Table 14.3). Severe photodamage requires medium-depth or deep peeling procedures. Such patients may also require ablative resurfacing procedures in conjunction with lifting or rhytidectomies [10].

14.4 Therapeutic Intervention

14.4.1 Photoprotection

Prevention of photodamage requires a multifaceted approach. Photoprotection encompasses avoidance of sun exposure when possible, wearing protective clothing, and daily use of sunscreens (Table 14.3). Of the aforementioned strategies, sunscreens are the gold standard for skin protection from UV light. Sunscreens were initially developed to prevent UVB-induced sunburns. In the last 10–15 years, agents have been formulated which also absorb and/or block UVA radiation. Sunscreens are classified as organic or physical blocking agents. Organic sunscreens protect by absorbing UVB radiation, UVA radiation, or both. These sunscreen ingredients include octyl-dimethyl-PABA (UVB), 2-ethylhexyl-p-methoxycinnamate (UVB), octocrylene (UVA/UVB), octyl salicylate (UVB), benzophenones (UVB/UVA), and methyl anthranilate (UVA). Avobenzone/oxybenzone or Parsol 1789 and mexoryl, a benzylidene camphor, block UVA. Mexoryl is the most efficient of the UVA organic sunscreens [11].

Table 14.2 Glogau's classification of photoaging

Group	Clinical features
I (Mild)	Ages 20s–30s Early photoaging Mild dyschromia No keratoses Minimal wrinkling Minimal, no makeup Minimal, or no scarring
II (Moderate)	Late 30s–40s Early senile lentigines Dyschromia Early actinic keratoses Parallel smile lines Early wrinkling Some foundation worn Mild acne scarring
III (Advanced)	Usually aged 50–65 Dyschromia, telangiectasias Visible keratoses Wrinkling at rest Always wears makeup Moderate acne scarring
IV (Severe)	Patient age 60–75 Actinic keratoses Prior skin cancers Wrinkling throughout Makeup cakes and cracks Severe acne scarring

From Glogau [9]

Many sunscreen formulations combine ingredients to maximize photoprotection.

Physical agents include zinc oxide and titanium dioxide. These are the most effective sunscreens because they reflect UVA and UVB. When applied to the skin, they induce a white or ashen color, which many patients find cosmetically unacceptable. Micronized formulations of these agents are available which enhance cosmetic acceptability. Sunscreens should be worn regularly prior to chemical peeling procedures.

14.4.2 Retinoids

Retinoids mediate cellular responses primarily through activation of nuclear retinoid receptors [12]. There are two types of nuclear retinoic acid receptors: the retinoic acid receptors (RARs) and the retinoid X receptors. Each type of receptor contains three receptor subtypes: alpha, beta, and gamma [12, 13]. Among the commonly prescribed retinoids, tretinoin activates the RARs alpha, beta, and gamma directly, and the retinoid X receptors indirectly (through conversion of tretinoin to 9-cis-retinoic acid) [12, 14]. Conversely, tazarotenic acid, the metabolite of tazarotene, selectively binds to RARs beta and gamma and is unable to directly or indirectly activate retinoid X receptors [15]. This difference in receptor activity may explain the varying efficacies of the different retinoids in the treatment of dermatologic conditions. Retinoids show significant efficacy for treatment of photodamaged skin, and can also increase the depth and penetration of peeling agents.

In general, retinoids are also well tolerated in ethnic skin; however, retinoid dermatitis may cause postinflammatory hyperpigmentation. In addition, progressive hyperpigmentation can occur with retinoids without any clinical evidence of irritation.

14.4.2.1 Tretinoin

Multiple open-label and vehicle-controlled studies have documented the efficacy and safety of tretinoin for treatment of photodamage [13, 16–18]. Griffiths et al. [16] assessed the efficacy of various concentrations of tretinoin in 100 subjects with photodamage. Subjects were randomized into three treatment groups, treated with 0.1% tretinoin, 0.025% tretinoin, or vehicle cream. Treatment with 0.1% tretinoin or 0.025% tretinoin induced statistically significant improvements in photoaging changes compared to vehicle. There were no clinically significant differences in the two tretinoin formulations. However, the degree of irritation was significantly greater with the 0.1% formulation.

In a double-blind study of photodamaged skin, it has been demonstrated that papillary dermal collagen I formation was reduced by 56% in photodamaged skin compared with sun-protected skin [19]. Compared with vehicle, treatment with 0.1% tretinoin resulted in an 80% increase in Type I collagen formation, whereas the vehicle-treated areas showed a decrease in collagen formation.

In an evaluation of the efficacy of tretinoin in the treatment of hyperpigmented lesions associated with photoaging in Asian (Chinese and Japanese) patients, 45 photoaged Asian patients were randomized to treatment with tretinoin or vehicle for 40 weeks [17] . At the end of the treatment period, hyperpigmented lesions of the face and hands were lighter or much lighter in 90% of the tretinoin group, compared with

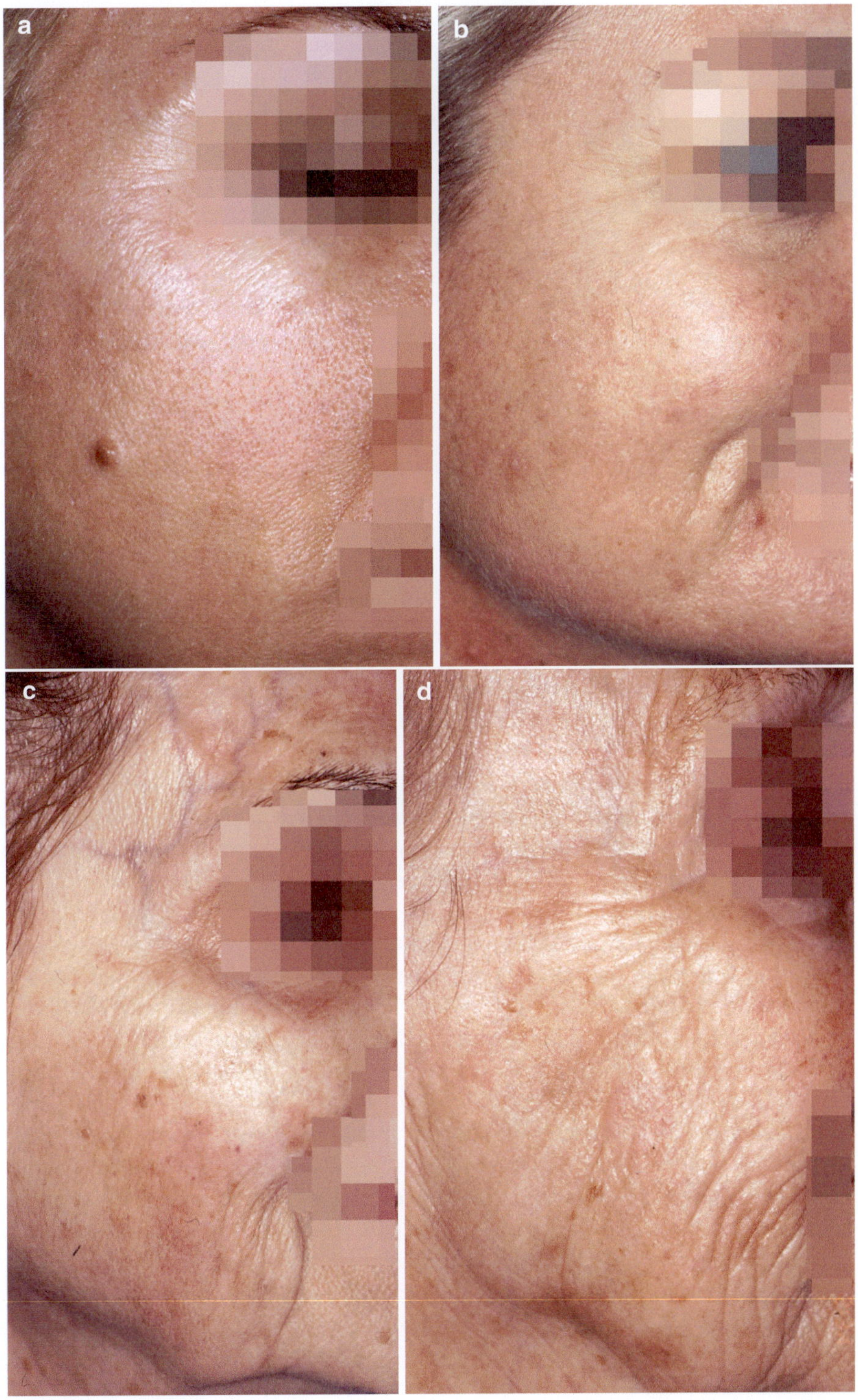

Fig. 14.3 (**a–d**) Series of patients showing Glogau's four photoaging groups: (**a**) mild photodamage, (**b**) moderate photodamage, (**c**) advanced photodamage, (**d**) severe photodamage

Table 14.3 Therapeutic approaches for photodamage

Topical agents	Resurfacing procedures
Broad spectrum sunscreens	Microdermabrasion
Retinoids • Tretinoin • Tazarotene • Adapalene • Retinol	Superficial chemical peeling Medium depth peeling Deep peeling Fractional resurfacing Ablative laser resurfacing
Vitamin C formulations	Nonablative laser resurfacing
Alpha hydroxy acids	Radio frequency therapy
Polyhydroxy acids	Facial lift
Beta hydroxy acids	Brow lift
Growth factors and peptides	
Bleaching agents • Hydroquinone • Kojic acid • Arbutin • Licorice • Azelaic acid	

33% of the vehicle group. Moreover, colorimetry demonstrated significant lightening of the lesions after tretinoin treatment compared with vehicle.

Tretinoin microsphere gel 0.1% has been assessed in a 6-month, randomized, double-blind, placebo-controlled study involving 45 patients with moderate-to-severe facial photodamage. After 6 months, the overall severity of photodamage was significantly improved with tretinoin, compared with placebo. Adverse effects included a higher frequency of increased cutaneous irritation at 1 month for tretinoin versus placebo; however, after 6 months, only peeling and dryness were significantly increased [20].

A long-term (2-year) placebo-controlled study of tretinoin emollient cream 0.05% has confirmed the beneficial effects of tretinoin on clinical signs of photoaging and overall severity. In addition, immunohistochemical analyses revealed a significant increase in facial procollagen 1 C terminal, a marker for procollagen synthesis, after 12 months of use [21]. A solution containing tretinoin 0.01% in combination with mequinol 2% has shown efficacy in the treatment of solar lentigines in a number of clinical trials in patients with all skin types [22–24].

14.4.2.2 Tazarotene

Tazarotene is a synthetic retinoid that mediates cell differentiation and proliferation [22]. Tazarotene, a pro-drug of tazarotenic acid, has been proven effective as a treatment for photodamaged skin [12, 25].

In a 1-year evaluation of 563 patients with facial photodamage, 0.1% tazarotene cream was applied to one-half of their faces and vehicle cream to the other half in a double-masked fashion for 24 weeks [26]. Patients then continued treatment with tazarotene for an additional 28 weeks. At week 24, compared with the vehicle cream, tazarotene treatment was associated with a significantly greater occurrence of treatment success (defined as at least 50% global improvement), and at least a 1-grade improvement in fine wrinkling, pore size, mottled hyperpigmentation, lentigines, elastosis, irregular depigmentation, roughness, and the overall assessment of photodamage. Moreover, Kang et al. also found tazarotene improved mottled pigmentation and fine wrinkles and that these improvements were comparable to those seen with tretinoin cream [12]. In a further study, Lowe at al. observed greater improvements in mottled hyperpigmentation and fine wrinkling at 16 weeks with tazarotene, compared with tretinoin [27]. On a histological level, study results suggest that tazarotene promotes normalization of cellular changes associated with photoaging and an increase in epidermal thickness [28].

14.4.2.3 Adapalene

Adapalene is a synthetic retinoid which is associated with less skin irritation than tretinoin. One clinical trial has investigated its efficacy for treating photodamage [29]. Kang and colleagues applied 0.1% or 0.3% adapalene gel or vehicle only to 83 Caucasian patients with actinic keratoses and solar lentigines. After 9 months of treatment, significant improvements in pigmentation of lentigines (reduced by 57% and 59% in the 0.1% and 0.3% adapalene groups, respectively), wrinkles, and other clinical features of photoaged skin were observed in the adapalene groups. Both formulations were well tolerated.

Retinol – All trans-retinol, also known as vitamin A1, is the predominant circulating retinoid in human tissue. Although retinol is believed to be a precursor of other retinoids, the metabolic pathways of the physiologic and pharmacologic effects are not well understood. Retinols are used extensively in cosmeceutical formulations for photoaging. They are generally recognized as safe ingredients in the United States and are widely used in cosmetics and toiletries, most often at a concentration of 0.1–1.0% [27, 28].

Kang et al. [29] compared the clinical, histologic, and molecular responses of normal human skin to topical retinol with that of retinoic acid. Application of retinol and retinoic acid produced epidermal thickening; however, retinol produced less erythema than retinoic acid. The authors suggest that these data are compatible with the idea that retinol may be a prohormone of retinoic acid.

The effects of a stabilized 0.1% retinol moisturizer versus its vehicle were tested in a double-blind, randomized, split-face study in women with moderate facial photodamage. Significant effects in a range of photodamage parameters were observed after 4 weeks, and the improvement continued to week 8 [30]. In two randomized, split-face studies, Kikuchi et al. investigated the effects of 0.075% and 0.04% retinol creams in middle-aged Japanese women with photoaged skin. The 0.075% retinol formulation was more effective than the lower concentration cream in reducing the appearance of fine wrinkling, but had greater irritancy potential [31].

14.4.3 Tyrosinase Inhibitors

14.4.3.1 Hydroquinone

Hydroquinone acts by inhibiting tyrosinase and preventing the conversion of tyrosine to dopa [32, 33]. It is commonly used in the treatment of melasma and postinflammatory hyperpigmentation, the dyschromia of photoaging, lentigines, and freckles. It has long been the gold standard for treating hyperpigmentation. Concerns over its safety in recent years have led to its removal from cosmetic products in the EU, Japan, and the United States, but it is still used in Rx products. Bleaching agents such as hydroquinone are often used in conjunction with retinoids and chemical peeling agents for photodamage (see peeling protocols).

Complications of hydroquinone therapy include acute and chronic reactions. Common acute reactions are irritant and allergic contact dermatitis, and postinflammatory hyperpigmentation. Lesional and perilesional hypopigmentation may occur. This is usually a temporary complication. With repeated application, hydroquinone may cause destruction of melanosomes, melanocyte organelles, and melanocyte necrosis [32]. A novel formulation of hydroquinone 4% plus retinol 0.15%, in which most of the hydroquinone and all of the retinol are encapsulated into macroporous beads, allows gradual delivery of hydroquinone into the skin, minimizing the effects of skin irritation [34–36].

The major long-term concern regarding the use of hydroquinone is ochronosis. This condition is most often observed in African patients who have used products containing high concentrations of hydroquinone for prolonged periods [37, 38]. In contrast, cases in the United States are rare and are predominantly associated with the use of hydroquinone 2%. Clinically, ochronosis is characterized by reticulated, sooty hyperpigmentation of the face. Ochronosis is often considered permanent. The author has treated cases with topical retinoids and topical corticosteroids combined with a series of superficial salicylic acid chemical peels, achieving moderate to excellent improvement. Bellew and Alster [39] reported the efficacy of the 755 nm Q-Switched Alexandrite laser for exogenous ochronosis in two patients.

14.4.3.2 Azelaic Acid

Azelaic acid is a naturally occurring dicarboxylic acid (1,7-heptanedicarboxylic acid) that has demonstrated beneficial therapeutic effects in the treatment of acne and several disorders of hyperpigmentation [40]. There are minimal effects on normally pigmented human skin, freckles, senile lentigines, and nevi. The cytotoxic and antiproliferative effects of azelaic acid may be mediated via inhibition of mitochondrial oxidoreductase activity and DNA synthesis. Disturbance of tyrosinase synthesis by azelaic acid may also influence its therapeutic effects. Azelaic acid can be used as a hypopigmenting agent in patients sensitive to hydroquinone.

14.4.3.3 Kojic Acid

Kojic acid (5-hydroxy-4 pyran 4-1-2 methyl) is a fungal derivative which inactivates tyrosinase via chelation of copper. Concentrations range from 2% to 4%. It can be used for monotherapy or in combination with retinoids or other cosmeceutical products such as glycolic acid. Compared to hydroquinone, these kojic acid formulations usually show less efficacy; however, they may be effective in patients who do not tolerate hydroquinone. In addition, they can be used as maintenance therapies for treatment of hyperpigmentation following 4–6 months of hydroquinone treatment. Use of kojic acid has been associated with contact dermatitis in sensitized individuals, however [41–43].

Vitamin C – Ascorbic acid (vitamin C) has been shown to protect against sunburn, delay the onset of skin tumors, and reduce ultraviolet-B radiation–induced skin wrinkling [44–47]. Ascorbic acid displays potent antioxidant properties and is the primary water-soluble nonenzymatic biologic antioxidant in human tissues [48–51]. Vitamin C is necessary for the normal formation and maintenance of collagen and is a cofactor for several hydroxylating enzymes [52–54]. The topical application of vitamin C has been suggested in order to maximize its antioxidant properties and stimulate collagen production, as oral administration is believed incapable of generating adequate tissue ascorbic acid levels for these tissue effects [45]. The efficacies of various topical vitamin C preparations have been extensively evaluated and have been found to improve photodamage and stimulate new collagen formation [55]. Ascorbyl palmitate, a fat-soluble synthetic ester of vitamin C, has also been shown to reduce redness associated with sunburn 50% sooner than areas on the same patient that were left untreated [56]. In one double-blind, placebo-controlled study by Humbert et al., 5% vitamin C cream was applied to photodamaged skin on the neck and arm over a period of 6 months. The researchers observed significant clinical improvement, favorable effects on skin topography, and histological evidence of tissue repair [57]. Vitamin C formulations are typically nonirritating when applied topically and have also been shown to improve hyperpigmentation [58].

14.4.3.4 Alpha-Hydroxy Acids

The alpha-hydroxy acids (AHAs) are organic carboxylic acids having one hydroxyl group attached to the alpha position of the carboxylic carbon atom. Alpha-hydroxy acids are naturally occurring products present in sugar cane juice, sour milk, tomato juice, grapes, and apples. Glycolic acid, the smallest of the AHA compounds, has gained widespread acceptance as a superficial exfoliant and peeling agent [59, 60].

AHAs induce changes in the epidermis and dermis. They cause exfoliation of the stratum corneum. Dermal effects have also been demonstrated. Studies in human skin specimens have demonstrated that glycolic acid promotes collagen synthesis by fibroblasts. In addition, glycolic acid was shown to modulate matrix degradation and induce epidermal and dermal remodeling [61, 62].

In a study by Ditre et al. [63], patients applied a lotion containing 25% glycolic, citric, or lactic acid to one forearm and a placebo lotion to the other for 6 months. Thickness of forearm skin was measured throughout the study. Treatment with AHAs caused an approximate 25% increase in skin thickness. The epidermis was thicker and papillary dermal changes included increased thickness, increased acid mucopolysaccharides, improved quality of elastic fibers, and increased density of collagen. No inflammation was evident. Treatment with AHAs produced significant reversal of epidermal and dermal markers of photoaging. Glycolic acid improves the tone and texture of the skin. It is used as a monotherapy, or in combination with retinoids and other bleaching agents for photodamage.

14.4.3.5 Polyhydroxy Acids

PHAs provide similar effects to AHAs, but do not cause the sensory irritation responses that limit the use of AHAs. PHAs have also been found to have some additional benefits including humectant and moisturizing properties. They have been shown to improve photodamage when combined with retinyl acetate and retinoic acid [64]. PHAs are also well tolerated when treating photodamage in dark skin.

14.4.3.6 Other Tyrosinase Inhibitors

Concerns about the safety of hydroquinone have energized the search for alternative tyrosinase inhibitors. Recent research into primarily natural-product derived substances, including polyphenols, benzaldehyde and benzoate derivatives, and long-chain lipids and steroids, has been extensively reviewed [65–67]. A number of these compounds have demonstrated potent in vitro activity, and some have also been tested successfully in small clinical trials.

Ellagic acid, a polyphenol present in pomegranates and berry fruits, has demonstrated improvements in signs of photoaging in vitro and significant reductions in pigmentation in patients with melasma [68, 69]. The latter study obtained similar results with the glycosylated hydroquinone, arbutin. Serine proteases extracted from soybeans provided significantly better improvement of mottled pigmentation, blotchiness, dullness, fine lines, overall texture, overall skin tone, and overall appearance in patients who received a novel soy-based moisturizer compared with patients who received vehicle only [70].

Niacinamide has been reported to improve the appearance and elasticity of aging skin [71]. Tested in a 4% cosmetic formulation, it showed efficacy relative to placebo in reducing periorbital wrinkles [72].

14.4.4 Other Agents

Undecylenoyl phenylalanine is a possible antagonist of alpha-melanocyte-stimulating hormone. When applied to solar lentigines on the hands of 30 patients, it provided moderate-to-marked improvements in pigmentation with minor adverse events [73].

Boswellic acids, which are pentacyclic triterpenes derived from the gum resin of a tropical tree, *Boswellia serrata*, have also recently shown promise in ameliorating signs of photoaging in facial skin [74].

Growth factors, peptides, and pentapeptides also show significant progress in the treatment of photodamage [75].

14.5 Chemical Peels for Photoaging

In 1982, Stegman reported the histologic effects of three peeling agents, including TCA, full-strength phenol, Baker's phenol, and dermabrasion on normal and sun-damaged skin of the neck. This study demonstrated that 40–60% TCA caused epidermal necrosis, papillary dermal edema, and homogenization to the midreticular dermis 3 days after peeling. Findings were similar in sun-damaged compared to non–sun-damaged skin. Ninety days after peeling, he observed an expanded papillary dermis which he defined as the Grenz zone. The thickness of the Grenz zone increased as the depth of peeling increased. The investigative work of Stegman and others facilitated our understanding of the capacity of medium-depth and deep peeling agents to improve photodamage [76–78]. Superficial, medium-depth, and deep peeling agents are currently utilized according to the degree of photodamage.

14.5.1 Superficial Peeling Agents

The benefits of superficial peeling agents have been reported for mild to moderate photodamage. Following the pioneering work of Van Scott and Yu on the effects of alpha-hydroxy acids [79], these agents were popularized as peeling agents for photodamage [80–82]. Moy et al. [81], in a mini pig model, showed that application of 50% and 70% glycolic acid was comparable to TCA 50% in stimulating collagen production.

Given the depth of injury induced by glycolic acid peeling, other investigators have reported no benefit when using a series of four 70% glycolic acid peels to treat moderate photodamage [83].

Several studies have reported the efficacy of salicylic acid peeling for treatment of photodamage. Kligman and Kligman [84] ushered salicylic acid into the modern arena of superficial peeling agents. They treated 50 women with mild to moderate photodamage, reporting improvement in pigmented lesions, surface roughness, and reduction in fine lines. Gladstone et al [85] subsequently assessed the efficacy of hydroquinone cream 4% used alone or in combination with serial 20% and 30% salicylic acid peeling for treatment of moderate to advanced photodamage of the neck and chest. Nineteen women were treated. Of that group, nine were treated with 4% hydroquinone and serial salicylic acid peeling. Both groups showed improvement in photodamage; however, there were no significant differences between the two treatments.

14.5.2 Medium-Depth Peeling

Trichloroacetic acid and phenol peels (see peel sections) have been used extensively to treat photodamage [86, 87]. However, TCA peels in concentrations above 35% are unpredictable. Albeit efficacious for severe photodamage, phenol peels are associated with myriad side effects [87]. Hence, combination medium-depth peeling agents have become increasingly popular for treatment of photodamage. Monheit and Coleman [88, 89] popularized the concept of combination peeling procedures using Jessner's solution or glycolic acid in combination with TCA 35%. The application of Jessner's solution prior to TCA peeling was effective in destroying the epidermal barrier allowing for deeper penetration and more even application of the TCA peel. Similar results are achieved with application of 70% glycolic acid prior to TCA peeling. Tse et al. [90] in a split-face study of 13 patients with photodamage compared the efficacy of 70% glycolic acid and TCA 35% to Jessner's solution and TCA 35%. Clinical and histological assessments were performed at 7, 30, and 60 days after peeling. Clinically, the glycolic acid/TCA 35% peel was more effective for the treatment of actinic keratoses. It induced a slightly thicker Grenz zone, greater papillary dermal fibrosis, and neovascularization compared to Jessner's solution/TCA 35% (Figs. 14.4–14.7).

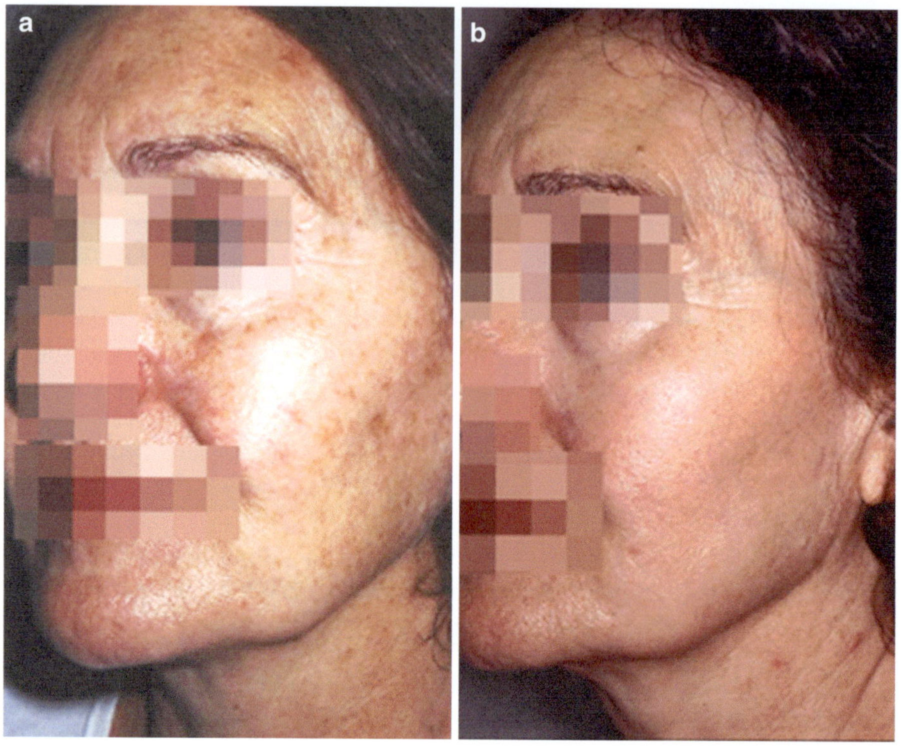

Fig. 14.4 (**a**, **b**) Moderate photodamage. Significant improvement after a 35% TCA peel (Dr. Mark Rubin)

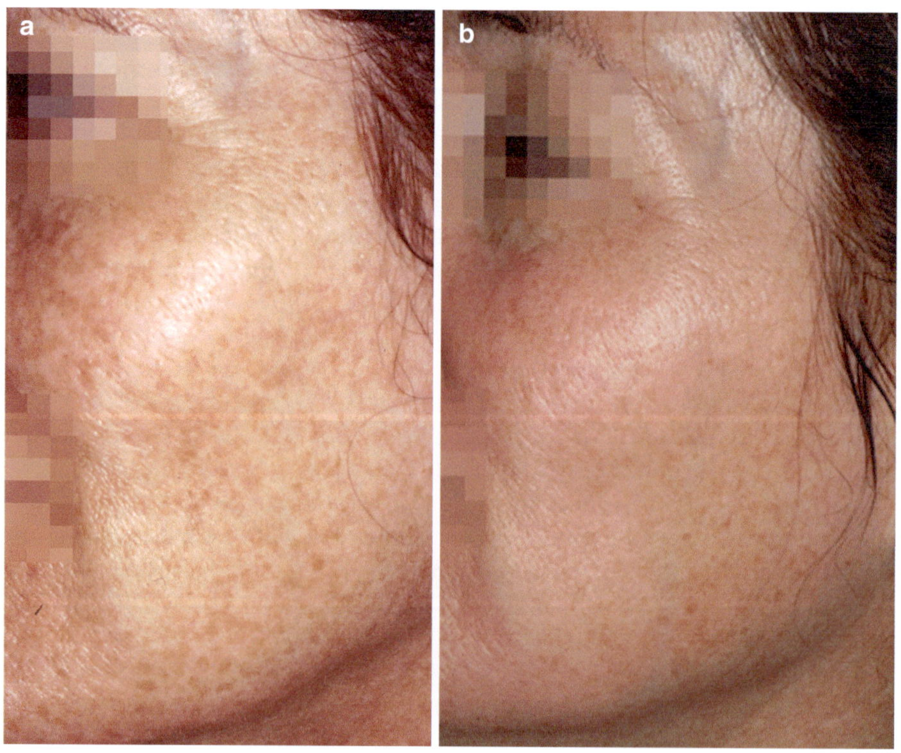

Fig. 14.5 (**a**, **b**) Fine wrinkles and mottled pigmentation before and after two 15% TCA peels

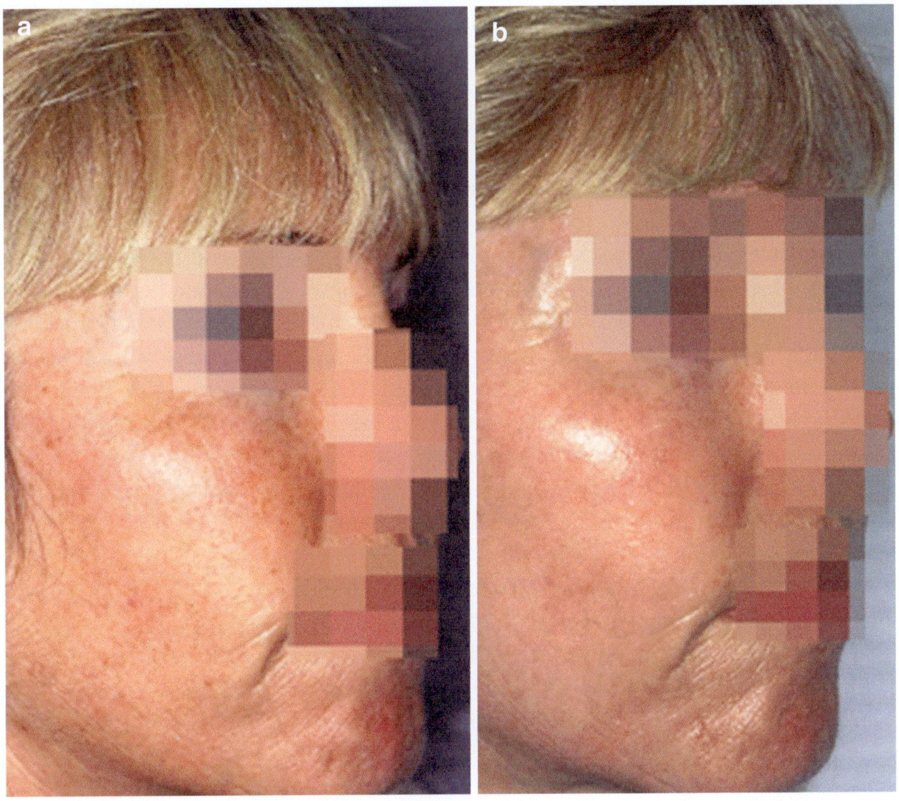

Fig. 14.6 (**a**, **b**) Before and after combination 35% TCA peeling (Mark Rubin, M.D.)

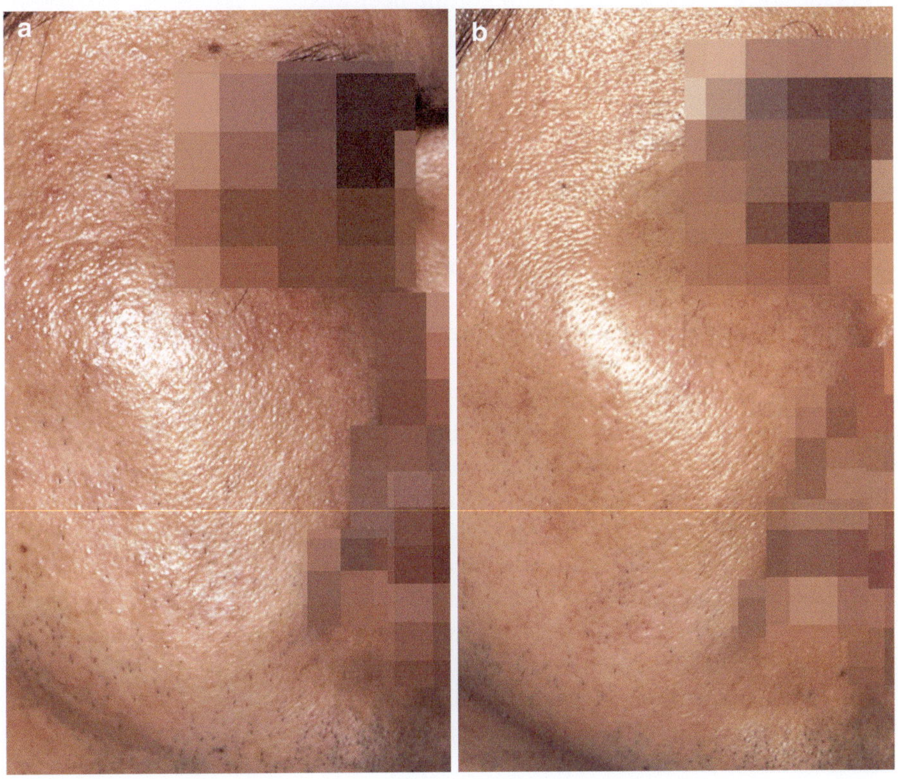

Fig. 14.7 (**a**, **b**) Texturally rough skin, a manifestation of photodamage, improved by a series of 5 salicylic acid 20%/30% peels

Samaby et al. [91] performed medium-depth peeling using 70% glycolic acid and 35% TCA in 5 patients with facial photodamage. Biopsies were performed at baseline, prior to chemical peeling, and at 3 months following the peel. Histological and ultrastructural assessments showed markedly decreased epidermal intracytoplasmic vacuoles, decreased elastic fibers, increased activated fibroblasts, and organized arrays of collagen fibrils suggesting that a combination medium-depth glycolic acid 70%/TCA 35% peel improves photodamage. These findings were confirmed by Sezer and colleagues, who found that glycolic acid 70%/TCA 35% gave results comparable to those achieved with cryotherapy [92]. They found that the peel was less painful and carried a lower risk of postprocedural hyperpigmentation than cryotherapy, although it was more time consuming.

Lawrence et al. [93], in a split-face study, compared the efficacy and safety of Jessner's solution and 35% TCA to 5% fluorouracil in the treatment of widespread facial actinic keratoses. Fifteen patients were treated. Both treatments reduced the number of visible actinic keratoses by 75%. Similarly, both caused equivalent reductions in keratinocyte atypia, hyperkeratosis, and parakeratosis. Compared to fluorouracil, only one application of the peel was necessary.

Pyruvic acid peels have also been used for treatment of photodamage. Pyruvic acid is an α-keto acid which is converted physiologically to lactic acid. It is used in concentrations of 40–70% in water/ethanol solutions. Ghersetich et al. [94] treated 20 patients with Glogau's photoaging types I and II. A series of 4 peels were performed at 4 week intervals. After pyruvic acid peeling, subjects demonstrated a smoother texture, less evident fine wrinkles, and lightening of areas of hyperpigmentation. Side effects were minimal. A modified 50% pyruvic acid peel, containing dimethyl isosorbide, propylene glycol, ethyl alcohol, dimethyl sulfone, ethyl lactate and water, has been used by Berardesca et al. in patients with photodamage, superficial scarring, and melasma. The treatment produced significant improvements in skin elasticity, wrinkling, and the degree of hyperpigmentation, with no reports of undue discomfort, persistent erythema, or postinflammatory hyperpigmentation. In addition, there was no negative impact of the treatment on patients' working and social lives [95].

14.6 Summary

In summary, multiple studies have documented the efficacy of topical agents (retinoids, antioxidants, and topical bleaching agents) used in combination with superficial and/or medium-depth or deep peeling agents for photodamage. The treatment of photodamage requires a multifaceted approach incorporating sun protection, antioxidants, exfoliating agents, retinoids, and resurfacing procedures. Despite the evolution of new and advanced laser technologies, chemical peeling remains a viable, efficacious, and cost-effective treatment for photodamage.

Disclaimer The author has no financial interest in any of the products or equipment mentioned in this article.

References

1. Bhawan J, Andersen W, Lee J, Labadie R, Solares G (1995) Photoaging versus intrinsic aging: a morphologic assessment of facial skin. J Cutan Pathol 22(2):154–159
2. Gilchrest BA (1996) A review of skin aging and its medical therapy. Br J Dermatol 135:867–875
3. Lavker RM (1995) Cutaneous aging: chronologic versus photoaging. In: Gilchrest BA (ed) Photodamage. Blackwell Science, Cambridge, pp 123–135
4. Vayalil PK, Mittal A, Hara Y, Elmets CA, Katiyar SK (2004) Green tea polyphenols prevent ultraviolet light-induced oxidative damage and matrix metalloproteinases expression in mouse skin. J Invest Dermatol 122(6):1480–1487
5. Kaczvinsky JR Jr, Grimes PE (2009) Practical applications of genomics research for treatment of aging skin. J Drugs Dermatol 8(7 Suppl):s15–s18
6. Spencer JM (2004) Premalignant manifestations of photoaging: actinic keratoses and atypical nevi. In: Goldberg DJ (ed) Photodamaged skin. Marcel Dekker, Inc, New York, pp 1–16
7. Grimes PE (2004) Benign manifestations of photodamage: ethnic skin types. In: Goldberg DJ (ed) Photodamaged skin. Marcel Dekker, Inc, New York, pp 175–196
8. Washington CV, Grimes PE (2003) Incidence and prevention of skin cancer. Cosmet Dermatol 16(S3):46–48
9. Glogau RG (1994) Chemical peeling and aging skin. J Geriatr Dermatol 2:30–35
10. Fulton JE, Porumb S (2004) Chemical peels: their place within the range of resurfacing techniques. Am J Clin Dermatol 5(3):179–187
11. Seite S, Colige A, Piquemal-Vivenot P, Montastier C, Fourtanier A, Lapiere C, Nusgens B (2000) A full-UV spectrum absorbing daily use cream protects human skin against biological changes occurring in photoaging. Photodermatol Photoimmunol Photomed 16(4):147–155
12. Kang S, Leyden JJ, Lowe NJ et al (2001) Tazarotene cream for the treatment of facial photodamage. Arch Dermatol 137:1597–1604

13. Chandraratna RAS (1996) Tazarotene: first of a new generation of receptor-selective retinoids. Br J Dermatol 135: 18–25
14. Weinstein GD, Nigra TP, Pochi PE et al (1991) Topical tretinoin for treatment of photodamaged skin: a multicenter study. Arch Dermatol 127:659–665
15. Levin AA, Sturzenbecker LJ, Kazmer S et al (1992) 9-cis Retinoic acid stereoisomer binds and activates the nuclear receptor RXR alpha. Nature 355:359–361
16. Griffiths CEM, Goldfarb MT, Finkel LJ et al (1994) Topical tretinoin (retinoic acid) treatment of hyperpigmented lesions associated with photoaging in Chinese and Japanese patients: a vehicle-controlled trial. J Am Acad Dermatol 30:76–84
17. Tadaki T, Watanabe M, Kumasaka K, Tanita Y, Kato T, Tagami H, Horii I, Yokoi T, Nakayama Y, Kligman AM (1993) The effect of topical tretinoin on the photodamaged skin of the Japanese. Tohoku J Exp Med 169(2):131–139
18. Griffiths CE, Kang S, Ellis CN, Kim KJ, Finkel LJ, Ortiz-Ferrer LC, White GM, Hamilton TA, Voorhees JJ (1995) Two concentrations of topical tretinoin (retinoic acid) cause similar improvement of photoaging but different degrees of irritation. A double-blind, vehicle-controlled comparison of 0.1% and 0.025% tretinoin creams. Arch Dermatol 131(9): 1037–1044
19. Griffiths CE, Russman AN, Majmudar G, Singer RS, Hamilton TA, Voorhees JJ (1993) Restoration of collagen formation in photodamaged human skin by tretinoin (retinoic acid). N Engl J Med 329(8):530–535
20. Weiss JS, Shavin JS, Nighland M, Grossman R (2006) Tretinoin microsphere gel 0.1% for photodamaged facial skin: a placebo-controlled trial. Cutis 78(6):426–432
21. Kang S, Bergfeld W, Gottlieb AB, Hickman J, Humeniuk J, Kempers S, Lebwohl M, Lowe N, McMichael A, Milbauer J, Phillips T, Powers J, Rodriguez D, Savin R, Shavin J, Sherer D, Silvis N, Weinstein R, Weiss J, Hammerberg C, Fisher GJ, Nighland M, Grossman R, Nyirady J (2005) Long-term efficacy and safety of tretinoin emollient cream 0.05% in the treatment of photodamaged facial skin: a two-year, randomized, placebo-controlled trial. Am J Clin Dermatol 6(4):245–253
22. Fleischer AB, Schwartzel EH, Colby SI, Altman DJ, the Depigmenting Solution Study Group (2000) The combination of 2% 4-hydroxyanisole (mequinol) and 0.01% tretinoin is effective in improving the appearance of solar lentigines and related hyperpigmented lesions in two double-blind multicenter clinical studies. J Am Acad Dermatol 42:459–467
23. Jarrett M (2004) Mequinol 2%/tretinoin 0.01% solution: an effective and safe alternative to hydroquinone 3% in the treatment of solar lentigines. Cutis 74:310–322
24. Draelos ZD (2006) The combination of 2% 4-hydroxyanisole (mequinol) and 0.01% tretinoin effectively improves the appearance of solar lentigines in ethnic groups. J Cosmet Dermatol 5:239–244
25. Kang S, Krueger GG, Tanghetti EA et al (2005) A multicenter, randomized, double-blind trial of tazarotene 0.1% cream in the treatment of photodamage. J Am Acad Dermatol 52:268–274
26. Sefton J, Kligman AM, Kopper SC, Lue JC, Gibson JR (2000) Photodamage pilot study: a double-blind, vehicle-controlled study to assess the efficacy and safety of tazarotene 0.1% gel. J Am Acad Dermatol 43:656–663
27. Cosmetic Ingredient Review (1987) Final report on the safety assessment of retinyl palmitate and retinol. J Am Coll Toxicol 6:279–320
28. Suzuki S, Miyachi Y, Niwa Y, Isshiki N (1989) Significance of reactive oxygen species in distal flap necrosis and its salvage with liposomal SOD. Br J Plast Surg 42:559–564
29. Kang S, Duell EA, Fisher GJ et al (1995) Application of retinol to human skin in vivo induces epidermal hyperplasia and cellular retinoid binding proteins characteristic of retinoic acid but without measurable retinoic acid levels or irritation. J Invest Dermatol 105:549–556
30. Tucker-Samaras S, Zedayko T, Cole C, Miller D, Wallo W, Leyden JJ (2009) A stabilized 0.1% retinol facial moisturizer improves the appearance of photodamaged skin in an eight-week, double-blind, vehicle-controlled study. J Drugs Dermatol 8(10):932–936
31. Kikuchi K, Suetake T, Kumasaka N, Tagami H (2009) Improvement of photoaged facial skin in middle-aged Japanese females by topical retinol (vitamin A alcohol): a vehicle-controlled, double-blind study. J Dermatolog Treat 20(5):276–281
32. Jimbow K, Obata H, Pathak MA et al (1974) Mechanism of depigmentation by hydroquinone. J Invest Dermatol 62: 436–449
33. Amer M, Metwalli M (1998) Topical hydroquinone in the treatment of some hyperpigmentary disorders. Int J Dermatol 37:449–450
34. Embil K, Nacht S (1996) The Microsponge Delivery System (MDS): a topical delivery system with reduced irritancy incorporating multiple triggering mechanisms for the release of actives. J Microencapsul 13:575–588
35. Grimes PE (2004) A microsponge formulation of hydroquinone 4% and retinol 0.15% in the treatment of melasma and postinflammatory hyperpigmentation. Cutis 74:362–368
36. Cook-Bolden FE, Hamilton SF (2008) An open-label study of the efficacy and tolerability of microencapsulated hydroquinone 4% and retinol 0.15% with antioxidants for the treatment of hyperpigmentation. Cutis 81:365–371
37. Findlay GH, Morrison JG, Simson IW (1975) Exogenous ochronosis and pigmented colloid milium from hydroquinone bleaching creams. Br J Dermatol 93(6):613–622
38. Mahe A, Ly F, Aymard G, Dangou JM (2003) Skin diseases associated with the cosmetic use of bleaching products in women from Dakar, Senegal. Br J Dermatol 148(3):493–500
39. Bellew SG, Alster TS (2004) Treatment of exogenous ochronosis with a Q-switched alexandrite (755 nm) laser. Dermatol Surg 30(4 Pt 1):555–558
40. Fitton A, Goa KL (1991) Azelaic acid. Drugs 41:780–798
41. Nakagawa M, Kawai K, Kawai K (1995) Contact allergy to kojic acid in skin care products. Contact Dermat 32:9–13
42. Mata TL, Sanchez JP, De La Cuadra Oyanguren J (2005) Allergic contact dermatitis due to kojic acid. Dermatitis 16:89
43. García-Gavín J, González-Vilas D, Fernández-Redondo V, Toribio J (2010) Pigmented contact dermatitis due to kojic acid. A paradoxical effect of a skin lightener. Contact Dermat 62:63–64
44. Bissett DL, Chatterjee R, Hannon DP (1990) Photoprotective effect of superoxide-scavenging antioxidants against ultraviolet radiation-induced chronic skin damage in the hairless mouse. Photodermatol Photoimmunol Photomed 7:56–62

45. Darr D, Combs S, Dunston S, Manning T, Pinnel S (1992) Topical vitamin C protects porcine skin from ultraviolet radiation-induced damage. Br J Dermatol 127:247–253
46. Black HS (1987) Potential involvement of free radical reactions in ultraviolet light mediated cutaneous damage. Photochem Photobiol 46:213–221
47. Eberlein-Konig B, Placzek M, Pryzbilla B (1998) Protective effect against sunburn of combined systemic ascorbic acid (vitamin C) and d-alpha-tocopherol (vitamin E). J Am Acad Dermatol 38:45–48
48. Colvin RM, Pinnell SR (1996) Topical vitamin C in aging. Clin Dermatol 14:227–234
49. Bachowski GJ, Girotti AW (1988) Light-stimulated formation of hydrogen peroxide and hydroxyl radical in the presence of uroporphyrin and ascorbate. Free Radic Biol Med 5:3–6
50. Bacq ZM, Fischer P (1957) The action of various drugs on the suprarenal response of the rat to total-body x-irradiation. Radiat Res 7:365–372
51. Frei B, England L, Amos B (1989) Ascorbate is an outstanding anti-oxidant in human blood plasma. Proc Natl Acad Sci USA 86:6377–6381
52. Koch CJ, Biaglow JE (1978) Toxicity, radiation sensitivity modification, and metabolic effects of dehydroascorbate and ascorbate in mammalian cells. J Cell Physiol 94:299–306
53. Bartlett MK, Jones CM, Ryan AE (1942) Vitamin C and wound healing: II. Ascorbic acid content and tensile strength of healing wounds in human beings. N Engl J Med 226: 474–481
54. Padh H (1990) Cellular functions of ascorbic acid. Biochem Cell Biol 68:1166–1173
55. Abt AF, von Schurching S (1961) Catabolism of L-ascorbic-1-C acid as a measure of its utilization in the intact and wounded guinea pig on scorbutic maintenance, and saturation diets. Ann NY Acad Sci 92:148–158
56. Fitzpatrick RE, Rostan EF (2002) Double blind, half-face study comparing topical vitamin C and vehicle for rejuvenation of photodamage. Dermatol Surg 28:231–236
57. Humbert PG, Haftek M, Creidi P, Lapière C, Nusgens B, Richard A, Schmitt D, Rougier A, Zahouani H (2003) Topical ascorbic acid on photoaged skin. clinical, topographical and ultrastructural evaluation: double-blind study vs. placebo. Exp Dermatol 12(3):237–244
58. Perricone NV (1993) The photoprotective and anti-inflammatory effects of topical ascorbyl palmitate. J Geriatr Dermatol 1:5–10
59. Moy LS, Murad H, Moy RL (1993) Glycolic acid peels for the treatment of wrinkles and photoaging. J Dermatol Surg Oncol 19:243–246
60. Murad H, Shamban AT, Moy RL (1995) The use of glycolic acid as a peeling agent. Dermatol Clin 13:285–3074
61. Bernstein EF, Lee J, Brown DB, Yu R, Van Scott E (2001) Glycolic acid treatment increases type I collagen mRNA and hyaluronic acid content of human skin. Dermatol Surg 27(5):429–433
62. Okano Y, Abe Y, Masaki H, Santhanam U, Ichihashi M, Funasaka Y (2003) Biological effects of glycolic acid on dermal matrix metabolism mediated by dermal fibroblasts and epidermal keratinocytes. Exp Dermatol 12(Suppl 2):57–63
63. Ditre CM, Griffin TD, Murphy GF, Sueki H, Telegan B, Johnson WC, Yu RJ, Van Scott EJ (1996) Effects of alpha-hydroxy acids on photoaged skin: a pilot clinical, histologic, and ultrastructural study. J Am Acad Dermatol 34(2 Pt 1): 187–195
64. Grimes PE, Green BA, Wildnauer RH, Edison BL (2004) The use of polyhydroxy acids (PHAs) in photoaged skin. Cutis 73(2 Suppl):3–13
65. Zhu W, Gap J (2008) The use of botanical extracts as topical skin-lightening agents for the improvement of skin pigmentation disorders. J Investig Dermatol Symp Proc 13:20–24
66. Chang T-S (2009) An updated review of tyrosinase inhibitors. Int J Mol Sci 10:2440–2475
67. Smit N, Vicanova J, Pavel S (2009) The hunt for natural skin whitening agents. Int J Mol Sci 10:5326–5349
68. Bae JY, Choi JS, Kang SW, Lee YJ, Park J, Kang YH (2010) Dietary compound ellagic acid alleviates skin wrinkle and inflammation induced by UV-B irradiation. Exp Dermatol 19(8):e182–e190
69. Ertam I, Mutlu B, Unal I, Alper S, Kivçak B, Ozer O (2008) Efficiency of ellagic acid and arbutin in melasma: a randomized, prospective, open-label study. J Dermatol 35: 570–574
70. Wallo W, Neybus J, Leyden JJ (2007) Efficacy of a soy moisturizer in photoaging: a double-blind, vehicle-controlled, 12-week study. J Drugs Dermatol 6:917–922
71. Bissett DL, Oblong JE, Berge CA (2005) Niacinamide: A B vitamin that improves aging facial skin appearance. Dermatol Surg 31(7 Pt 2):860–865, discussion 865
72. Kawada A, Konishi N, Oiso N, Kawara S, Date A et al (2008) Evaluation of anti-wrinkle effects of a novel cosmetic containing niacinamide. J Dermatol 35(10):637–642
73. Katoulis AC, Alevizou A, Bozi E, Makris M, Zafeiraki A, Mantas N, Kousta F, Mistidou M, Kanelleas A, Stavrianeas NG (2010) A randomized, double-blind, vehicle controlled study of a preparation containing undecylenoyl phenylalanine 2% in the treatment of solar lentigines. Clin Exp Dermatol 35(5):473–6
74. Calzavara-Pinton P, Zane C, Facchinetti E, Capezzera R, Pedretti A (2010) Topical Boswellic acids for treatment of photoaged skin. Dermatol Ther 23(Suppl 1):S28–S32
75. Ghersetich I, Troinano M, De Girogi V, Lotti T (2007) Receptors in skin ageing and antiageing agents. Dermatol Clin 25(4):655–662, xi. Review
76. Stegman SJ (1986) Medium-depth chemical peeling: digging beneath the surface. J Dermatol Surg Oncol 12(12): 1245–1246
77. Baker TJ, Gordon HL, Mosienko P et al (1974) Long-term histological study of skin after chemical face peeling. Plast Reconstr Surg 53:522
78. Behin F, Feuerstein SS, Marovitz WF (1977) Comparative histological study of minipig skin after chemical peel and dermabrasion. Arch Otolaryngol 103:271–277
79. Van Scott EJ, Yu RJ (1984) Hyperkeratinization, corneocyte cohesion, and alpha hydroxy acids. J Am Acad Dermatol 11(5 Pt 1):867–879
80. Moy LS, Howe K, Moy RL (1996) Glycolic acid modulation of collagen production in human skin fibroblast cultures in vitro. Dermatol Surg 22(5):439–441
81. Moy LS, Peace S, Moy RL (1996) Comparison of the effect of various chemical peeling agents in a mini-pig model. Dermatol Surg 22(5):429–432
82. Newman N, Newman A, Moy LS, Babapour R, Harris AG, Moy RL (1996) Clinical improvement of photoaged skin

with 50% glycolic acid. A double-blind vehicle-controlled study. Dermatol Surg 22(5):455–460
83. Piacquadio D, Dobry M, Hunt S, Andree C, Grove G, Hollenbach KA (1996) Short contact 70% glycolic acid peels as a treatment for photodamaged skin. A pilot study. Dermatol Surg 22(5):449–452
84. Kligman D, Kligman AM (1998) Salicylic acid peels for the treatment of photoaging. Dermatol Surg 24(3):325–328
85. Gladstone HB, Nguyen SL, Williams R, Ottomeyer T, Wortzman M, Jeffers M, Moy RL (2000) Efficacy of hydroquinone cream (USP 4%) used alone or in combination with salicylic acid peels in improving photodamage on the neck and upper chest. Dermatol Surg 26(4):333–337
86. Dinner MI, Artz JS (1998) The art of the trichloroacetic acid chemical peel. Clin Plast Surg 25(1):53–62
87. Matarasso SL, Glogau RG (1991) Chemical face peels. Dermatol Clin 9(1):131–150
88. Monheit GD (1989) The Jessner's + TCA peel: a medium-depth chemical peel. J Dermatol Surg Oncol 15(9): 945–950
89. Coleman WP 3rd, Futrell JM (1994) The glycolic acid trichloroacetic acid peel. J Dermatol Surg Oncol 20(1): 76–80
90. Tse Y, Ostad A, Lee HS, Levine VJ, Koenig K, Kamino H, Ashinoff R (1996) A clinical and histologic evaluation of two medium-depth peels. Glycolic acid versus Jessner's trichloroacetic acid. Dermatol Surg 22(9):781–786
91. El Samahy MH, Ghoz MM, Ramzy N (1998) Morphological investigation of chemical peel on photodamaged facial skin. Int J Cosmet Sci 20(5):269–282
92. Zezer E, Erbil H, Kurumlu Z, Tastan HB, Etikan I (2007) A comparative study of focal medium-depth chemical peel versus cryosurgery for the treatment of solar lentigo. Eur J Dermatol 17:26–29
93. Lawrence N, Cox SE, Cockerell CJ, Freeman RG, Cruz PD Jr (1995) A comparison of the efficacy and safety of Jessner's solution and 35% trichloroacetic acid vs. 5% fluorouracil in the treatment of widespread facial actinic keratoses. Arch Dermatol 131:176–181
94. Ghersetich I, Brazzini B, Peris K, Cotellessa C, Manunta T, Lotti T (2004) Pyruvic acid peels for the treatment of photoaging. Dermatol Surg 30(1):32–36
95. Berardesca E, Cameli N, Primavera G, Carrera M (2006) Clinical and instrumental evaluation of skin improvement after treatment with a new 50% pyruvic acid peel. Dermatol Surg 32(4):526–531

Melasma

15

Evangeline B. Handog and Maria Juliet E. Macarayo

15.1 Definition

Melasma is a chronic recurrent acquired symmetric cutaneous hypermelanosis, representing a dysfunction of the pigmentary system. Characterized by irregular brown, grayish brown, or tan macules and patches occurring on sun-exposed skin areas, it mostly involves the forehead, malar eminences, mandibular areas, and cutaneous part of the upper lip. Melasma develops slowly, can last for many years, worsens in summer and improves in colder seasons. It may be called "chloasma" and "mask of pregnancy" but the widely accepted term for this entity is melasma.

15.2 Epidemiology

The true incidence of melasma, up to this date, remains unknown [68, 123].

It is approximated that 5–6 million individuals in the United States alone are afflicted with this pigmentary problem, with a higher incidence worldwide [98].

E.B. Handog (✉)
Department of Dermatology,
Asian Hospital and Medical Center,
2205, Civic Drive, Room 316 Medical Office Building,
Filinvest Corporate City, Alabang, Muntinlupa City,
Metro Manila, Philippines
e-mail: vangee@handog.net

Ma. J.E. Macarayo
Department of Dermatology,
Angeles University Foundation Medical Center,
Angeles City, Pampanga, Philippines
e-mail: julietmacarayomd@yahoo.com

Considered a dyschromia most commonly observed in females, it also affects 5–10% of the males [45, 68, 106, 135]. Though all racial and ethnic groups are variedly affected, melasma is more prevalent among darker skin phototypes IV-VI, most especially those with extensive exposure to ultraviolet radiation.

15.3 Etiology

The exact etiology of melasma maybe uncertain but a multitude of factors have been implicated as causative agents, all of which significantly increase the activity of tyrosinase in melanin production:

15.3.1 Ultraviolet Radiation (UVA and UVB) Exposure

- Most important factor in the genesis of melasma for both sexes.
- Predisposed to melasma are sun-exposed areas.
- Increased incidence of melasma in geographic areas with high levels of UV light.
- Worsening or complete relapse of melasma lesions from one episode of UV exposure; single exposure to UV radiation increases size of melanocytes and increases tyrosinase activity [16].
- Repeated exposure to UV radiation increases the number of stage IV melanosome transfer to keratinocytes and increases the number of active melanocytes; the density of melanocytes is twice greater in sun-exposed areas [40].

A. Tosti et al. (eds.), *Color Atlas of Chemical Peels*,
DOI 10.1007/978-3-642-20270-4_15, © Springer-Verlag Berlin Heidelberg 2012

- Improvement of degree of melasma during periods of sun avoidance and colder season.
- Signaling growth factors (MSH, c-kit, and endothelin-1) secreted by the keratinocyte in response to UV are found to be deranged in the setting of melasma [67, 75].
- Increased solar radiation induced dermal changes in the cohort with the diagnosis of melasma [120].

15.3.2 Genetic Predisposition

- As many as 54% of patients have a family history of melasma [115].
- Found to be a significant etiologic factor among males with melasma [146].
- One pair of identical twins reported developing melasma, while other siblings under similar conditions did not [63].
- Increase in pigmentation following exposure to UV radiation may be a consequence of DNA repair [120].

15.3.3 Hormonal Influences

- Pregnancy
  - Found in 50–70% in pregnant women [115]
- Oral contraceptives [68, 98, 123]
- Hormone replacement therapies [120, 145]
  - Hyperpigmentation on the forearms developed in menopausal and postmenopausal women on HRT [145]
- Ovarian dysfunctions
  - Elevated levels of LH, FSH [123]
  - Lowered levels of estradiol [123]
  - Tumors [98]
- Increased expression of estrogen receptors in melasma-affected skin [95]
- Thyroid dysfunctions [68, 98, 99, 123]

15.3.4 Others

- Hepatic diseases [41]
- Altered nutrition [41]
- Oral medications
  - Phototoxic/photoallergic medications [41, 60]
  - Antiseizure (phenytoin) [41, 45, 68, 115]
- Nutritional supplements (containing estrogen- and progesterone-like properties) [126]
- Cosmetic chemicals (perfumes) [41, 45, 68, 115]

15.4 Clinical Types

Bilateral symmetric uniformly hyperpigmented lesions are seen in three clinical patterns [68, 98, 123, 126]:

Centrofacial (63–64%) – cheeks, forehead, upper lip, nose, and chin

Malar (21–27%) – cheeks and nose

Mandibular (9–16%) – ramus of the mandible

Other areas which may be involved are the dorsal forearms [68], rarely on the nipples and external genitalia [8]. Melasma does not involve the mucous membranes [123].

15.5 Diagnostic Criteria

Pigmentary distribution in the skin layers is important in the diagnosis and treatment of melasma.

Clinically, four types of melasma have been described [20, 68, 127]:

Epidermal – light brown

Dermal – dark brown to gray

Mixed – dark brown

Indeterminate – melasma in skin phototype V-VI

By Wood's lamp (365 nm), enhancement of pigment is only seen in the epidermal type [68, 98, 126]. Though it may determine the depth of melanin in the skin, it is not useful for phototypes V-VI [50]. Sanchez et al. [127], in his study, classified melasma using Wood's lamp into:

Epidermal (70%) – enhancement or accentuation of color contrast between affected and normal skin (most common)

Dermal (10–15%) – no enhancement of color contrast

Mixed (20%) – both enhancement and no color accentuation in different areas on the same patient

Indeterminate – in very dark-skinned individuals, one cannot see the lesions under Wood's light

Histopathologically and ultrastructurally, normal skin presents with melanin confined to the basal layer. Melasma lesions have more melanin in the whole epidermis, with increased number of melanocytes and widely dispersed melanosomes in the keratinocytes [19, 77, 126]. Dermal solar elastosis is likewise evident in lesional areas [19, 77].

Epidermal type – increased melanin in the basal, suprabasal, and stratum corneum layers [19, 68, 123, 126, 127]; dermal melanophages present [19, 47].

Dermal type – melanin increase in the superficial and deep dermis; melanin-laden macrophages and melanosomes within the superficial dermis and perivascularly in the middermis [19, 68, 123, 126, 127].

Mixed type – both the epidermal and dermal melanin are increased [19, 68, 126, 127].

Although this histopathological classification of melasma is widely accepted [45], Kang et al.'s study suggested that there may not be a true dermal type since the melanophages in the dermis of this type of melasma may actually be undiagnosed acquired bilateral nevus of Ota-like macules (ABNOM) or Hori's macules [77].

The *MELASMA AREA AND SEVERITY INDEX (MASI)* is a subjective classification [85] that divides the face into four areas:

F (forehead) 30%, MR (malar, right) 30%, ML (malar, left) 30%, C (chin) 10%

In each of these areas, melasma is graded as to:

A (total area of involvement) 0–6, D (darkness) 0–4 and H (homogeneity of hyperpigmentation) 0–4

Calculation of MASI:

$$30\%\,(DF + HF)\,AF + 30\%\,(DMR + HMR)\,AMR + 30\%\,(DML + HML)\,AML + 10\%\,(DC + HC)\,AC$$

Maximum value of MASI is 48, correlating with severe hyperpigmentation.

It is imperative to establish the clinical and histologic type of melasma before starting therapy. Though a simple skin examination can lead to the diagnosis, Wood's lamp examination is still helpful. Skin biopsy has been mainly done to differentiate melasma from other conditions but its specificity for all skin phototypes makes it a more reliable diagnostic tool.

15.6 Differential Diagnosis

- *Erythema dyschromicum perstans or ashy dermatosis*
  Ashen gray to brown-blue macules and patches, variably shaped and sized, seen on both sun-exposed and sun-protected areas, affecting mostly young adults
- *Riehl's melanosis*
  Reticular gray-brown to almost black hyperpigmentation, affecting darker skin types such as Mexicans and Asians; main histopathology is epidermal basal layer liquefaction degeneration with consequent pigment incontinence
- *Hori's Nevus*
  Also termed as acquired bilateral nevus of Ota-like macules (ABNOM); presents with blue-brown to slate gray facial hyperpigmentation mostly on the malar regions, affecting mostly Asian females
- *Bilateral nevus of Ota*
  Congenital blue to slate gray macular hyperpigmentation on areas innervated by the trigeminal nerve, affecting mostly Asian females; may be associated with ocular and mucosal melanosis
- *Postinflammatory Hyperpigmentation* (PIH)
  Hypermelanosis usually seen on areas of previous inflammatory or traumatic event; symmetry may or may not be present
- *Exogenous Ochronosis*
  Hyperpigmentation that may be seen not only on the face but also on the neck, back, and extremities; results from use of medications like antimalarials and products containing hydroquinone, resorcinol, phenol, mercury, and picric acid; histopathologically presents with yellowish brown banana-shaped globules in the papillary dermis
- *Minocycline pigmentation*
  Homogenous hyperpigmentation presenting histopathologically with dermal macrophages containing iron-staining pigment (siderophages)

Medical history and clinical examination are important in arriving at the diagnosis of melasma. Its symmetry and bilateral distribution set it apart from the other hyperpigmentary disorders.

15.7 5-Point Strategy for Melasma Therapy

Melasma therapy aims to eradicate existing pigments and prevent formation of new pigments by retarding the proliferation and growth of melanocytes and inhibiting the formation of melanosomes [68, 98].

Therapeutic success does not end with the initial outcome of decreasing or eliminating the pigmentation. Optimal treatment must revolve around maintaining that initial outcome and continuously avoiding the triggering and aggravating factors.

A 5-point strategy is offered:

- Protection from the Sun
- Reduction of melanocyte activity
- Inhibition of melanin synthesis
- Removal of melanin
- Disruption of melanin granules

15.7.1 Protection from the Sun

Broad-spectrum sunscreens (SPF of ≥ 30 + UVA filters) are the gold standard for skin protection from UV light. Consistent usage is a must in order to prevent worsening of melasma and to maintain results of treatment.

Photoprotection against UVB, UVA, and Visible Light Range is essential [104, 149].

Application should be daily, both indoors and outdoors.

UVB absorbers are chemicals that absorb in the 290–320 nm and include PABA and its derivatives, the salicylates, cinnamates, and camphor derivatives (i.e., octyldimethyl PABA, octyl salicylate, 2-ethoxyethyl-p-methoxycinnamate).

UVA absorbers take in the 320–400 nm region of the UV spectrum and include parsol 1789, terephthalylidene dicamphor sulfonic acid and derivatives of benzophenone, dibenzoylmethane, and anthranilate (i.e., oxybenzone, methyl anthranilate).

Physical UVA and UVB absorbers are insoluble materials such as zinc oxide and titanium dioxide that either scatter or absorb light [147].

A variety of systemic drugs are also photoprotectives [118]:

UVA – chloroquine, polypodium leucotomos [1, 89, 102]

UVB – indomethacin, vitamins C and E, green tea

UVA and Visible Light – beta carotene

UVA and UVB – fish oil

15.7.2 Reduction of Melanocyte Activity

This can be achieved by knowing and avoiding the factors that may trigger or aggravate melasma.

15.7.3 Inhibition of Melanin Synthesis

This constitutes the use of depigmenting compounds which can be categorized according to their action in the melanin synthesis. These agents act either through interference with tyrosinase transcription or glycosylation, inhibition of tyrosinase by different modalities or reduction of by-products and posttranscriptional control [17].

Pre-melanin synthesis via inhibition of	
Transcription	Tretinoin
Glycosylation	Calcium-D-pantetheine-S-sulfonate (PaSSO3Ca) and N-acetyl glucosamine (NAG)
Melanin synthesis proper via	
Tyrosinase inhibition	hydroquinone (HQ), azelaic acid, kojic acid (KA) Others: 4-OH-anisole (Mequinol), 4-S-Cystaminylphenol (4-S-CAP) and derivatives, methyl gentisate, ellagic acid, paper mulberry extract, 4-n-butyl-resorcinol (rucinol), arbutin, aloesin, resveratrol, oxyresveratrol, licorice extract, bearberry, acerola, cinnamic acid, macelignan, sophora extract
Peroxidase inhibition	methimazole, phenols/cathecols, topical indomethacin, green tea
ROS scavengers/ Reduction agents	ascorbic acid and its palmitate Mg-L-ascorbyl-2-PO4 (VC-PMG), thioctic acid, alpha-tocopherol (a-Toc) and its ferulate (D, L-a TF), hydrocoumarins, glutathione, pyc nogenol, tetrahydrocurcumin
Inhibition of inflammation-induced melanogenic response	topical corticosteroids, tranexamic acid, M. chamomilla, glabridin
Post-melanin synthesis via	
Tyrosinase degradation	linoleic acid, a-linolenic acid
Melanosome transfer inhibition	serine protease inhibitors, lectins and neoglycoproteins, niacinamide, soybean/milk extracts, octadecene dioic acid (ODA)
Skin turnover acceleration	lactic acid (LA), liquiritin, retinoic acid, linoleic acid, glycolic acid (GA), mandelic acid, lactobionic acid

15.7.4 Removal of Melanin

Procedural options that aim to remove melanin are chemical peeling and microdermabrasion.

15.7.5 Disruption of Melanin Granules

Lasers, light therapy, and fractional resurfacing aim to disrupt melanin granules and thus decrease the degree of pigmentation.

15.8 Depigmenting Agents

A variety of topical depigmenting agents are at hand for the dermatologists to choose from. Setback however is the length of time needed to effect treatment and patient compliance.

Using the Level of Evidence set by Stevens and Raferty [137] where A, B, C respectively represent good, fair, and poor evidence to support the use of a procedure, and D, E respectively represent fair and good evidence to support rejection of the use of a procedure, Rendon et al. [122] graded the use of the different topical treatments in the different studies as follows:

A	HQ 4%+tretinoin (RA) 0.05%+fluocinolone acetonide 0.01% [140, 142]
B	HQ 4% alone [6, 31, 51] or combined with GA 5% [39] or GA 10% [49]; RA 0.1% [44, 85]; adapalene [28]; azelaic acid 20% [6]; KA 4%+GA 5% [39]; modified Kligman+GA 30–40% Peel [128]
C	HQ 2% alone or in combination with KA 2% and/or GA 10%; HQ 3%+RA 0.1%; HQ 5%+RA 0.1–0.4%+ LA 7%/ascorbic acid 10%; HQ 5%+RA 0.1%+Hydrocortisone 1%; Modified Kligman alone; RA 0.05% alone or combined with azelaic Acid 20%; isotretinoin 0.05%; N-acetyl-4-S-CAP 4%

15.9 Tyrosinase Inhibitors

15.9.1 Hydroquinone

Hydroquinone (HQ) is the most commonly used bleaching agent and the gold standard for melasma treatment: A phenolic derivative that inhibits tyrosinase, it also inhibits RNA and DNA synthesis in melanotic cells, degrades melanosomes, and destroys melanocytes [71, 114]. With side effects including mostly irritant and rarely allergic contact dermatitis, nail discoloration, postinflammatory hyperpigmentation, and cutaneous ochronosis [94], 2–4% concentrations are the safest to use at once-nightly application. As far as carcinogenicity or mutagenicity is concerned, there are, by far, no known associations of cancer development in humans related to the use of topical HQ.

As a prime melasma therapeutic agent, it has been used alone or in combination for more than 50 years. From Kligman and Willis' (1975) combination of HQ 5%, tretinoin 0.1% and dexamethasone 0.1% [86], several variations from the concentration of each component to substitution of different corticosteroids evolved. In the combination formula, the three components act synergistically. The tretinoin disperses pigment granules in keratinocytes, interferes with pigment transfer, accelerates epidermal transfer and cell turnover, and decreases transfer rate of melanosomes to the keratinocytes. It suppresses the atrophy and antimitotic effect of the steroid and prevents HQ oxidation, facilitating its epidermal penetration [98]. The steroid suppresses melanin production, devoid of melanosome destruction thru suppression of the melanocytes' biosynthetic and secretory functions [78, 86, 101]. It antagonizes the thinning effect and irritation from tretinoin.

A variation of this combination employing hydrocortisone 1% produced clinical and histological improvement of pigmentation but with a higher rate of irritant dermatitis [76]. Retaining hydrocortisone 1% but lowering HQ to 4% and tretinoin to 0.05% led to a faster notable improvement within 3 weeks of application with maximum results in 5–7 weeks [116]. With these findings, a triple combination formula consisting of HQ 4%, tretinoin 0.05%, and fluocinolone acetonide 0.01% (Triluma cream, Galderma) has been made available commercially. It has undergone extensive multiracial multicenter clinical trials and has been shown to be effective in the treatment of melasma at once-nightly application, up to the present time [7, 21, 48, 76, 140–142].

Westerhof's formula is another variation using N-acetylcysteine 4.7%, HQ 2%, and triamcinolone acetonide 0.1%. N-acetylcysteine aims at increasing intercellular glutathione concentration, stimulating pheomelanin instead of eumelanin synthesis. Significant bleaching was evident within 4–8 weeks [107].

HQ 4% combined with GA 10% in a cream containing vitamins C, E and sunscreen showed a significant decrease in pigmentation compared to sunscreen alone [49].

15.9.2 Azelaic Acid [6, 68, 128, 148, 152]

Azelaic acid is a non-phenolic derivative (1,7-heptanedicarboxylic acid) acting as a weak tyrosinase inhibitor and producing antiproliferative and cytotoxic effects on abnormal melanocytes. It has anti-inflammatory, antibacterial, and anti-keratinizing activities. At 10–20% concentration, twice-daily application may treat melasma with minimal side effects (allergic reactions). Its efficacy is comparable if not better than HQ 2–4%.

Sequential therapy involving clobetasol proprionate cream 0.05% for 8 weeks followed by azelaic acid cream 20% for 16 weeks revealed excellent clearance of melasma compared to azelaic acid 20% monotherapy. Better results are also obtained if a glycolic acid cream is applied sequentially to azelaic acid treatment.

Dual combination cream containing azelaic acid 20% and tretinoin 0.05% was compared with azelaic acid monotherapy in 50 Asian patients over a 24-week period. Though 73% yielded good to excellent results for both treatments, the combination cream showed a faster response with a more pronounced improvement during the first 12 weeks and a higher rate of excellent results by the end of the trial [42]. Combination with 15–20% glycolic acid lotion was as effective as 4% hydroquinone in the treatment of moderate or severe melasma in darker-skinned patients, with only a slightly higher rate of mild local irritation [72].

Azelaic acid may be used as a depigmenting agent in those sensitive to hydroquinone at 1–2× daily application.

15.9.3 Kojic Acid [39, 68, 96, 98]

Kojic acid (KA) is a fungal metabolite (5-hydroxy-4 pyran 4–1-2 methyl) known to inhibit tyrosinase by copper chelation and is used to treat melasma at a concentration of 2–4% twice a day. Though a more stable compound compared to HQ, it was shown to be less effective than the latter, added to its high sensitizing potential.

A triple combination of KA2%, GA10%, and HQ2% was compared and shown to be superior to a double combination of GA10% and HQ2% [96]. In a comparative study among 39 melasma patients, the use of KA4%/GA5% gel on one side of the face and HQ4%/GA5% gel on the other side applied daily for 3 months showed equivalent results in pigment reduction [39].

15.9.4 4-OH-Anisole (Mequinol)

Used in combination with tretinoin, mequinol was shown to be effective in the treatment of melasma in men [34, 81].

15.9.5 Licorice Extract

Licorice extract (active ingredient: 10–40% glabridin) was shown to be 16× more efficacious than HQ with no cytotoxicity [61].

15.9.6 Rucinol

Rucinol, a resorcinol derivative, is the first substance shown to inhibit both tyrosinase and TRP-1. In 28 melasma patients, a 12-week application significantly lessened pigmentation than vehicle, producing good to fair efficacy in 78% of patient population. It significantly reduces pigmentation scores compared to controls [82].

15.9.7 Other Compounds Showing Inhibition of Tyrosinase

4-S-Cystaminylphenol (4-S-CAP) and derivatives [70], acerola (*Malpighia emarginata* contains carotenoids, bioflavonoids, and high vitamin C) [53], aloesin [24], arbutin [22], bearberry, cinnamic acid [87], ellagic acid [155], macelignan (from *Myristica fragrans* HOUTT) [23], methyl gentisate (MG) [15], paper mulberry extract, resveratrol [113], oxyresveratrol (exhibited 150 fold greater potency than resveratrol) [84], sophora extract (kurarinol, kuraridinol, and trifolirhizin) [66].

15.10 Peroxidase Inhibitors

Topical indomethacin was shown to be effective for epidermal type melasma particularly on the cutaneous upper lip of women [117]. In the author's experience, a study done on 48 Filipino women with epidermal and mixed melasma showed that 8% topical indomethacin applied twice daily for 12 weeks on melasma areas was effective and safe, with a significant difference on mexameter readings between the treatment and placebo groups [57].

Green tea and methimazole likewise act on the premise of peroxidase inhibition.

15.11 Ros Scavengers/Reduction Agents

15.11.1 Ascorbic Acid

The importance of L-ascorbic acid in the treatment of melasma lies in its ability to reduce the enzymatically generated *o*-quinones, thus reducing melanin synthesis. It prevents the production of free radicals that trigger melanogenesis. In addition to being an antioxidant, it has a photoprotective effect, preventing the absorption of both UVA and UVB radiation. In a study on 16 females with idiopathic melasma, ascorbic acid cream 5% was compared to HQ 4%. Both produced significant improvement with better results for the HQ group but significantly lesser side effects for the ascorbic acid group [33]. Quickly oxidized in aqueous solution, magnesium l-ascorbyl-2-phosphate is a more stable derivative [74].

15.11.2 Pycnogenol

With its active ingredient proanthocyanidins, it is a potent antioxidant 50× more powerful than vitamin E and 20× more than vitamin C. It recycles vitamin C, regenerates vitamin E, and increases the endogenous antioxidant enzyme system [110].

Thirty women with melasma were given 75-mg daily dose of French Maritime Pine Bark Extract (FMPBE) for 30 days. There was a statistically significant decrease in MASI score and pigmentary intensity index, a general efficacy rate of 80% with no observed side effects [105]. In an RCT involving 30 melasma patients (phototypes III-V), 80-mg dose of FMPBE given daily for 60 days produced a significant improvement in the degree of lightening of the skin in the treatment group compared to the placebo group [131]. In the author's recently concluded RCT [56] involving 60 Filipino females with epidermal melasma (phototypes III-V), 48-mg daily procyanidin with vitamins A, C, E for 8 weeks resulted in a significant improvement in mexameter readings and MASI scores, with minimal adverse events.

15.11.3 Tetrahydrocurcumin

Curcumin is a polyphenol antioxidant derived from the turmeric root. Its hydrogenated form tetrahydrocurcumin (THC) was found to significantly lighten skin color [151]. In a local double-blind placebo-controlled study done at Research Institute for Tropical Medicine, Philippines, the depigmenting effects of 0.25% THC and 4% HQ were shown to be comparable throughout the 4 week trial in 50 subjects. No adverse reactions were noted from 0.25% THC whereas reactions were mild to moderate with 4% HQ [119].

Other agents in this category are glutathione, hydrocoumarins, thioctic acid (α-lipoic acid) [111], alpha-tocopherol (a-Toc), and its ferulate (D, L-a TF) [38, 134].

15.12 Inhibitors to Melanosome Transfer

15.12.1 Niacinamide [12, 13, 52]

Niacinamide was shown to significantly decrease hyperpigmentation and increase skin lightness after 4 weeks of use compared to vehicle alone. This may be attributed to its capacity to inhibit melanosome transfer in a keratinocyte/melanocyte coculture model by 35–68%. Studies have shown the effectiveness of niacinamide 3.5% combined with retinyl palmitate for the improvement of hyperpigmentation.

15.12.2 Octadecene Dioic Acid (ODA)

ODA is a monounsaturated dicarboxylic acid derived by biofermentation from oleic acid.

Tested for once-daily spot treatment of darker pigmented facial areas for 8 weeks on 20 melasma patients, a 42.3% decrease in MASI score was shown [130].

15.12.3 Soybeans Extract [29, 58, 112]

Hermanns and colleagues first documented clinical skin-lightening activity by the non-denatured soybeans extracts. It is considered an alternative to HQ for treatment of PIH and melasma.

15.13 Skin Turnover Accelerators

15.13.1 Retinoic Acid (Tretinoin) [44, 68, 109, 122]

Generally used at a concentration of 0.05–0.1% with minimal side effects (erythema and desquamation), retinoic acid is usually applied once nightly. It does not suppress melanogenesis, but accelerates epidermal turnover.

As monotherapy, facial melasma showed statistically significant improvement with the use of tretinoin 0.1% for 40 weeks even in darker skin patients [85]. Sequential [154] or dual combination with HQ [79] provided good to excellent results with mild to moderate reactions to tretinoin that lessened as therapy was continued.

Other retinoids used in melasma include isotretinoin, tazarotene, and adapalene.

Adapalene, a synthetic naphthoic acid derivative with potent retinoic acid receptor activity, has been documented to be a safe and efficacious monotherapy in the treatment of melasma, with a lower potential for skin-irritation compared with topical tretinoin [28].

15.13.2 Alpha-Hydroxy Acids [49, 144]

Glycolic acid (GA) 5–10% decreases pigmentation by many mechanisms, including thinning of the stratum corneum and enhancing epidermolysis. An additive inhibitory effect on melanin synthesis through tyrosinase activity in melanoma cells was noted.

Melasma was also shown to improve up to 50% after a month of using mandelic acid 10% lotion. Lactobionic acid belongs to a newer polyhydroxy acid group that effects a decrease in pigmentation in a similar manner but with lesser irritant effect.

Lactic acid, linoleic acid, and Liquiritin [2] also act as skin turnover accelerators.

Calcium-D-Pantetheine-S-Sulfonate (PaSSO3Ca) [35] and N acetyl glucosamine (NAG) [14] act as inhibitors to glycosylation. Inhibitors to inflammation-induced melanogenic response are *M. chamomilla*, topical corticosteroids, glabridin [153], and tranexamic acid. Linoleic and alpha-linolenic acid [4] degrade tyrosinase after melanin has been synthesized.

15.14 Chemical Peeling

Chemical peeling is the most common office-based procedure done by dermatologists, according to the 1995–2003 audit of the National Ambulatory Medical Care Survey data in the United States [62]. In 2007, it landed 6th among the top 10 nonsurgical procedures performed in the United states, done mostly for the 19–64 year olds, women outnumbering men [3].

Done for the right indication and chosen for the correct patient, chemical peeling remains as an alternative modality for patients with melasma. It becomes more effective when combined with medical therapy since the peels mechanically remove the melanin while topical medications inhibit melanocytes or melanogenesis.

Melasma can either be treated with superficial or medium-depth peels. Though medium-depth peels can yield good results if done with utmost care, superficial peels are currently the preferred and most frequently performed peels. It is effective and safer to use for all skin phototypes (Fitzpatrick 1–6) but with precautionary measures and care for darker skin [30, 125]. Intense pulsed light, laser resurfacing, and dermabrasion have essentially supplanted medium-depth and deep peels [9].

Different agents have been studied and depicted effectual in achieving a superficial depth peel. Among these, preferred for use are alpha-hydroxy acids (AHAs), beta-hydroxy acid (BHA), Jessner's original and modified solutions, and trichloroacetic acid (TCA).

Rendon et al. [122] evaluated the use of different chemical peeling agents in different studies, using the Level of Evidence set by Stevens and Raferty [137] as follows:

B	GA 20–30% + HQ 4% [65]; GA 70% [91]
C	GA 10–50% [69]; GA 10%/HQ 2% + GA 20–70% [97]; Jessner's solution [91]; salicylic acid 20–30% [46]; RA 1–5% [26]

15.14.1 Alpha-Hydroxy Acids [30, 69]

- From the smallest to biggest molecular size: GLYCOLIC acid, LACTIC acid, PYRUVIC acid, MALIC acid, TARTARIC acid, and CITRIC acid (GALAPAMATACA)
- Small molecular sizes per volume are more active and penetrate the skin more deeply

- ↑Bioavailability of AHAs as the pH↓ [desirable pH 2.8–4.8]
- The only peels that are time dependent and can be neutralized easily

15.14.1.1 Glycolic Acid (GA) [9, 25, 65, 69, 97, 98, 129]

- The depth of a GA peel is a function of the concentration, volume, and duration of application.
- Being a weak acid with a pKa of 3.8, it has to be neutralized by water or a weak buffer as sodium bicarbonate.
- It is one of the most frequently used superficial peeling agents for epidermal melasma.
- Stable, not light sensitive, inexpensive.
- Easy to administer, with generally little or no downtime.
- Generally safe; scarring uncommon; persistent erythema and postpeel hyperpigmentation rarely seen.

When used alone, it yields moderate to good response [69]. Serial glycolic acid peels (20–70%), combined with a variety of topical depigmenting agents (modified Kligman's formula, azelaic cream, adapalene, HQ 2% – GA 10% cream, HQ 2–4%, tretinoin 0.05–1%, KA 10%), achieve better results compared to using each modality alone [25, 32, 91, 97, 129]. Its effects are comparable to Jessner's solution [91]. It can be applied every 2, 3, or 4 weeks, for a series of 3–6 peels. Side effects are minimal but PIH must always be in mind when treating darker-skinned patients [69].

15.14.1.2 Lactic Acid

A 92% pH 3.5 lactic acid solution used as a peeling agent was found to have effects comparable to Jessner's solution in the treatment of melasma. It can be applied every 3 weeks for up to six sessions until the desired response was achieved [25, 132, 133].

15.14.1.3 Pyruvic Acid

Pyruvic acid, an alpha-keto acid physiologically converted to lactic acid, penetrates down to the papillary dermis resulting in an increased production of collagen and elastic tissue. It must not be used in full-strength concentration to avoid potential for scarring. A gel form (40%) applied once monthly for 4–5 sessions has been used with success in the treatment of melasma. It has a more pleasant smell, is easier to apply and remove, provides homogeneity, releases pyruvic acid more gradually, and produces a more uniform erythema [9, 10, 18, 27, 108].

15.14.1.4 Mandelic Acid [138]

- As a chemical agent, 30–50% is used.
- With a pKa of 3.41, it is stronger than glycolic acid.
- Its larger molecular weight slows the penetration, making it less irritant.

15.14.2 Beta-Hydroxy Acid (BHA)

15.14.2.1 Salicylic Acid (SA)

- pKa 3
- Lipophilic

BHA affects the arachidonic acid cascade, thereby exhibiting anti-inflammatory capabilities. This allows SA peels to be effective while inducing less irritation than AHA peels [9]. Salicylic acid (20–30%) peels used alone to treat melasma resulted in moderate to significant improvement with minimal side effects, after a total of five peels done every 2 weeks [46].

Combined peel using salicylic acid 25% in alcoholic solution and TCA 10% gel, in 3–4 settings at 4–5-week intervals, showed regression of epidermal melasma with no relapse even after 6 months post peels; significant pigmentation reduction was noted in cases of mixed melasma. With the absence of inflammatory reaction that may lead to PIH, it is safe for patients with darker skin phototypes [143].

15.14.3 Beta-Lipohydroxy Acid (LHA)

LHA up to 10% is widely used in Europe. A derivative of salicylic acid (SA) with an additional fatty chain, its lipophilicity is increased. Even with a lowered concentration, its keratolytic effect is three times more potent than SA. It possesses a superficial desquamating effect and it increases the ration of cycling keratinocytes as part of an overall boosting of epidermal turnover [11, 93].

15.14.4 Jessner's Solution

- Combe's formula: 14 g each of resorcinol, salicylic acid, and lactic acid in 200-proof ethanol to make 100 mL [30, 103].

- Modified formula: 17% lactic acid, 17% salicylic acid, and 8% citric acid in 200-proof ethanol is preferred in the presence of resorcinol allergic contact dermatitis [37].

Even with a light superficial peel, it affects the full thickness of epidermis.

For melasma, one coat of the solution every 2–3 weeks will avoid exacerbating the hyperpigmentation.

15.14.5 **Trichloroacetic Acid (TCA)** (Fig. 15.1 and 15.2)

- Versatile, stable, inexpensive.
- Self-neutralizing, hence not absorbed in the systemic circulation.
- A stronger acid with pKa of 0.26.
- Concentrations above 35% can cause scarring and PIH.

At 10–25%, TCA produces an injury superficial to the papillary dermis. Applied every 2 weeks for patients with recalcitrant melasma, it provided a more favorable response as to time and degree of improvement, compared with 55–75% GA peel. However, relapse was noted to be more common with TCA compared to GA [73]. Combined with topical therapy (5% ascorbic acid), results were superior compared to TCA alone in treating epidermal melasma [136]. TCA 35% applied in conjunction with GA or Jessner's solution achieves a midlevel peel, with healing time between 7 and 10 days [9, 25].

15.14.6 Tretinoin

Tretinoin 1% peel applied at weekly intervals for 12 weeks was shown to be as effective as 70% GA peel in lightening moderate to severe melasma. It was better tolerated with less erythema and desquamation [83].

15.14.7 Recommended Chemical Peeling Agents for Superficial Depth Peel [30, 80, 103, 108, 121, 156]

Frequency: once weekly, once biweekly, or once monthly

- α-OH acids (GA) 30–70% variable time
- TCA 10–35%
- JESSNER'S solution 4–10 coats
- RESORCINOL 40–50% 30–60 min

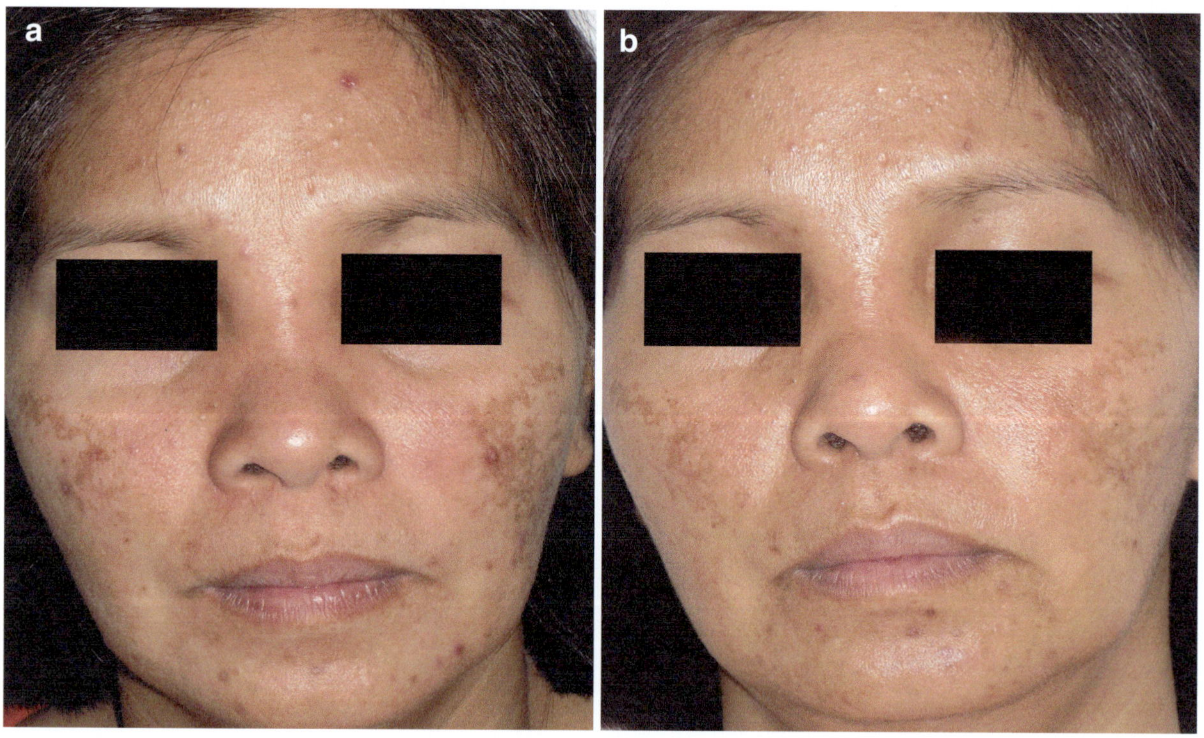

Fig. 15.1 (**a**, **b**) Patient with moderately severe melasma responding mildly with 20% TCA after a month. (Photos courtesy of E.B.Handog, MD, Manila, Philippines)

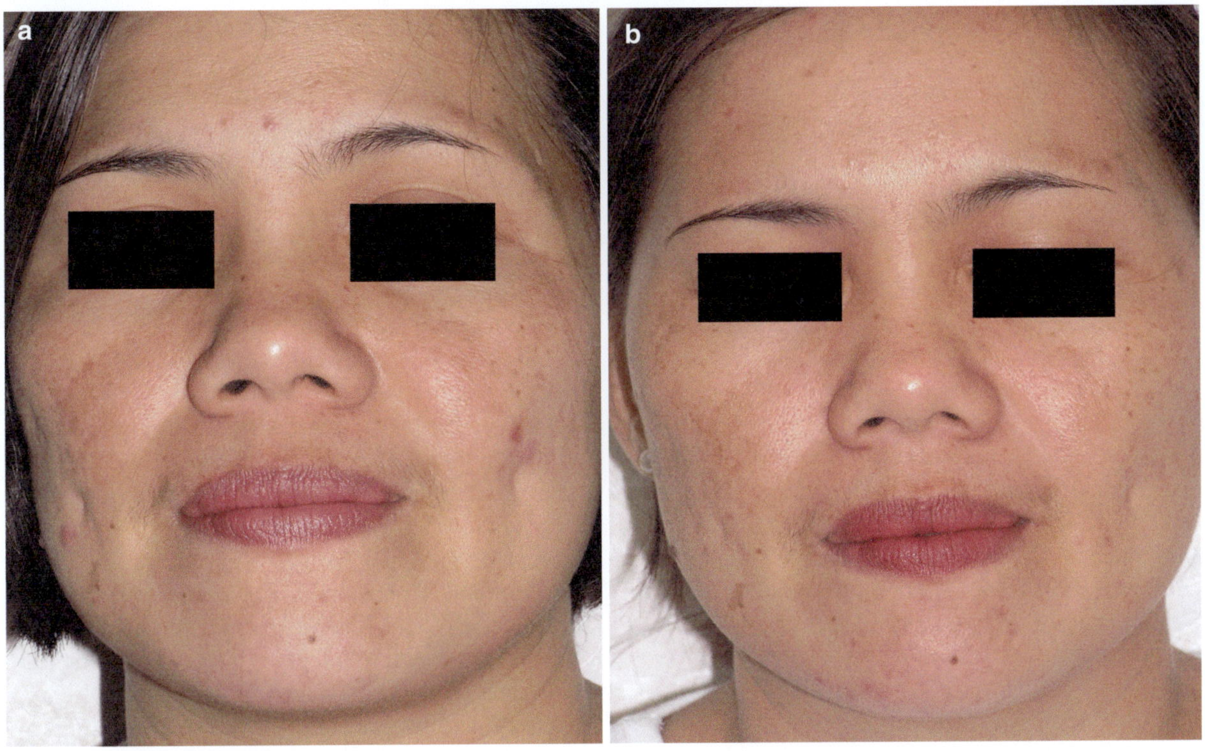

Fig. 15.2 (**a**, **b**) Patient with mild melasma improving significantly with Jessner's solution after a month. (Photos courtesy of E.B. Handog, MD, Manila, Philippines)

- SALICYLIC ACID 20–30% solution, 50% ointment
- TRETINOIN

In the authors' experience and practice, strong peels are generally avoided since PIH is a common adverse event among our patient population. The choice would generally revolve around Jessner's solution, glycolic acid, or salicylic acid. Frequency would generally be every 2–4 weeks until desired result is reached. Pretreatment for 2 weeks with a mild hypoallergenic cleanser twice daily, sunscreen SPF≥30 in the morning, a depigmenting agent (0.05% RA cream±4% HQ±KA±GA) with or without a light moisturizer at night is recommended. Immediately after the peel and 2 days thereafter, a light moisturizer is advised twice daily with or without betamethasone cream. Sunscreen is resumed. On the third day after the peel, the patient can go back to her usual regimen. Astringent/toner solutions are definitely not advised.

15.14.8 Relative Contraindications for All Chemical Peels [30]

- Previous recent (2–6 months) facial undermining surgery (blepharoplasty, rhytidectomy, brow lift, liposuction) in the treatment area, except for the most superficial peels
- Active viral, fungal, or bacterial infection or inflammatory dermatoses in treatment area
- Current medications (photosensitizing drugs)
- Immunocompromising diseases (possibility of delayed healing, increased susceptibility to infection, or excessive pigmentation after peeling)
- Previous facial radiation therapy that might impair the ability of the skin to regenerate
- Recent oral isotretinoin treatment (may be a contraindication to peeling based on type of peel and on dose and duration of treatment with isotretinoin)
- Keloid susceptibility
- Patients with unrealistic expectations or are uncooperative

15.15 Other Procedural Options

15.15.1 Microdermabrasion

Microdermabrasion is a multi-session mechanical peeling method that can be used in conjunction with other procedural modalities like chemical peels. Compared to dermabrasion, it is safer for patients with skin of color since it produces a more superficial injury. It alters the skin barrier, resulting in improved penetration and efficacy of topical agents. Though microdermabrasion removes only the stratum corneum and not viable epidermis [36, 59], the procedure followed by a combination skin-lightening agent containing hydroquinone, tretinoin, and fluocinolone was efficacious in melasma patients [124].

15.15.2 Dermabrasion

Dermabrasion abrades the skin down to the level of the upper or middermis. Though it may have achieved good results in one study in melasma patients, it has also been associated with an increased incidence of PIH and other more serious adverse skin changes [90].

15.15.3 Iontophoresis

IONTOPHORESIS is an effective and painless method of delivering medication to a localized tissue area by applying electrical current to a solution of the medication.

Vitamin C is known to inhibit melanin formation and reduce oxidized melanin. Iontophoresis with vitamin C is being used to enhance penetration of the vitamin in the skin. In Chung-Hun and colleagues' study involving 29 females with melasma, luminance value was shown to significantly decrease compared to control sites [64].

But in the author's experience on two different studies, using vitamin C or tretinoin 0.1% gel iontophoresis, the Filipino women with epidermal and mixed melasma obtained lightening of their pigmentation whether they were in the treatment or placebo group [54, 55].

15.15.4 Lasers

Lasers can and has been tried for pigmented lesion removal, in as much as the melanin, the chromophore, can absorb wider range of light. This modality has been used with varying degrees of success, if not worsening of cases.

A 510-nm pigmented lesion dye laser (PLDL) and a Q-switched (QS) ruby laser used for the management of melasma caused little to no improvement [43, 88, 139] and even worsening of the hyperpigmentation in some cases. This may be due to the presence of an increase in the activity of melanogenic enzymes resulting in hyperactive melanocytes. There is increased synthesis and transfer of melanosomes but with decreased degradation of keratinocytes [77]. Laser damage to these labile melanocytes may cause an increase in melanin production leading to PIH.

Comparing the QS laser with the long-pulsed 532-nm Nd:YAG laser in the treatment of melasma, the latter produced less PIH because it lacks the photomechanical effects of the QS laser [126]. QS alexandrite laser or PLDL combined with 15–25% TCA peel and/or Jessner's solution was shown to be effective, safe, and relatively inexpensive treatment modalities in the recalcitrant pigmentary disorders [92]. Combination of QS alexandrite and ultrapulse CO_2 lasers yielded statistically significant result in improving refractory melasma compared to QS alexandrite laser alone [5]. Erbium:YAG used on patients with skin phototypes II-V may have demonstrated improvement but transient PIH developed 3–6 weeks after laser treatment [100].

15.15.5 Fractional Resurfacing

Using a mid-infrared 1,550 nm laser produced a low incidence of pigmentary changes associated with traditional resurfacing techniques. There was minimal downtime and erythema. For darker skin patients with epidermal melasma, long-pulsed 532 nm QS laser and the nonablative 1,540 nm CO_2 laser may prove safer and efficacious, with care in the choice of fluence and spot size [126].

15.15.6 Light Therapy

Intense pulsed light (IPL) has recently been shown to manifest previously subclinical melasma. Even with the use of bleaching agents and sunscreens for 6 weeks to 3 months prior to this light therapy, PIH was still reported in the study of Wang and colleagues [150].

15.16 Management of the Patient

There remains no single treatment for melasma. Being an equally serious entity that affects perception of oneself, therapy must entail a multisectoral approach:

- *Physician's dedication (3 E's)*
  - Exploration of the possible causative factor(s) of the patient's melasma
  - Explanation of the treatment choices
  - Exposition of outcomes and expectations: patient education
- *Patient's continuous cooperation (3 A's)*
  - Avoidance of aggravating factors
  - Adherence to therapy
  - Adaptation to changes effective to improve quality of life
- *5-Point strategy to treat melasma*
  - Protection from the Sun
  - Reduction of melanocyte activity
  - Inhibition of melanin synthesis
  - Removal of melanin
  - Disruption of melanin granules
- *Mandatory Sun protection*
  - Continuous use of daily broad-spectrum topical sunscreen ± oral photoprotective agents
  - Physical protection (wide-brimmed hats, dark sunglasses, umbrellas, protective clothings, tight woven textiles, tinted automobile windows)
- *Reduction of melanocyte activity*
  - Avoid exposure to sunlight and even indoor lights
  - Precautionary measures on melasma-inducing factors such as OCPS, scented cosmetics, phototoxic drugs, and pregnancy.
- *Initial treatment of melasma until evident clearance, if not improvement*
  - First line – choose from a variety of topical depigmenting agents, either alone or in combination
  - Second line – therapy using both topical medications and chemical peeling
  - Third line – topical medications and other procedural therapies (laser and light therapy, microdermabrasion, iontophoresis) with utmost consideration of the skin phototype
- *Maintenance treatment with a chosen topical agent (s)*

References

1. Alfonso-Lebrero JL et al (2003) Photoprotective properties of a hydrophilic extract of the fern polypodium leucotomos on human skin cells. J Photochem Photobiol B 70(1):31–37
2. Amer M, Metwalli M (2000) Topical liquiritin improves melasma. Int J Dermatol 39:299–301
3. American Society of Aesthetic Plastic Surgery 1997–2007 statistics found at http://www.surgery.org/download/2007stats.pdf. Accessed October 22, 2009
4. Ando H, Ryu A, Hashimoto A et al (1998) Linoleic and α-linoleic acid lightens ultraviolet-induced hyperpigmentation of the skin. Arch Dermatol Res 290:375–381
5. Angsuwarangsee S, Polnikorn N (2003) Combined ultrapulse CO_2 laser and Q-switched alexandrite laser compared with Q-switched alexandrite laser alone for refractory melasma: split-faced design. Dermatol Surg 29:59–64
6. Balina LM, Graupe K (1991) The treatment of melasma: 20% azelaic acid versus 4% hydroquinone cream. Int J Dermatol 30:893–895
7. Balkrishnan R, Kelly AP, McMichael A et al (2004) Improved quality of life with effective treatment of facial melasma: the Pigment trial. J Drugs Dermatol 3:377–381
8. Baran R, Maibach HL (1998) Textbook of cosmetic dermatology, 2nd edn. Martin Dunitz, London
9. Baumann L, Saghari S (2009) Chemical peels. In: Bauman L (ed) Cosmetic dermatology principles and practice, 2nd edn. McGraw Hill, New York
10. Berardesca E, Cameli N, Primavera G et al (2006) Clinical and instrumental evaluation of skin improvement after treatment with a new 50% pyruvic acid peel. Dermatol Surg 32:526–531
11. Berson DS, Cohen JL, Rendon MI et al (2009) Clinical role and application of superficial chemical peels in today's practice. J Drugs Dermatol 8(9):803–811
12. Bissett DL, Miyamoto K, Sun P et al (2004) Topical niacinamide reduces yellowing, wrinkling, red blotchiness, and hyperpigmented spots in aging facial skin. Int J Cosmet Sci 26(5):231–238
13. Bissett DL, Oblong JE, Berge CA (2005) Niacinamide: a B vitamin that improves aging facial skin appearance. Dermatol Surg 31(7):860–865
14. Bissett DL, Robinson LR, Raleigh PS et al (2007) Reduction in the appearance of facial hyperpigmentation by topical N-acetyl glucosamine. J Cosmet Dermatol 6(1):20–26
15. Bocchietto E, Pecis L, D'Abrosca F et al (2001) In vitro testing of innovative depigmenting and low toxicity topic compositions. Pigment Cell Res 14:405
16. Bolognia JL, Pawelek JM (1988) Biology of hypopigmentation. J Am Acad Dermatol 19:217–255
17. Briganti S, Camera E, Picardo M (2003) Chemical and instrumental approaches to treat hyperpigmentation. Pigment Cell Res 16(2):101–110
18. Brody HJ (1996) Chemical peeling and resurfacing, 2nd edn. Mosby Year Book, New York
19. Casintahan FA (2008) Correlation of Wood's lamp and histologic findings in the classification of melasma among Filipinos. Presented in the 3rd Meeting of the Pigmentary Disorders Advisory Board of the Philippines May 2008. unpublished
20. Cestari T, Arellano I, Hexsel D et al (2009) Melasma in Latin America: options for therapy and treatment algorithm. J Eur Acad Dermatol Venereol 23:760–772
21. Cestari TF, Hexsel D, Viegas ML et al (2007) Validation of a melasma quality of life questionnaire for Brazilian Portuguese language: the MelasQoL-BP study and improvement of QoL of melasma patients after triple combination therapy. Br J Dermatol 156(S1):13–20

22. Chakraborty AK, Funasaka Y, Komoto M et al (1998) Effect of arbutin on melanogenic proteins in human melanocytes. Pigment Cell Res 11:206–212
23. Cho Y, Kim KH, Shim JS et al (2008) Inhibitory effects of Macelignan isolated from *Myristica fragrans* HOUTT. on melanin biosynthesis. Biol Pharm Bull 31(5):986–989
24. Choi S, Park YI, Lee SK et al (2002) Aloesin inhibits hyperpigmentation induced by UV radiation. Clin Exp Dermatol 27(6):513–515
25. Cotellessa C, Peris K, Onorati MT et al (1999) The use of chemical peelings in the treatment of different cutaneous hyperpigmentations. Dermatol Surg 25:450–454
26. Cuce LC, Bertino MC, Scattone LK et al (2001) Tretinoin peeling. Dermatol Surg 27:12–14
27. De Padova MP, Bellavista S, Tosti A (2007) Peel with pyruvic acid: the new formulation in gel. J Am Acad Dermatol 56(S2):AB17
28. Dogra S, Kanwar AJ, Parsad D (2002) Adapalene in the treatment of melasma: a preliminary report. J Dermatol 29:539–540
29. Draelos Z (2007) Skin lightening preparations and the hydroquinone controversy. Dermatol Ther 20:308–313
30. Drake LA, Brody HJ (1995) American Academy of Dermatology: guidelines of care for chemical peeling. J Am Acad Dermatol 33:497–503
31. Ennes SBP, Paschoalick RC, De Avelar M et al (2000) A double-blind, comparative, placebo-controlled study of the efficacy and tolerability of 4% hydroquinone as a depigmenting agent in melasma. J Dermatol Treat 11:173–179
32. Erbil H, Sezer E, Tastan B et al (2007) Efficacy and safety of serial glycolic acid peels and a topical regimen in the treatment of recalcitrant melasma. J Dermatol 34(1):25–30
33. Espinal-Perez LE, Moncada B, Castanedo-Cazares JP (2004) A double-blind randomized trial of 5% ascorbic acid versus hydroquinone in melasma. Int J Dermatol 43:604–607
34. Fleischer AB, Schwartzel EH, Colby SI et al (2000) The combination of 2% 4-hydroxyanisole (Mequinol) and 0.01% tretinoin is effective in improving the appearance of solar lentigines and related hyperpigmented lesions in two double-blind multicenter clinical studies. J Am Acad Dermatol 42:459–467
35. Franchi J, Coutadeur MC, Marteau C et al (2000) Depigmenting effects of calcium D-Pantetheine-S-Sulfonate on human melanocytes. Pigment Cell Res 13:165–171
36. Freedman BM, Rueda-Pedraza E, Waddell SP (2001) The epidermal and dermal changes associated with microdermabrasion. Dermatol Surg 27:1031–1033
37. Fulton JE Jr (2006) Jessner's peel. In: Rubin MG (ed) Chemical peels. Elsevier Saunders, Philadelphia
38. Funasaka Y, Komoto M, Ichihashi M (2000) Depigmenting effect of alpha-tocopheryl ferulate on normal human melanocytes. Pigment Cell Res 13(S8):170–174
39. Garcia A, Fulton JE Jr (1996) The combination of glycolic acid and hydroquinone or kojic acid for the treatment of melasma and related conditions. Dermatol Surg 22: 443–447
40. Gilchrest BA, Blog FB, Szabo G (1979) Effects of aging and chronic sun exposure on melanocytes in human skin. J Invest Dermatol 73:141–143
41. Goh CL, Diova CN (1999) A retrospective study on the clinical presentation and treatment outcome of melasma in a tertiary Dermatological Referral Centre in Singapore. Sing Med J 40:455–458
42. Graupe K, Verallo-Rowell VM, Verallo V et al (1996) Combined use of 20% azelaic acid cream and 0.05% tretinion cream in the topical treatment of melasma. J Dermatol Treat 7:235–237
43. Grekin RC, Shelton RM, Geisse JK et al (1993) 510 nm pigmented lesion dye laser: its characteristics and clinical uses. J Dermatol Surg Oncol 19:380–387
44. Griffiths CEM, Finkel LJ, Ditre CM et al (1993) Topical tretinoin (retinoic acid) improves melasma: a vehicle-controlled, clinical trial. Br J Dermatol 129:415–421
45. Grimes PE (1995) Melasma: etiologic and therapeutic considerations. Arch Dermatol 131:1453–1457
46. Grimes PE (1999) The safety and efficacy of salicylic acid chemical peels in darker racial-ethnic groups. Dermatol Surg 25:18–22
47. Grimes PE, Yamada N, Bhawan J (2005) Light microscopic, immunohistochemical, and ultrastructural alterations in patients with melasma. Am J Dermatopath 27:96–101
48. Grimes P, Kelly P, Toork H et al (2006) Community-based trial of a triple-combination agent for the treatment of facial melasma. Cutis 77:177–184
49. Guevara IL, Pandya AG (2003) Safety and efficacy of 4% hydroquinone combined with 10% glycolic acid, antioxidants, and sunscreen in the treatment of melasma. Int J Dermatol 42:966–972
50. Gupta LK, Singhi MK (2004) Wood's lamp. Indian J Dermatol Venereol Leprol 70:131–135
51. Haddad AL, Matos LF, Brunstein F et al (2003) A clinical, prospective, randomized, double-blind trial comparing skin whitening complex with hydroquinone vs. placebo in the treatment of melasma. Int J Dermatol 42:153–156
52. Hakozaki T, Minwalla L, Ang JZ et al (2002) The effect of niacinamide on reducing cutaneous pigmentation and suppression of melanosome transfer. Br J Dermatol 147: 20–31
53. Hanamura T, Uchida E, Aoki H (2008) Skin-lightening effect of a polyphenol extract from Acerola (Malpighia emarginata DC.) fruit on UV-induced pigmentation. Biosci Biotechnol Biochem 72(12):3211–3218
54. Handog EB et al (2005) A prospective randomized double blind placebo controlled trial on the efficacy of vitamin C solution applied using iontophoresis technology in the treatment of melasma in Filipino women. RITM, Philippines, unpublished
55. Handog EB et al (2005) A prospective randomized double blind placebo controlled trial on the efficacy of Tretinoin 0.1% gel applied using iontophoresis technology in the treatment of melasma in Filipino women. RITM, Philippines, unpublished
56. Handog EB, Galang DA, De Leon-Godinez MA et al (2009) A randomized double-blind placebo controlled trial of oral procyanidin with vitamins A, C, E for melasma among Filipino women. Int J Dermatol 48(8):896–901
57. Handog EB, Vitug RL, Masa EJ et al (2005) A prospective, randomized, double-blind, placebo controlled trial on the efficacy of 8% indomethacin cream in the treatment of melasma in Filipino women. RITM, Philippines
58. Hermanns JF, Petit L, Pierard-Franchimont C et al (2002) Assessment of topical hypopigmenting agents on solar lentigines of Asian women. Dermatology 204: 281–286

59. Hernández-Perez E, Ibiett EV (2001) Gross and microscopic findings in patients undergoing microdermabrasion for facial rejuvenation. Dermatol Surg 27:637–648
60. Ho SGY, Chan HL (2009) The Asian dermatologic patient: review of common pigmentary disorders and cutaneous diseases. Am J Clin Dermatol 10(3):153–168
61. Holloway VL (2003) Ethnic cosmetic products. Dermatol Clin 21:743–749
62. Housman TS, Hancox JG, Mir MR et al (2008) What specialties perform the most common outpatient cosmetic procedures in the United States? Dermatol Surg 34(1):1–7
63. Hughes BR (1987) Melasma occurring in twin sisters. J Am Acad Dermatol 17:841
64. Huh CH, Seo KI, Park JY et al (2003) A randomized double blind placebo controlled trial of vitamin C iontophoresis in melasma. Dermatology 206:316–320
65. Hurley ME, Guevara IL, Gonzales RM et al (2002) Efficacy of glycolic acid peels in the treatment of melasma. Arch Dermatol 138:1578–1582
66. Hyun SK, Lee WH, Jeong DM et al (2008) Inhibitory effects of kurarinol, kuraridinol, and trifolirhizin from *Sophora flavescens* on tyrosinase and melanin synthesis. Biol Pharm Bull 31(1):154–158
67. Im S, Kim J, On WY et al (2002) Increased expression of alpha melanocyte-stimulating hormone in the lesional skin of melasma. Br J Dermatol 146:165–167
68. Iorizzo M, Tosti A, De Padova M (2006) Melasma. In: Tosti AT, Grimes PE, De Padova MP (eds) Color atlas of chemical peels. Springer, New York
69. Javaheri SM, Handa S, Kaur I et al (2001) Safety and efficacy of glycolic acid facial peel in Indian women with melasma. Int J Dermatol 40:354–357
70. Jimbow K (1991) N-acetyl-4-S-cystaminylphenol as new type of depigmenting agent for the melanoderma of patients with melasma. Arch Dermatol 127:1528–1534
71. Jimbow K, Obata H, Pathak MA et al (1974) Mechanism of depigmentation by hydroquinone. J Invest Dermatol 62:436–449
72. Kakita LS, Lowe NJ (1998) Azelaic acid and glycolic acid combination therapy for facial hyperpigmentation in darker-skinned patients: a clinical comparison with hydroquinone. Clin Ther 20:960–970
73. Kalla G, Garg A, Kachlawa D (2001) Chemical peeling – glycolic acid versus trichoracetic acid in melasma. Indian J Dermatol Venereol Leprol 67(2):82–84
74. Kameyama K, Sakai C, Kondoh S et al (1996) Inhibitory effect of magnesium l -ascorbyl-2-phosphate (VC-PMG) on melanogenesis in vitro and in vivo. J Am Acad Dermatol 34:29–33
75. Kang HY, Hwang JS, Lee JY et al (2006) The dermal stem cell factor and c-kit are over expressed in melasma. Br J Dermatol 154:1094–1099
76. Kang WH, Chun SC, Lee S (1998) Intermittent therapy for melasma in Asian patients with combined topical agents retinoic acid, hydroquinone and hydrocortisone: clinical and histological studies. J Dermatol 25:587–596
77. Kang WH, Yoon KH, Lee ES et al (2002) Melasma: histopathological characteristics in 56 Korean patients. Br J Dermatol 146:228–237
78. Kanwar AJ, Dhar S, Kaur S (1994) Treatment of melasma with potent topical corticosteroids. Dermatology 188:170–172
79. Kauh YC, Zachian TF (1999) Melasma. Adv Exp Med Biol 455:491–499
80. Kauvar ANB, Dover JS (2001) Facial skin rejuvenation: laser resurfacing or chemical peel: choose your weapon. Dermatol Surg 27:209–212
81. Keeling J, Cardona L, Benitez A et al (2008) Mequinol 2%/Tretinoin 0.01% topical solution for the treatment of melasma in men: a case series and review of the literature. Cutis 81:179–183
82. Khemis A, Kaiafa A, Queille-Roussel C et al (2007) Evaluation of efficacy and safety of rucinol serum in patients with melasma: a randomized controlled trial. Br J Dermatol 156:997–1004
83. Khunger N, Sarkar R, Jain RK (2004) Tretinoin Peels versus glycolic acid peels in the treatment of melasma in dark skinned patients. Dermatol Surg 30:756–760
84. Kim YM, Yun J, Lee CK et al (2002) Oxyresveratrol and hydroxystilbene compounds. Inhibitory effect on tyrosinase and mechanism of action. J Biol Chem 277(18): 16340–16344
85. Kimbrough-Green CK, Griffiths CEM, Finkel LJ et al (1994) Topical retinoic acid (tretinoin) for melasma in black patients. A vehicle-controlled clinical trial. Arch Dermatol 130:727–733
86. Kligman AM, Willis I (1975) A new formula for depigmenting human skin. Arch Dermatol 111:40–48
87. Kong YH, Jo YO, Cho CW et al (2008) Inhibitory effects of cinnamic acid on melanin biosynthesis in skin. Biol Pharm Bull 31(5):946–948
88. Kopera D, Hohenleutner U (1995) Ruby laser treatment of melasma and postinflammatory hyperpigmentation. Dermatol Surg 21:990–995
89. Kullavanijaya P, Lim HW (2005) Photoprotection. J Am Acad Dermatol 52(6):937–958
90. Kunachak S, Leelaudomlipi P, Wongwaisayawan S (2001) Dermabrasion: a curative treatment for melasma. Aesthetic Plast Surg 25:114–117
91. Lawrence N, Cox SE, Brody HJ (1997) Treatment of melasma with Jessner's solution versus glycolic acid: a comparison of clinical efficacy and evaluation of the predictive ability of Wood's light examination. J Am Acad Dermatol 36:589–593
92. Lee GY, Kim HJ, Whang KK (2002) The effect of combination treatment of the recalcitrant pigmentary disorders with pigmented laser and chemical peeling. Dermatol Surg 28:1120–1123
93. Leveque JL, Corcuff P, Rougier A et al (2002) Mechanism of action of lipophilic salicyclic acid derivative on normal skin. Eur J Dermatol 12(4):XXXV–XXXVIII
94. Levin C, Maibach H (2001) Exogenous ochronosis: an update on clinical features, causative agents and treatment options. Am J Clin Dermatol 2:213–217
95. Liberman R, Moy L (2008) Receptor Expression in melasma: results from facial skin of affected patients. J Drugs Dermatol 7(5):463–465
96. Lim JTE (1999) Treatment of melasma using kojic acid in a gel containing hydroquinone and glycolic acid. Dermatol Surg 25:282–284
97. Lim JTE, Tham SN (1997) Glycolic acid peels in the treatment of melasma among Asian women. Dermatol Surg 23(3):177–179

98. Lin JY, Lim JT, Chan HL (2009) Treatment of melasma. In: Alam M, Bhatia AC, Kundu RV et al (eds) Cosmetic dermatology in skin of colour. McGraw-Hill, New York
99. Lufti RJ, Fridmanis M, Misiunas AL et al (1985) Association of melasma with thyroid autoimmunity and other thyroidal abnormalities and their relationship to the origin of the melasma. J Clin Endocrinol Metab 61:8–31
100. Manaloto RM, Alster T (1999) Erbium:YAG laser resurfacing for refractory melasma. Dermatol Surg 25:121–123
101. Menter A (2004) Rationale for the use of topical corticosteroids in melasma. J Drugs Dermatol 3(2):169–174
102. Middelkamp-Hup MA, Pathak MA, Parrado C et al (2004) Orally administered polypodium leucotomos extract decreases ultraviolet induced damage of human skin. J Am Acad Dermatol 51(6):910–918
103. Monheit GD, Kayal JD (2003) Chemical peeling. In: Nouri K, Leal-Khouri S (eds) Techniques in dermatologic surgery. Mosby, Philadelphia
104. Moseley H, Cameron H, MacLeod T et al (2001) New sunscreens confer improved protection for photosensitive patients in the blue light region. Br J Dermatol 145:789–794
105. Ni Z, Mu Y, Gulati O (2002) Treatment of melasma with Pycnogenol. Phytother Res 16:567–571
106. Nicolaidou E, Antoniou C, Katsambas AD (2007) Origin, clinical presentation, and diagnosis of facial hypermelanoses. Dermatol Clin 25:321–326
107. Njoo MD, Menke HE, Pavel S et al (1997) N-acetylcystein as a bleaching agent in the treatment of melasma. J Eur Acad Dermatol Venereol 9:86–87
108. Ogden S, Griffiths TW (2008) A review of minimally invasive cosmetic procedures. Br J Dermatol 159(5):1036–1050
109. Ortonne JP (2006) Retinoid therapy of pigmentary disorders. Dermatol Ther 19:280–288
110. Packer L, Rimbach G, Virgili F (1999) Antioxidant activity and biologic properties of a procyanidin-rich extract from pine (pinus maritima) bark. Free Radic Biol Med 27:702–724
111. Packer L, Witt H, Tritscheler H (1995) Lipoic acid as a biological antioxidant. Free Radic Biol Med 19:227–250
112. Paine C et al (2001) An alternative approach to depigmentation by soybean extracts via inhibition of the PAR-2 pathway. J Invest Dermatol 116(4):587–595
113. Palmieri L, Mameli M, Ronca G (1999) Effect of resveratrol and some other natural compounds on tyrosine kinase activity and on cytolysis. Drugs Exp Clin Res 25:79–85
114. Palumb A, Ischia M, Misuraca G et al (1991) Mechanism of inhibition of melanogenesis by hydroquinone. Biochim Biophys Acta 1073:85–90
115. Pandya AG, Guevara IL (2000) Disorders of pigmentation. Dermatol Clin 18:91–98
116. Perez-Bernal A, Munoz-Perez MA, Camacho F (2000) Management of facial hyperpigmentation. Am J ClinDermatol 1:261–268
117. Piamphongsant T (1998) Treatment of melasma: a review with personal experience. Int J Dermatol 37:897–903
118. Piamphongsant T (2002) Practical dermatology. Year Book Publisher, Bangkok
119. Pineda RT, Chan G, Gabriel T (2006) A randomized double blind placebo controlled comparative study on the safety and efficacy of 0.25% tetrahydrocurcumin (Turmeric) cream as depigmenting agent against 4% hydroquinone cream. RITM, Philippines, unpublished
120. Ponzio HA, Favaretto AL, Rivitti EA (2007) Proposal of a quantitative method to describe melasma distribution in women. J Cosmet Dermatol 20:103–111
121. Rabe et al (2006) Photoaging: mechanisms and repair. J Am Acad Dermatol 55:1–19
122. Rendon M, Berneburg M, Arellano I et al (2006) Treatment of melasma. J Am Acad Dermatol 54(5):S272–S281
123. Rigopoulos D, Gregoriou S, Katsambas A (2007) Hyperpigmentation and melasma. J Cosmet Dermatol 6: 195–202
124. Roberts WE (2002) Microdermabrasion dual therapy. Microdermabrasion Skin and Allergy News 33:42
125. Roberts WE (2004) Chemical peeling in ethnic/dark skin. Dermatol Ther 17:196–205
126. Roberts WE (2009) Melasma. In: Kelly AP, Taylor SC (eds) Dermatology for skin of color. McGraw-Hill, New York
127. Sanchez NP, Pathak MA, Sato SS et al (1982) Circumscribed dermal melaninoses: classification, light, histochemical, and electron microscopic studies on three patients with the erythema dyschromicum perstans type. Int J Dermatol 21:25–31
128. Sarkar R, Bhalla M, Kanwar AJ (2002) A comparative study of 20% azelaic acid cream monotherapy versus a sequential therapy in the treatment of melasma in dark-skinned patients. Dermatology 205:249–254
129. Sarkar R, Kaur C, Bhalia M et al (2002) The combination of glycolic acid peels with a topical regimen in the treatment of melasma in dark skinned patients: a comparative study. Dermatol Surg 28:828–832
130. Scherdin U, Burger A, Bielfeldt S et al (2008) Skin-lightening effects of a new face care product in patients with melasma. J Cosmet Dermatol 7:68–75
131. Shahrir M, Saadiah S, Sharifah I et al (2004) The efficacy and safety of French Maritime pine bark extract in the form of MSS Complex Actinosome on melasma. Int Med J 3(2):130–132
132. Sharquie KE, Al-Tikreety MM, Al-Mashhadani SA (2005) Lactic acid as a new therapeutic peeling agent in melasma. Dermatol Surg 31:149–154
133. Sharquie KE, Al-Tikreety MM, Al-Mashhadani SA (2006) Lactic acid chemical peels as a new therapeutic modality in melasma in comparison to Jessner's solution chemical peels. Dermatol Surg 32:1429–1436
134. Shimizu K, Kondo R, Sakai K et al (2001) Novel vitamin E derivative with 4-substituted resorcinol moiety has both antioxidant and tyrosinase inhibitory properties. Lipids 36(12):1321–1326
135. Sialy R, Hasan I, Kaur I et al (2000) Melasma in men: a hormonal profile. J Dermatol 27:64–65
136. Soliman MM, Ramadan SA, Bassiouny DA et al (2007) Combined trichoracetic acid peel and topical ascorbic acid versus trichloracetic acid peel alone in the treatment of melasma: a comparative study. J Cosmet Dermatol 6(2): 89–94
137. Stevens A, Raferty J (1997) Health care needs assessment. Radcliffe Medical Press, New York
138. Taylor MB (1999) Summary of mandelic acid for the improvement of skin conditions. Cosmet Dermatol 12:28
139. Taylor CR, Anderson RR (1994) Ineffective treatment of refractory melasma and post-inflammatory hyperpigmentation by Q-switched ruby laser. J Dermatol Surg Oncol 20:592–597

140. Taylor SC, Torok H, Jones T et al (2003) Efficacy and safety of a new triple-combination agent for the treatment of facial melasma. Cutis 72:67–72
141. Torok H (2005) A large 12 month extension study of an 8-week trial to evaluate the safety and efficacy of triple combination (TC) cream in melasma patients previously treated with TC cream or one of its dyads. J Drugs Dermatol 4:592–597
142. Torok HM, Jones T, Rich P et al (2005) Hydroquinone 4%, tretinoin 0.05%, fluocinolone acetonide 0.01%: a safe and efficacious 12-month treatment for melasma. Cutis 75: 57–62
143. Tosti A, De Padova MP, Venturo N et al (2005) New combined peel in Melasma. J Am Acad Dermatol 52(3):169
144. Usuki A, Ohashi A, Sato H et al (2003) The inhibitory effect of glycolic acid and lactic acid on melanin synthesis in melanoma cells. Exp Dermatol 12:43–50
145. Varma S, Roberts DL (1999) Melasma of the arms associated with hormone replacement therapy. Br J Dermatol 141:592
146. Vazquez M, Maldonado H, Benmaman C et al (1988) Melasma in men: a clinical and histologic study. Int J Dermatol 27:25–27
147. Verrallo-Rowell VM (2001) Facial hyperpigmentation problems common to multi-heritage Asian skin phototypes in the tropics: melasma, freckles, PIH, liver spots and warts: Q&A. In: Skin in the tropics. The House Printers, Philippines
148. Verallo-Rowell VM, Verallo V, Graupe K et al (1989) Double-blind comparison of azelaic acid and hydroquinone in the treatment of melasma. Acta Derm Venereol Suppl (Stockh) 143(suppl):58–61
149. Verallo-Rowell VM et al (2002) SPF and PFA of colored cosmetics. In: Skin in the tropics: sunscreens and hyperpigmentations. Anvil, Philippines
150. Wang CC, Hui CY, Sue YM et al (2004) Intense pulsed light for the treatment of refractory melasma in Asian persons. Dermatol Surg 30:1196–1200
151. Wanitphakdeedecha R, Eimpunth S, Manuskiatti W (2009) The effects of tetrahydrocurcumin in curmin cream on the hydration, elasticity, and color of human skin. J Am Acad Dermatol 60(3):AB83
152. Westerhof W, Njoo MD (2003) Bleaching agents. In: Katsambas AD, Lotti TM (eds) European handbook of dermatological treatments, 2nd edn. Springer, Berlin
153. Yokota T, Nishio H, Kubota Y et al (1998) The inhibitory effect of glabridin from liquorice extracts on melanogenesis and inflammation. Pigment Cell Res 11:355–361
154. Yoshimura K, Momosawa A, Alba E et al (2003) Clinical trial of bleaching treatment with 10% all trans retinol gel. Dermatol Surg 29:155–160
155. Yoshimura M, Watanabe Y, Kasai K et al (2005) Inhibitory effect of an ellagic acid-rich pomegranate extract on tyrosinase activity and ultraviolet-induced pigmentation. Biosci Biotechnol Biochem 69(12):2368–2373
156. Zakapoulu N, Kontochristopoulos MD, Kontochristopoulos G (2006) Superficial chemical peels. J Cosmet Dermatol 5:246–253

Senile Lentigo

16

Matilde Iorizzo

16.1 Definition

Benign hyperpigmented, sometimes irregular, flat spot on chronically sun-exposed areas of the skin. They are also called solar lentigos, liver spots, or age spots. The chronic sun exposure causes an increased number of pigment-producing cells in the skin.

Histologically, senile lentigo shows a hyperpigmented basal layer and an elongation of the rete ridges, which seem to drive deeply into the dermis. The epidermis contains clusters of keratinocytes, which retained and accumulated the melanin pigment [1, 2].

16.2 Epidemiology

Senile lentigo is present in 90% of Caucasians older than 60% years of age and is rare among individuals with dark-pigmented skin [3].

16.3 Diagnostic Criteria

Senile lentigo can be easily diagnosed by clinical examination of the skin. Dermoscopy can be a useful tool to aid the clinician in performing the correct diagnosis, and histopathology is usually limited to doubtful cases.

M. Iorizzo
Private Dermatologist, Lugano, Switzerland
e-mail: matildeiorizzo@gmail.com

16.4 Differential Diagnosis

Lentigo maligna: ill defined and variably pigmented skin spot precursor of malignant melanoma. Histopathology is mandatory for the correct diagnosis revealing the spreading of atypical melanocytes.

16.5 Treatment

Senile lentigo does not require treatment, unless the patient requests treatment for cosmetic reasons.

Treatment or not, long-term sun protection using adequate SPF is useful to prevent further spreading of the lesions.

Topical depigmenting agents (hydroquinone, tretinoin, kojic acid, azelaic acid, L-ascorbic acid) are the most commonly used home treatment, but several months are required to see results and very often the pigmentation recurs after discontinuation of treatment [4].

Chemical peeling (trichloroacetic acid) [5, 6], cryotherapy (liquid nitrogen) [7], and laser surgery (Q-switched lasers/KTP/IPL) [8] are the most effective and rapid treatments to treat senile lentigos.

All of them destroy the outer layer of the skin creating, in a week, mild erythema and fine crusts that peel off more or less in 2 weeks.

16.6 Chemical Peeling

Chemical peeling with trichloroacetic acid (TCA) is a good choice to treat senile lentigos. The application of this agent on the skin causes protein denaturation

A. Tosti et al. (eds.), *Color Atlas of Chemical Peels*,
DOI 10.1007/978-3-642-20270-4_16, © Springer-Verlag Berlin Heidelberg 2012

(white frost) and for this reason is very important to find the best concentration of the agent in order to treat and not to damage the skin. According to several studies, 25–35% TCA is the best concentration for senile lentigos.

Preparation of the skin before and between the peelings, so as the anatomic site to treat, is also an important factor to take into consideration to avoid injuries.

As a rule, non-facial skin takes much longer to heal and is at much greater risk of scarring than when using a similar concentration on the face.

Home treatment started at least 1 month before the first peeling is helpful to achieve better results. Photoprotection (high SPF), topical tretinoin, and topical exfoliants (lactic acid, glycolic acid) are the three agents to be used every day, also between one session of peeling and the other.

Photoprotection is useful to reduce the risk of postinflammatory hyperpigmentation; tretinoin and the exfoliants reduce skin thickness, improving the efficacy of TCA (better and more homogeneous penetration).

Prior to the application of TCA, a thorough cleaning is mandatory for defatting the skin, thus allowing a better penetration of the peeling agent.

Once TCA is applied, it is very important to observe the degree of frosting and its duration before proceeding to the next area. If the desired level of frosting is not reached within 2–3 min, an additional application of the agent should be performed. Once the desired frost is achieved, the skin can be rinsed off with water and moisturized with an emollient cream.

TCA peelings can be repeated every 4–6 weeks.

References

1. Noblesse E, Nizard C, Cario-André M et al (2006) Skin ultrastructure in senile lentigo. Skin Pharmacol Physiol 19: 95–100
2. Pierard GE, Pierard-Franchimont C, Laso Dosal F et al (1991) Pigmentary changes in skin senescence. J Appl Cosmetol 9:63–67
3. Nordlund JJ, Boissy RE, Hearing VJ et al (2006) The pigmentary system, 2nd edn. Blackwell Publishing, Oxford, p 829
4. Katsambas AD, Stratigos AJ (2001) Depigmenting and bleaching agents: coping with hyperpigmentation. Clin Dermatol 19:483–488
5. Humphreys TR, Werth V, Dzubow L, Klingman A (1996) Treatment of photodamaged skin with TCA and topical tretinoin. J Am Acad Dermatol 34:638–644
6. Sezer E, Erbil H, Kurumulu Z et al (1997) A comparative study of focal medium-depth chemical peel versus cryosurgery for the treatment of solar lentigo. Eur J Dermatol 17: 26–29
7. Zouboulis CC, Rosenberger AD, Adler Y, Orfanos CE (1999) Treatment of solar lentigo with cryosurgery. Acta Derm Venereol 79:489–490
8. Rinaldi F (2008) Lasers: a review. Clin Dermatol 26: 590–601

Postinflammatory Hyperpigmentation

17

Teresa Soriano and Pearl E. Grimes

17.1 Definition

Postinflammatory hyperpigmentation is the acquired presence of darker macules and patches of skin occurring at sites of previous cutaneous inflammatory conditions. The processes preceding the altered skin color include mechanical injuries, allergic reactions, primary inflammatory skin disorders, and therapeutic interventions.

17.2 Epidemiology

Postinflammatory hyperpigmentation is one of the most common causes of altered skin color. Although it can manifest in various skin types, it is more frequently seen with greater intensity and persistence in darker skin types [1, 2] (Fig. 17.1). Its incidence is equal in males and females.

17.3 Etiology

Postinflammatory hyperpigmentation can be seen after endogenous or exogenous inflammatory conditions. Essentially any disease with cutaneous inflammation can potentially result in postinflammatory hyperpigmentation in individuals capable of producing melanin.

P.E. Grimes
Division of Dermatology, Department of Medicine, David Geffen School of Medicine, University of California—Los Angeles, Vitiligo and Pigmentation Institute of Southern California, 5670 Wilshire Blvd., Suite 650, Los Angeles, CA 90036, USA
e-mail: pegrimesmd@earthlink.net

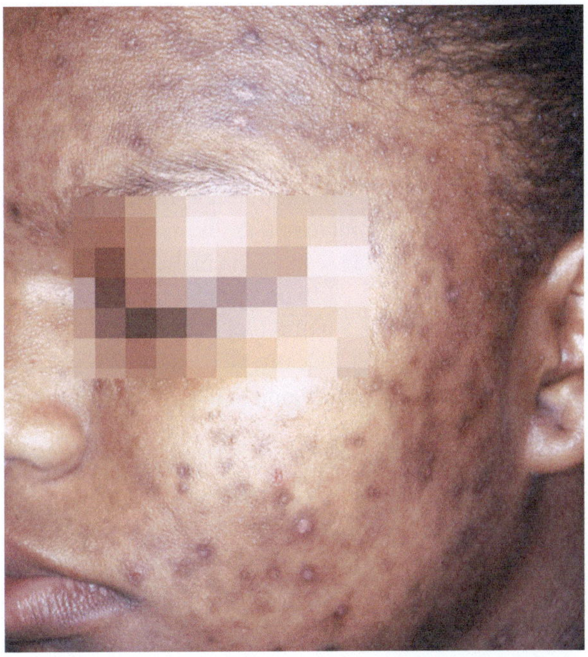

Fig. 17.1 Severe postinflammatory hyperpigmentation caused by acne vulgaris

Several skin disorders such as acne, atopic dermatitis, allergic contact dermatitis, incontinenti pigmenti, lichen planus, lupus erythematosus, and morphea have postinflammatory hyperpigmentation as a predominant feature. Exogenous stimuli, both physical and chemical, can cause injury to the skin followed by PIH. These include mechanical trauma, ionizing and nonionizing radiation, heat, contact dermatitis, and phototoxic reactions and laser therapies [2, 3, 4].

In postinflammatory hyperpigmentation, there appears to be an increase in melanin production and/or an abnormal distribution of pigment. However, the exact

A. Tosti et al. (eds.), *Color Atlas of Chemical Peels*,
DOI 10.1007/978-3-642-20270-4_17, © Springer-Verlag Berlin Heidelberg 2012

pathophysiology linking cutaneous inflammation and altered pigmentation is not fully understood. Different stimuli may involve different mechanisms [5, 6].

Some have proposed that arachidonic acid–derived chemical mediators may play a role in inducing postinflammatory hyperpigmentation of the skin by stimulating increased melanin production and transfer to surrounding keratinocytes [6–9]. Tomita et al. [8, 9] demonstrated that human epidermal melanocytes became more dendritic with an increase in tyrosinase when cultured with several arachidonic acid metabolites, including prostaglandin D2, leukotriene (LT) B4, LTC4, LTD4, LTE4.

17.4 Clinical Types

In postinflammatory hyperpigmentation, cutaneous pigmentary changes can be observed primarily in the epidermis, or in both the epidermis and dermis. In both instances, epidermal melanin is increased. In the epidermal/dermal type of PIH, pigment is seen within melanophages in the superficial dermis [2, 3]. Wood's light, by accentuating epidermal melanin, is a useful tool in defining the extent of pigment alteration. Clinically, heavy deposition of dermal pigment can be challenging to bleach.

17.5 Diagnostic Criteria

The diagnosis of postinflammatory hyperpigmentation is often made by history and clinical presentation. It is characterized by macules and patches of varying shades of hyperpigmentation limited to the sites of inflammed skin lesions. Lesions of the preceding inflammatory process may be present at various stages of evolution and at other anatomic areas, and thus, helpful with the diagnosis.

Although the diagnosis is relatively straightforward when a patient provides a history of a preceding coetaneous eruption, it can be more challenging when no specific history of inflammation is noted. If the diagnosis is unclear, a skin biopsy can be performed. Histologically, postinflammatory hyperpigmentation is characterized by increased epidermal melanin. In addition, a sparse superficial perivascular infiltrate with melanophages in the dermis can be seen [2, 3]. Basal cell vacuolation and band-like deposition of mucin have also been observed in some cases of PIH [10].

17.6 Differential Diagnosis

The differential diagnosis for postinflammatory hyperpigmentation includes the following: fixed drug eruption, systemic drug-induced hyperpigmentation, macular amyloid, ashy dermatosis, melasma, and tinea versicolor. Medications, such as tetracyclines, antimalarial drugs, arsenic, bleomycin, and doxorubicin, can result in hyperpigmentation of the skin.

17.7 Therapy

The management of postinflammatory hyperpigmentation involves prevention of further pigment deposition and diminishing altered discoloration. First and foremost, treatment or removal of the etiologic insult is essential to avert development of new lesions. Protecting the areas from sun exposure is also critical to prevent darkening of existing lesions. In some circumstances, the above measures along with a tincture of time result in the resolution of postinflammatory hyperpigmentation. However, in cases of incomplete or slow resolution, other treatment modalities can aid in the management of PIH.

17.8 Topical Agents

Monotherapy with topical retinoids has been shown to facilitate resolution of PIH. A randomized, double-blind, vehicle-controlled study using tretinoin 0.1% cream for 40 weeks to treat facial PIH in black patients demonstrated significant lightening with tretinoin 0.1% cream compared with vehicle [11]. The overall improvement was initially noted after 4 weeks of therapy. Fifty percent (12 of 24) of the tretinoin-treated patients experienced erythema and desquamation; however, none had any further hyperpigmentation or depigmentation as a side effect. In another double-blind, randomized, vehicle-controlled study, Grimes and Callender [12] reported the efficacy of once-daily tazarotene 0.1% cream in the treatment of PIH from acne in patients with Fitzpatrick skin types IV–VI. Significant advantage over vehicle was noted at 10 weeks of therapy, and only trace levels of erythema, burning, and peeling were reported throughout the study. An open-label study of darker-skinned patients with acne showed the utility of adapalene 0.1% gel to reduce PIH [13].

The concomitant use of various bleaching agents has also been shown to improve PIH. In 1975, tretinoin in combination with hydroquinone and dexamethasone was reported as an effective treatment for PIH [14]. In a small study, the application of 2% hydroquinone and 10% glycolic acid gel twice daily and 0.05% tretinoin cream at night has been shown to provide benefit for darker-skinned patients with PIH [15]. Similarly, Yoshimura et al. [16] suggested efficacy of the tretinoin combined with hydroquinone and lactic acid in reducing PIH. More recently, Cook-Bolden [17] reported significant improvement of PIH with the use of a combination bleaching cream (Glyquin®) containing hydroquinone 4%, buffered glycolic acid 10%, vitamin C, vitamin E, and sunscreen. In this study, 35 patients with skin types IV–VI experienced clinical improvement after 12 weeks of twice-daily treatment.

17.9 Chemical Peels

Chemical peeling can be a useful adjunct in treating cases of persistent postinflammatory hyperpigmentation and those unresponsive to topical bleaching agents [18, 19]. As many cases of postinflammatory hyperpigmentation occur in darker-skinned individuals, one must be aware of the inherent differences between light and darker skin types when considering the use of chemical peeling agents. Although no quantitative differences in melanocytes are seen in various ethnic groups, melanocytes of darker-skinned individuals produce greater quantities of melanin and demonstrate exaggerated responses to cutaneous injury. This translates clinically to an increased susceptibility to irritation and to a greater risk of further pigment alteration in darker-skinned individuals. To decrease the potential risk of exacerbation of hyperpigmentation, the authors' protocol in peeling darker skin types includes pretreatment for 2 weeks with bleaching agents, such as hydroquinone 4% cream. In addition, tretinoin is discontinued 1–2 weeks prior to and during the series of chemical peels performed at 2- to 4-week intervals [18].

Superficial chemical peels, including salicylic acid, glycolic acid, and Jessner's peels, target the stratum corneum to the papillary dermis and can safely be used to facilitate the resolution of PIH. These agents facilitate the resolution of PIH (Figs. 17.2a, b to 17.5a, b).

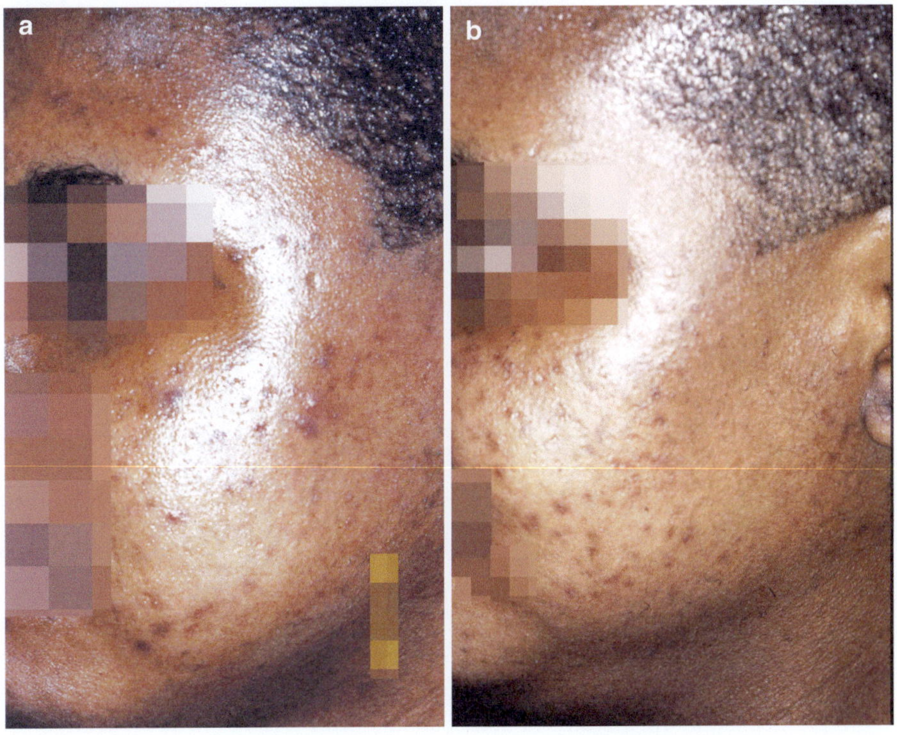

Fig. 17.2 (**a**) Postinflammatory hyperpigmentation from acne vulgaris. (**b**) After a series of salicylic acid peels and hydroquinone 4%

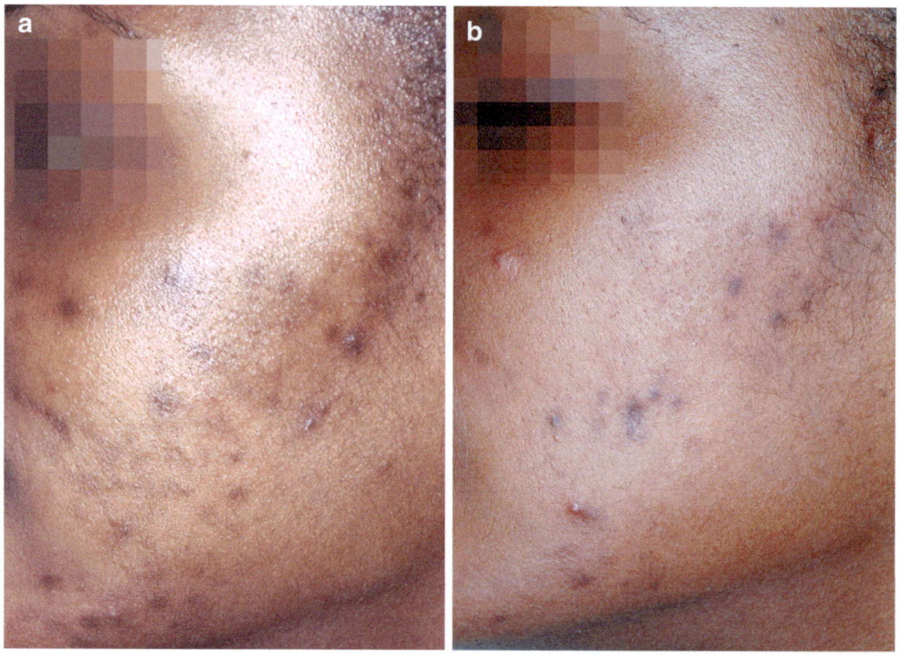

Fig. 17.3 (**a**) Severe recalcitrant postinflammatory hyperpigmentation secondary to acne excorians. (**b**) After a series of four salicylic acid 20% and 30% peels and 10% hydroquinone cream

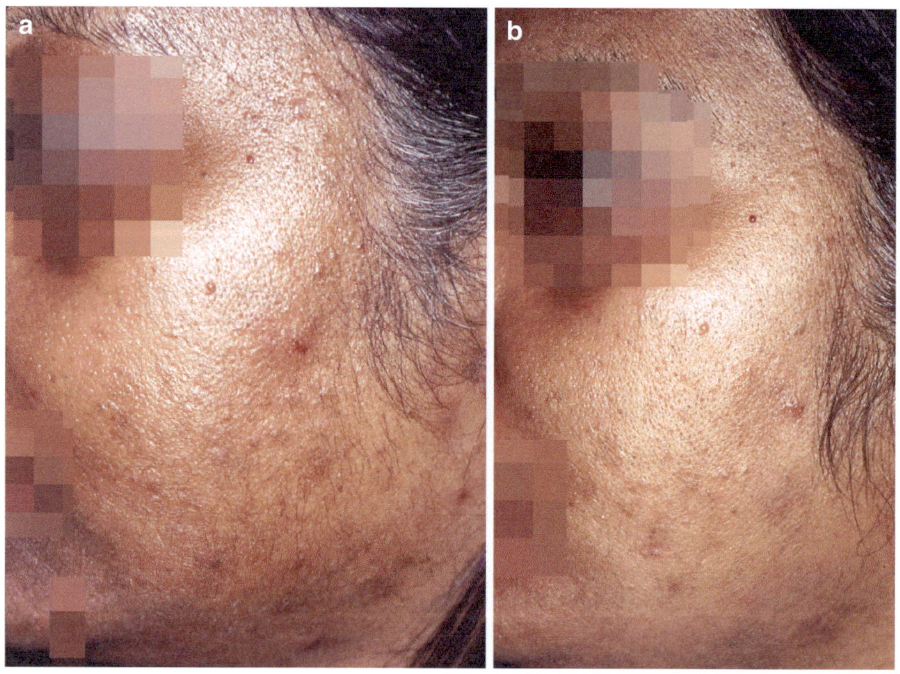

Fig. 17.4 (**a**) Post-inflammatory hyperpigmentation from unknown topical irritant. (**b**) Cleared after a series of two gylcolic acid peels (20% and 35%)

To assess for variability in response and limit further PIH, chemical peels should be started at the lower concentration and titrated up as tolerated and necessary.

Superficial salicylic acids have been shown to be safe and efficacious for treatment of postinflammatory hyperpigmentation. In a study of five patients with skin types V and VI with PIH, pretreatment for 2 weeks with hydroquinone 4% cream followed by a series of five 20–30% salicylic acid chemical peels (B-lift®) at 2-week intervals resulted in 51–75% improvement in one patient and 75% improvement in four patients [20]. No adverse effect was noted.

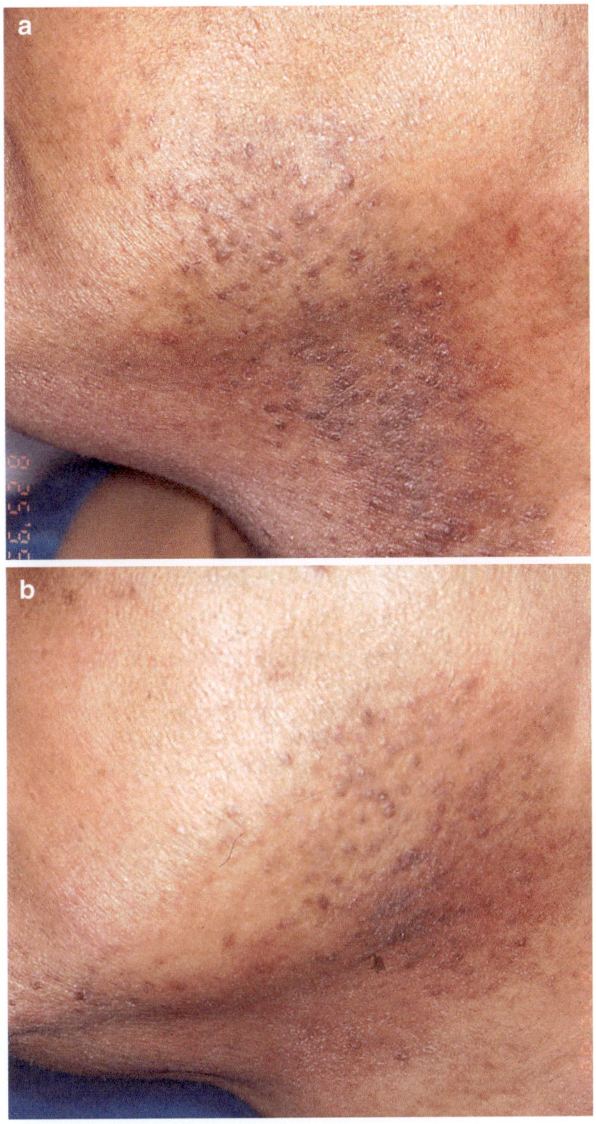

Fig. 17.5 (**a**) Pseudofolliculitis barbae and postinflammatory hyperpigmentation. (**b**) After two Jessner's peels

Glycolic acid peels can also be used to facilitate resolution of PIH. Burns et al. [15] demonstrated greater and more rapid improvement with the addition of glycolic acid peels to a topical regimen of topical combination of hydroquinone, glycolic acid gel, and tretinoin. In this study, patients with Fitzpatrick IV, V, and VI who received six serial glycolic acid peels in addition to the topical regimen were found to have additional benefit with minimal adverse effects compared to the patients who were treated with the topical regimen alone.

17.10 Laser Therapy

In general, lasers are not routinely used to treat postinflammatory hyperpigmentation as lasers can be the culprit of PIH especially in darker skin types. PIH is one of the most common side effects following treatment of pigmented lesions, laser hair removal, traditional skin resurfacing, and fractional resurfacing [21–23]. The use of potent topical corticosteroids 10 min prior to laser treatment and 5 days after laser hair removal treatment reduced the duration of postinflammatory hyperpigmentation in one study in darker skin types [24].

One report showed some efficacy in using a 1064 nm QS Nd:Yag as a second-line treatment for PIH. Three Korean patients developed PIH after intense pulsed light and/or QS laser treatment of facial pigmented lesions. After failing topical bleaching agents, the patients received five weekly treatments of a 1064 nm QS Nd:Yag laser at low fluences with improvement of their lesions [25].

17.11 Summary

Optimal treatment for PIH includes prevention of further pigment deposition and clearing of the deposited pigment. Chemical peels work best when used in combination with topical bleaching regimens. Laser therapy should be used with extreme caution and care. Given the propensity of darker-skin types to develop postinflammatory hyperpigmentation, superficial peels work best, while minimizing complications.

Disclaimer The author has no financial interest in any of the products or equipment mentioned in this article

References

1. Halder RM, Grimes PE, McLaurin CI, Kreiss MA, Kenney JA (1983) Incidence of common dermatoses in a predominantly black dermatologic practice. Cutis 32:378–380
2. Pandya AG, Guevara IL (2000) Disorders of hyperpigmentation. Dermatol Clin 18(1):91–98
3. Epstein JH (1989) Postinflammatory hyperpigmentation. Clin Dermatol 7(2):55–65
4. McBurney EI (2002) Side effects and complications of laser therapy. Dermatol Clin 20(1):165–176
5. Nordlund JJ, Abdel-Malek ZA (1988) Mechanisms of postinflammatory hyperpigmentation and hypopigmentation. Prog Clin Biol Res 256:219–236

6. Johansson O, Ljungberg A, Han SW, Vaalasti A (1991) Evidence for gamma-melanocyte stimulating hormone containing nerves and neutrophilic granulocytes in the human skin by indirect immunofluorescence. J Invest Dermatol 96(6):852–856
7. Morelli JG, Yohn JJ, Lyons MB, Murphy RC, Norris DA (1989) Leukotrienes C4 and D4 as potent mitogens for cultures human neonatal melanocytes. J Invest Dermatol 93(6):719–722
8. Tomita Y, Iwamoto M, Masuda T, Tagami H (1987) Stimulatory effect of prostaglandin E2 on the configuration of normal human melanocytes in vitro. J Invest Dermatol 89(3):299–301
9. Tomita Y, Maeda K, Tagami H (1992) Melanocyte-stimulation properties of arachidonic acid metabolites: possible role of post-inflammatory pigmentation. Pigment Cell Res 5(5 pt 2):357–361
10. Noto G, Pravata G, Arico M (1998) Reticulate postinflammatory hyperpigmentation with band-like mucin deposition. Int J Dermatol 37(11):829–832
11. Bulengo-Ransby SM, Griffiths C, Kimbrough-Green CK, Finkel LJ, Hamilton TA, Ellis CN, Voorhees JJ (1993) Topical tretinion (retinoic acid) therapy for hyperpigmented lesions caused by inflammation of the skin in black patients. N Engl J Med 328:1438–1443
12. Grimes PE, Callender VD (2003) Tazarotene cream 0.1% in the treatment of facial post-inflammatory hyperpigmentation associated with acne vulgaris: a two-center, double-blind, randomized, vehicle – controlled study. Poster presentation at the 61st annual meeting of the American Academy of Dermatology, San Francisco, 21–26 March 2003
13. Jacyk WK, Mpofu P (2001) Adapalene gel 0.1% for topical treatment of acne vulgaris in African patients. Cutis 68:48–54
14. Kligman AM, Willis I (1975) A new formula for depigmenting human skin. Arch Dermatol 111:40–48
15. Burns R, Prevost-Blank PL, Lawry MA, Lawry TB, Faria DT, Fivenson DP (1999) Glycolic acid peels for postinflammatory hyperpigmentation in black patients. Dermatol Surg 25:18–22
16. Yoshimura K, Harii K, Aoyama T, Iga T (2000) Experience with a strong bleaching treatment for skin hyperpigmentation in Orientals. Plast Reconstr Surg 105:1097–1110
17. Cook-Bolden FE (2004) The efficacy and tolerability of a combination cream containing 4% hydroquinone in the treatment of postinflammatory hyperpigmentation in skin types IV-VI. J Cosmet Dermatol 17(3):149–155
18. Grimes PE (2000) Agents for ethnic skin peeling. Dermatol Ther 30:159–164
19. Callender VD (2004) Acne in ethnic skin: special considerations for therapy. Dermatol Ther 17:184–195
20. Grimes PE (1999) The safety and efficacy of salicylic acid chemical peels in darker racial-ethnic groups. Dermatol Surg 25:18–22
21. Nanni CA, Alster TS (1999) Laser-assisted hair removal: side effects of Q-switched Nd:Yag, long-pulsed ruby, and alexandrite lasers. J Am Acad Dermatol 41(2 pt1):165–171
22. Tanzi EL, Alster TS (2003) Single-pass carbon dioxide versus multiple-pass Er:YAG laser skin resurfacing: a comparison of postoperative wound healing and side-effect rates. Dermatol Surg 29(1):80–84
23. Graber EM, Tanzi EL, Alster TS (2008) Side effects and complications of fractional laser photothermolysis: experience with 961 treatments. Dermatol Surg 34(3):301–305
24. Aldraibi MS, Touma DJ, Khachemoune A (2007) Hair removal with the 3-mec alexandrite laser in patients with skin types IV-VI: efficacy, safety, and the role of topical steroids in preventing side effects. J Drugs Dermatol 6(1):60–66
25. Cho SB, Park SJ, Kim JS, Kim MJ, Bu TS (2009) Treatment of post-inflammatory hyperpigmentation using a 1064 nm QS Nd:Yag laser with low fluence: report of three cases. J Eur Acad Dermatol Venereol 23:1206–1207

Deep Chemical Peels for Post-acne Scarring

18

Marina Landau

18.1 History and Classification

Acne is a common disease affecting almost 100% of youngsters [1, 2]. Acne settles in the vast majority by 20–25 years of age but 1% of males and 5% of females exhibit acne lesions at 40 years of age [3]. Scarring occurs early in the course of acne and may affect to some degree 95% of patients from both sexes [4]. Differences in the cell-mediated immune response are involved in the personal tendency to develop post-acne scarring [5].

Acne scars are debilitating and socially disabling for the individual. Treatment of acne scars presents a challenge for a treating physician. Usually, they cannot be effectively corrected by a single treatment modality because of their widely varied depth, width, and structure [6].

A few morphologic acne scar classifications have been proposed to assess the efficacy of different therapeutic options based on the scar types. Standard classification includes three basic types of scars: icepick scars, rolling scars, and boxcar scars [7, 8]. Icepick scars are narrow (<2 mm), deep sharply marginated epithelial tracts that extend vertically to the deep dermis or subcutaneous tissue (Fig. 18.1). Rolling scars occur from dermal tethering of otherwise relatively normal-appearing skin and are usually wider (4–5 mm) (Fig. 18.2). The subdermal tether precludes treatment from the surface above; thus, correction of subdermal

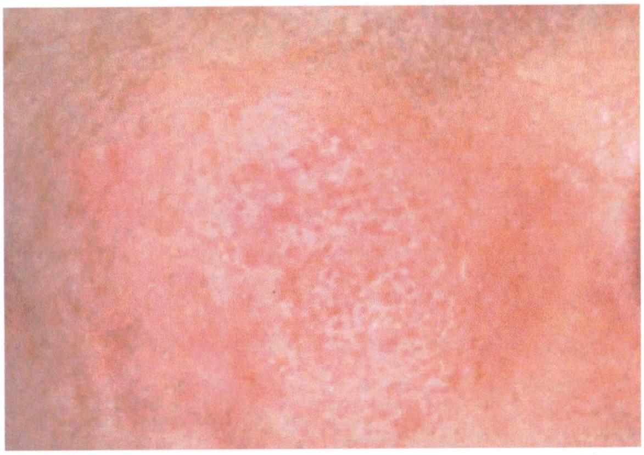

Fig. 18.1 Icepick scars

component is essential. Boxcar scars are round to oval depressions with demarcated vertical edges, similar to varicella scars (Fig. 18.3). They may be shallow or deep. Other less common scars are sinus tracts, hypertrophic scars, and keloidal scars.

According to the other classification, acne scars are divided into elevated, dystrophic, or depressed. Elevated scars are subdivided into hypertrophic, keloidal, and papular, while depressed scars are subdivided into distensible and non-distensible (Fig. 18.4). Quantitative global acne scarring assessment tool assigns points depending on the type of scar and the number of scars present [9].

As far back as 1905, surgical methods have been used to improve skin that has been scarred by facial acne. One hundred years ago, two New York dermatologists, George MacKee and Florentine Karp, began using phenol peels for post-acne scarring [10]. Thereafter methods used to correct acne scars included dermatome dermaplaning [11, 12], dermabrasion [13–15], collagen

M. Landau
Wolfson Medical Center, 56 Joshua Ben Nun Street, Herzlia Pituach, 46763 Holon, Israel
e-mail: mlandau@zahav.net.il

A. Tosti et al. (eds.), *Color Atlas of Chemical Peels*,
DOI 10.1007/978-3-642-20270-4_18, © Springer-Verlag Berlin Heidelberg 2012

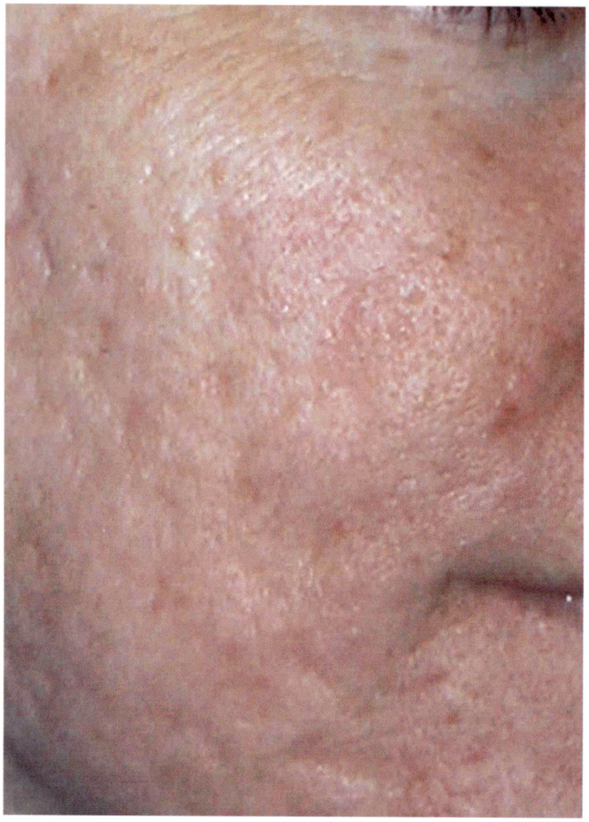

Fig. 18.2 Rolling scars

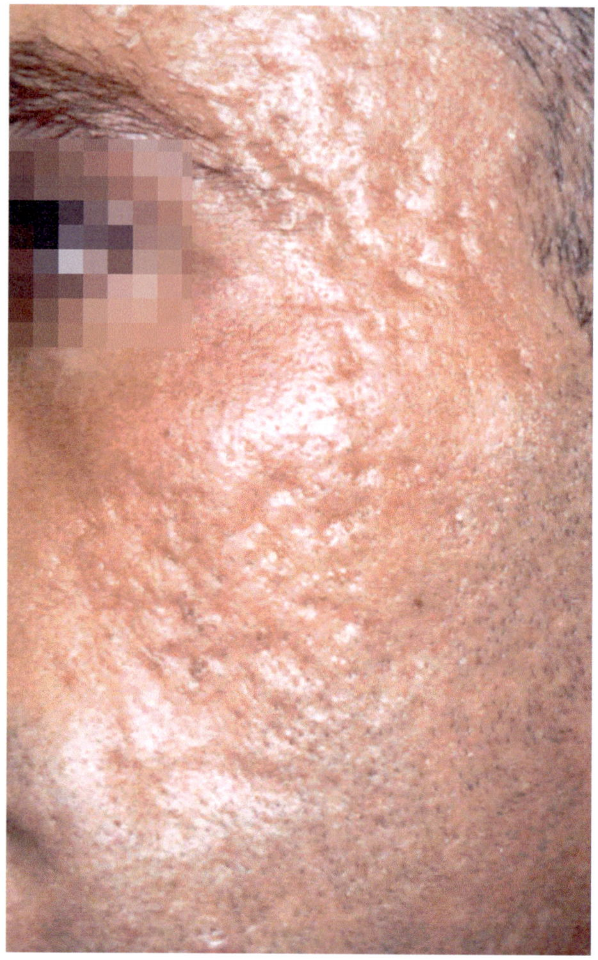

Fig. 18.3 Boxcar scars

implantation [16–18], dermal overgrafting [19], punch excision, grafting and elevation [20, 21], dermal grafting [22, 23], subcision [24], laser resurfacing [25–31], microdermabrasion [32], dermasanding [33], and their combinations [34–36].

But the mainstay of therapy for skin resurfacing continues to be chemical peels together with abrasion [37–42]. Chemical peels in use to improve facial scarring include alpha-hydroxy acid peels, trichloroacetic acid, and deep phenol-based methods [43–48]. In this chapter, we discuss deep chemical peels for post-acne scars treatment.

18.2 Indications

Generally, best results are achieved in depressed and atrophic or rolling and boxcar scars. Icepick scars always need to be preceded by punch excision. Our experience shows that in older ages, when skin is less elastic, it is possible to achieve more significant improvement of the scars. In male skin, the improvement is usually less cosmetically significant.

In general, it is important to manage patients' expectations, since, as mentioned previously, no complete elimination of acne scars of any type is possible.

18.3 Contraindications

It is important to obtain details regarding history of keloid or hypertrophic scar formation. Previously, we used to recommend delaying a procedure for a period of 6–12 months in patients being treated by isotretinoin [49]. This recommendation has been revised and changed by us and others, and currently we peel patients, especially those with thick and oily skin, on low-dosage isotretinoin (up to 40 mg a week) with no increase in side-effect rate. Active acne is not a contraindication for chemical peel. In these cases, the peel is combined with systemic antibiotics for 2–3 weeks. It is always advisable to consider isotretinoin treatment after the peel to avoid acne flare and scars reappearance.

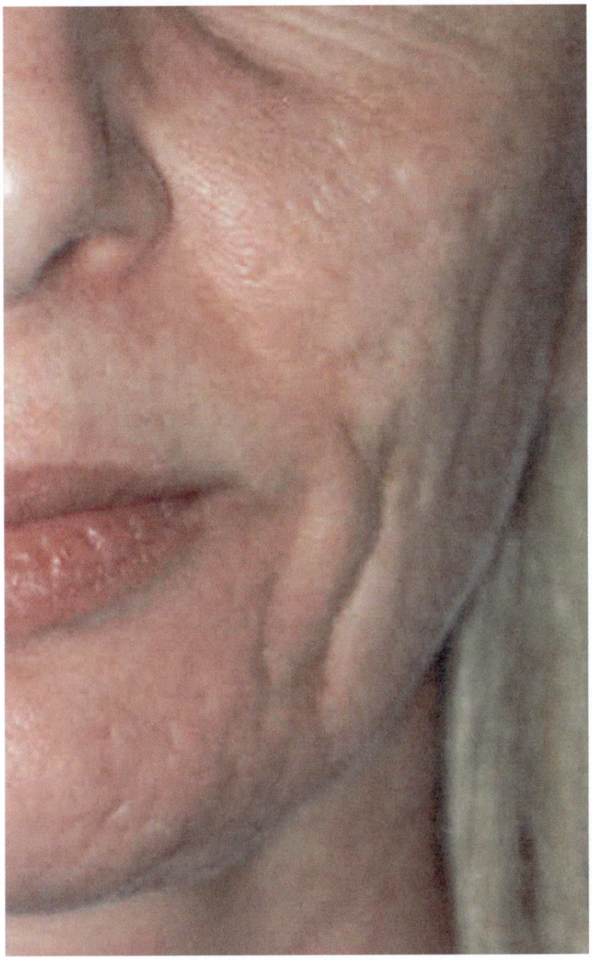

Fig. 18.4 Depressed distensible scars

There are a few absolute contraindications for deep peeling, mainly physical or mental instability. During pregnancy and lactation, any cosmetic intervention is considered to be undesirable. All patients are required to perform electrocardiogram and complete blood count prior to the procedure. Any heart disease requires special precautions and it is always recommended to work in cooperation with patient's cardiologist.

18.4 Pre-peeling Preparation

Treatment of acne scars must be individually tailored to address the specific findings. The patient has to understand that the scar revision process may require more than one surgical session. Punch excisions or elevations have to be performed 4–6 weeks before the peel, while subcision can be performed at the same session with the peel.

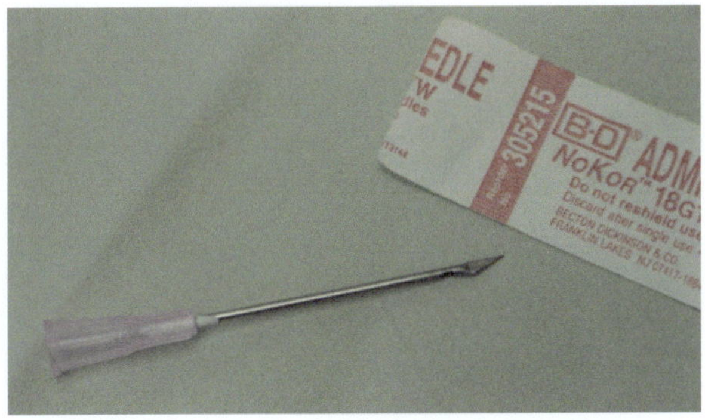

Fig. 18.5 NoKor Admix subcision needle

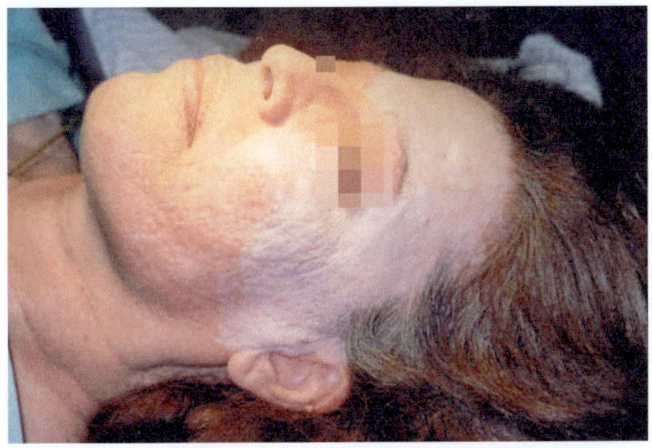

Fig. 18.6 Frosting after application of the peeling solution

Before the peel, prophylactic oral antivirals are given to patients with history of recurrent herpes simplex.

18.5 Peeling Technique

The full description of deep chemical peel procedure is found elsewhere. (Chapter 6). Before the peeling, the subcision (subcutaneous incision) technique is used to free the fibrous bands from the base of the scars. For this purpose, we use an 18-gauge 1.5 in. NoKor Admix needle (Becton Dickinson and Co). This needle has a triangular tip similar to No. 11 blade (Fig. 18.5). It allows smooth separation of fibrous cords. The needle is inserted through a skin surface, and its sharp edges are maneuvered under the defect to make subcutaneous cuts or incisions. The depression is lifted by the releasing action of the procedure, as well as from connective tissue that forms in the course of normal wound healing.

The Exoderm solution is applied evenly and gradually on the skin until full frosting is achieved (Fig. 18.6).

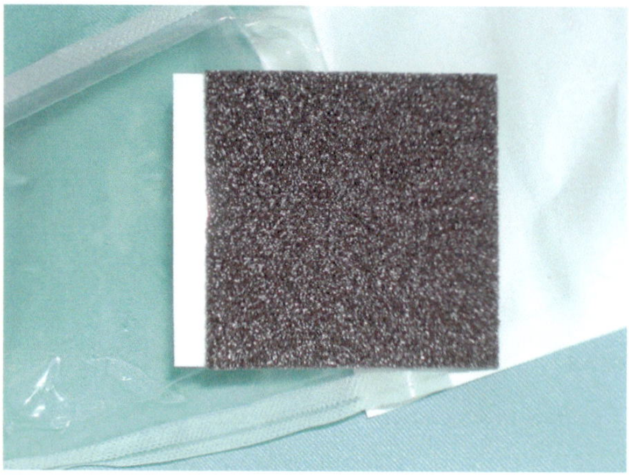

Fig. 18.7 Tipolisher

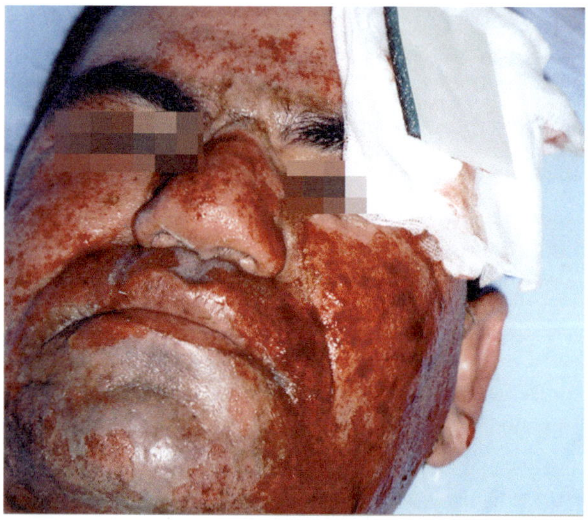

Fig. 18.8 Skin dermabrasion using tipolisher

At this stage, we combine mechanical skin dermabrasion by using a tipolisher, which is a sterile surgical equipment designed originally for cleaning cautery tips during operations (Fig. 18.7). This simple disposable tool is available in any standard operating setting. Another option is to use sterilized gentle sandpaper. At this stage, pint-point bleeding is observed. Reapplication of peeling solution coagulates most of the bleeding (Fig. 18.8). The face is covered with impermeable tape mask for 24 h. After 24 h, the tape mask is removed and the exudate is cleansed with sterile saline. Regional reapplication of peeling solution and re-taping of the scarred areas is performed and the tape is left for an additional 4–6 h and then removed by a patient. The face is covered with bismuth subgalate antiseptic powder for 7 days. The third phase of the treatment is regional re-peeling, being performed 6–8 weeks after the original treatment. This phase is optional for patients with residual scar areas.

18.6 Aftercare

After the procedure, the patient is advised to use water-based lotion creams and potent sunscreens. The erythema gradually resolves over about 2-month period. During this time, makeup foundation is encouraged. In dark skin patients (Fitzpatrick skin type 3 or 4), the application of Kligman preparation is recommended to prevent reactive hyperpigmentation. In after-procedural flare-ups, minocycline or systemic isotretinoin are prescribed immediately to avoid new scars creation.

18.7 Advantages

Combination of deep chemical peel with other minor surgical procedures, such as punch excision, elevation, and subcision, provides a possibility to tailor an effective treatment for each person.

18.8 Disadvantages

In spite of the fact that the final result is always significant, a complete elimination of all the scars is usually impossible. Patients need to be aware that use of multiple complementary techniques and time-consuming treatments is needed to produce optimal results.

Results of a combination of phenol-based peel with abrasion and subcision are shown below (Figs. 18.9–18.15).

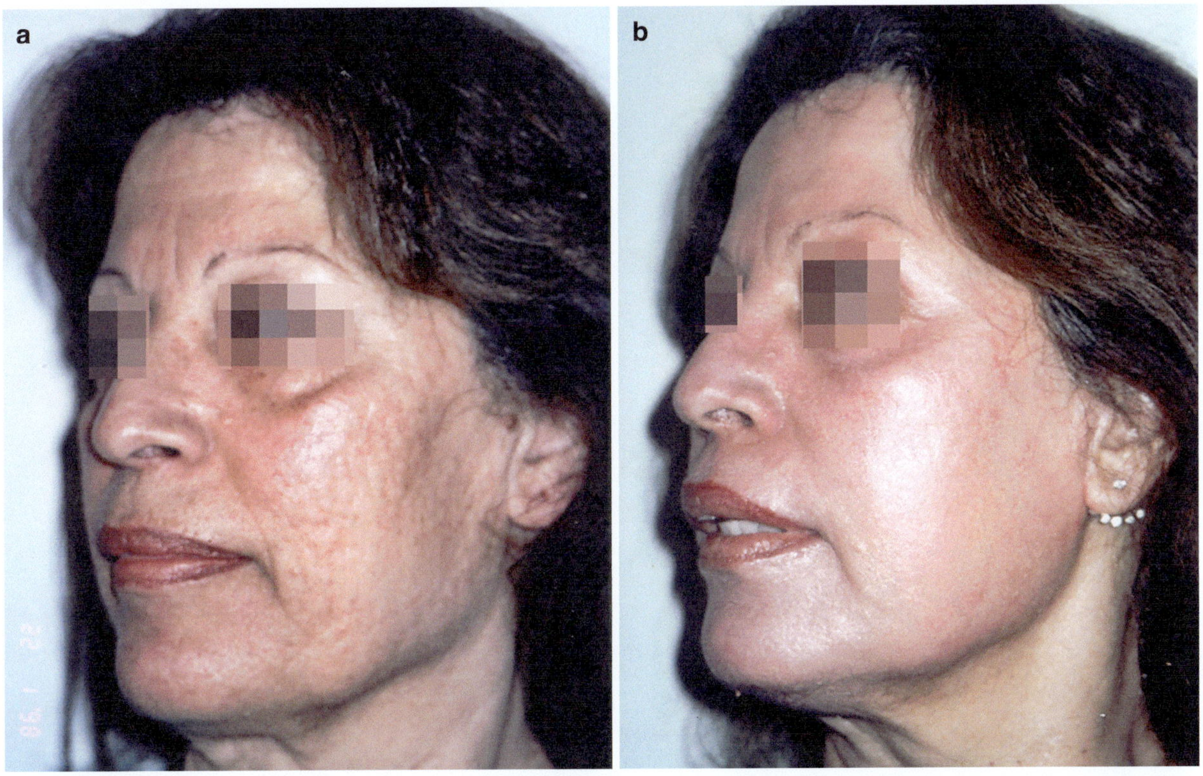

Fig. 18.9 A 52-year-old patient with boxcar acne scars. (**a**) Before. (**b**) One month after deep chemical peel and skin abrasion

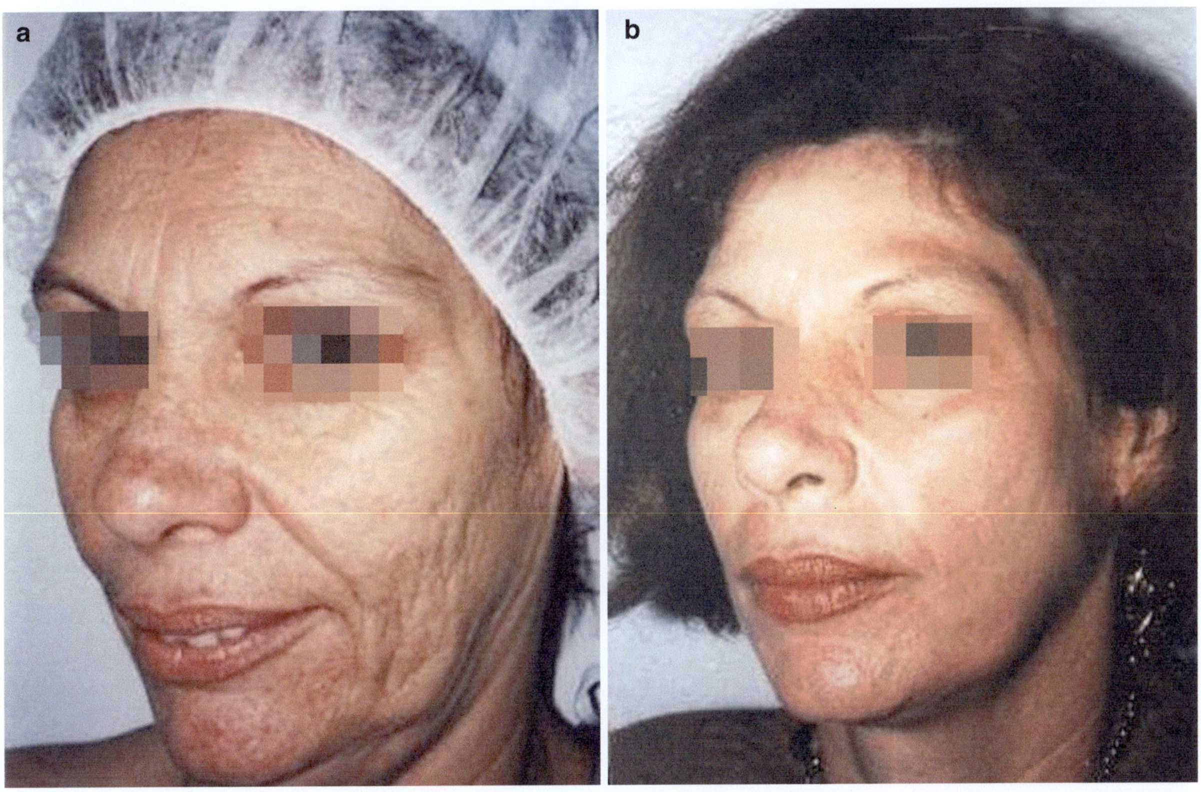

Fig. 18.10 A 48-year-old patient with acne scars and wrinkles. (**a**) Before. (**b**) Six months after deep chemical peel with skin abrasion

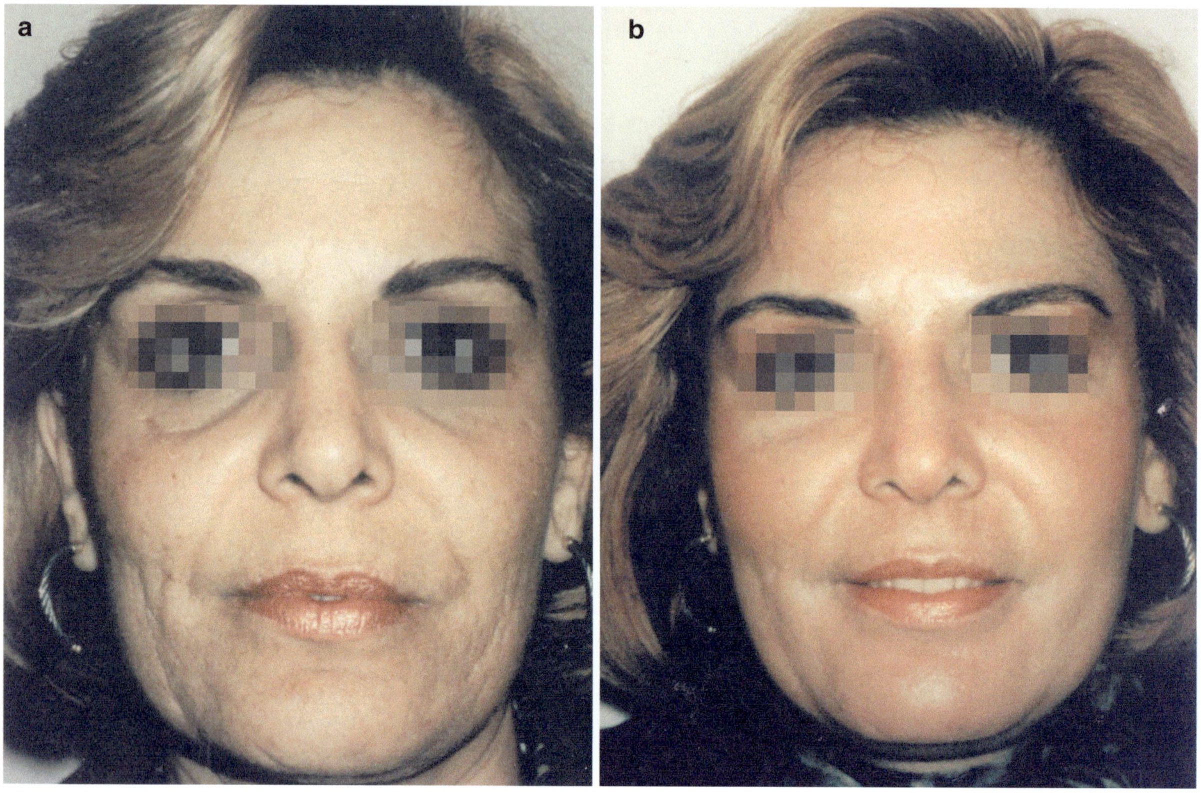

Fig. 18.11 A 44-year-old patient with rolling acne scars. (**a**) Before. (**b**) Three months after deep chemical peel combined with subcision and dermabrasion

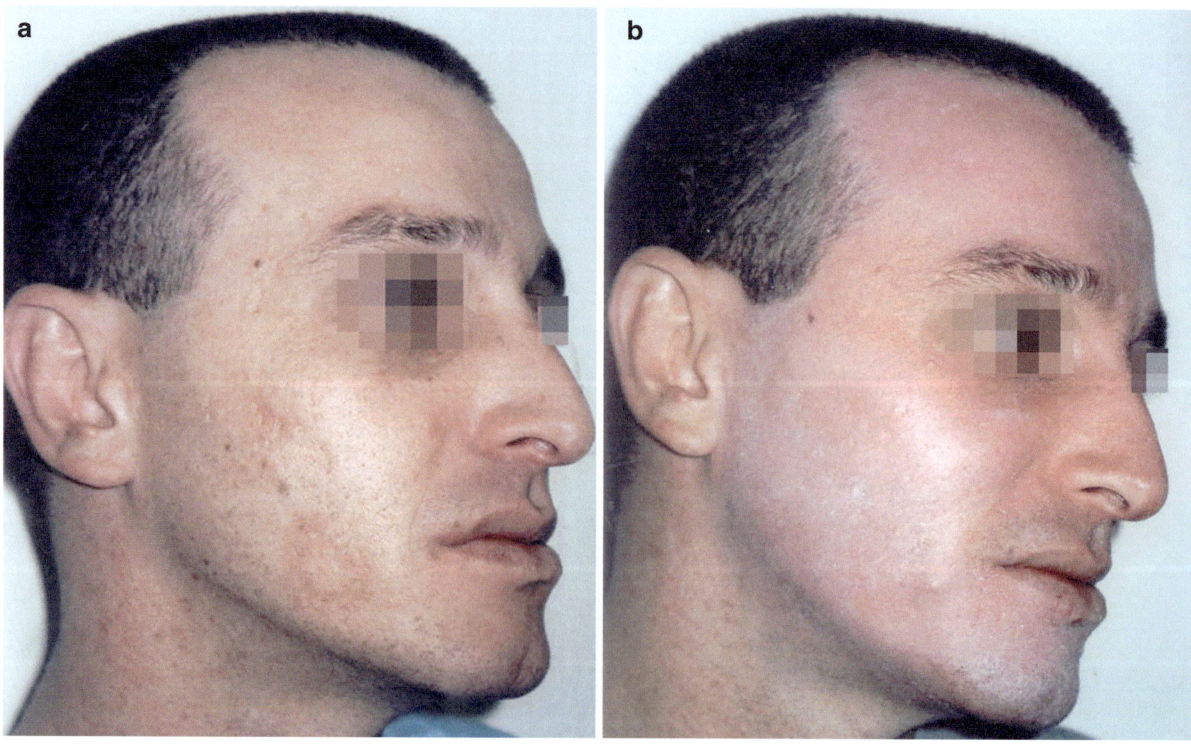

Fig. 18.12 A 42-year-old male patient with boxcar acne scars. (**a**) Before. (**b**) Two weeks after deep chemical peel and skin abrasion

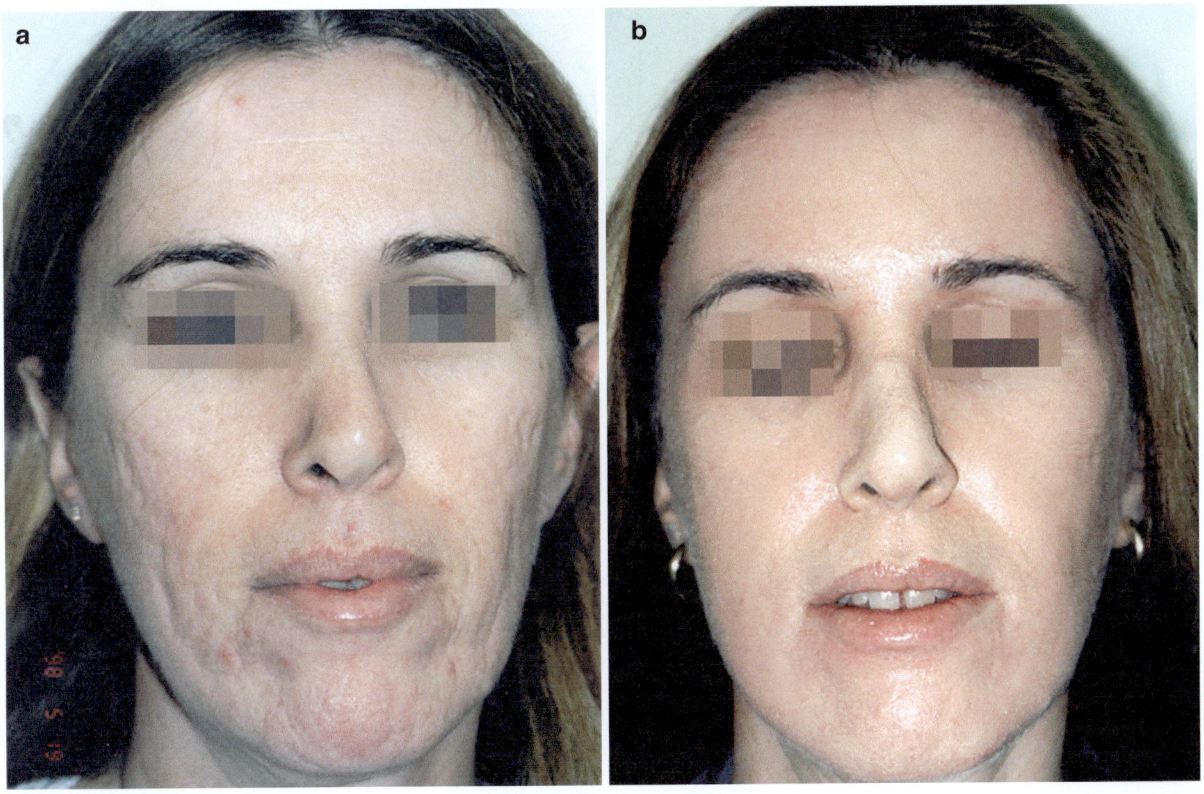

Fig. 18.13 A 38-year-old patient with rolling and depressed distensible scars. (**a**) Before. (**b**) One month after deep chemical peel combined with subcision and skin abrasion

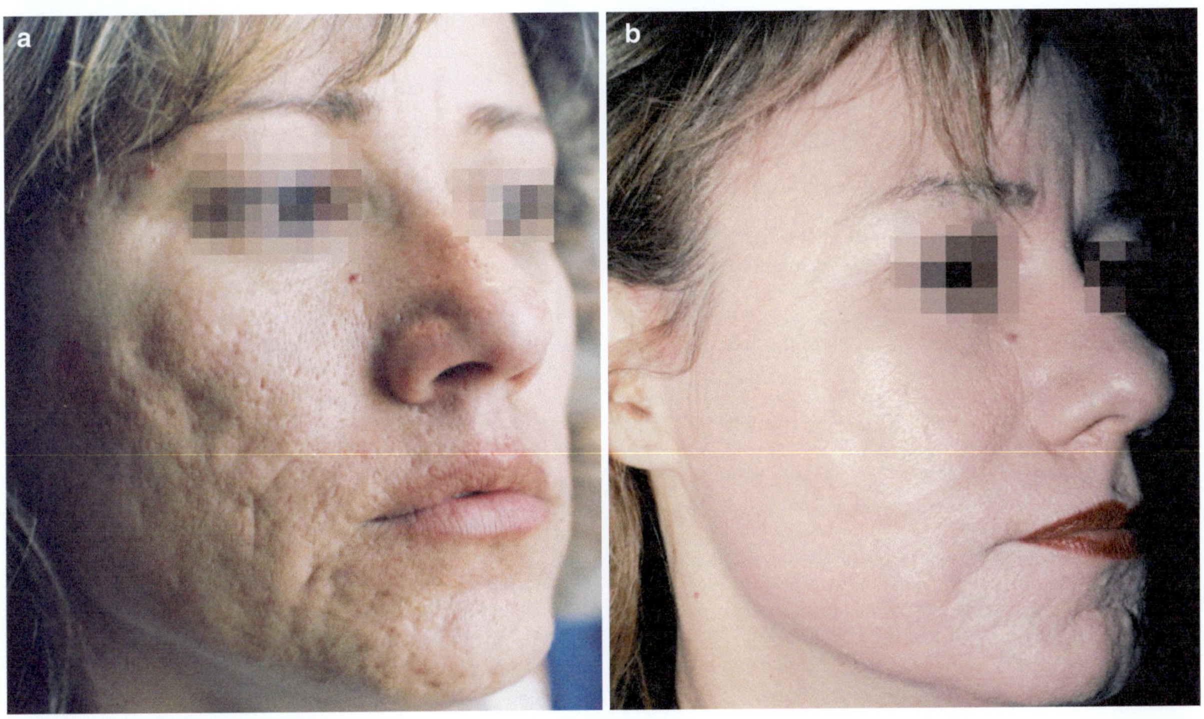

Fig. 18.14 A 51-year-old patient with severe facial scarring. (**a**) Before. (**b**) Two months after deep chemical peel combined with subcision and skin abrasion

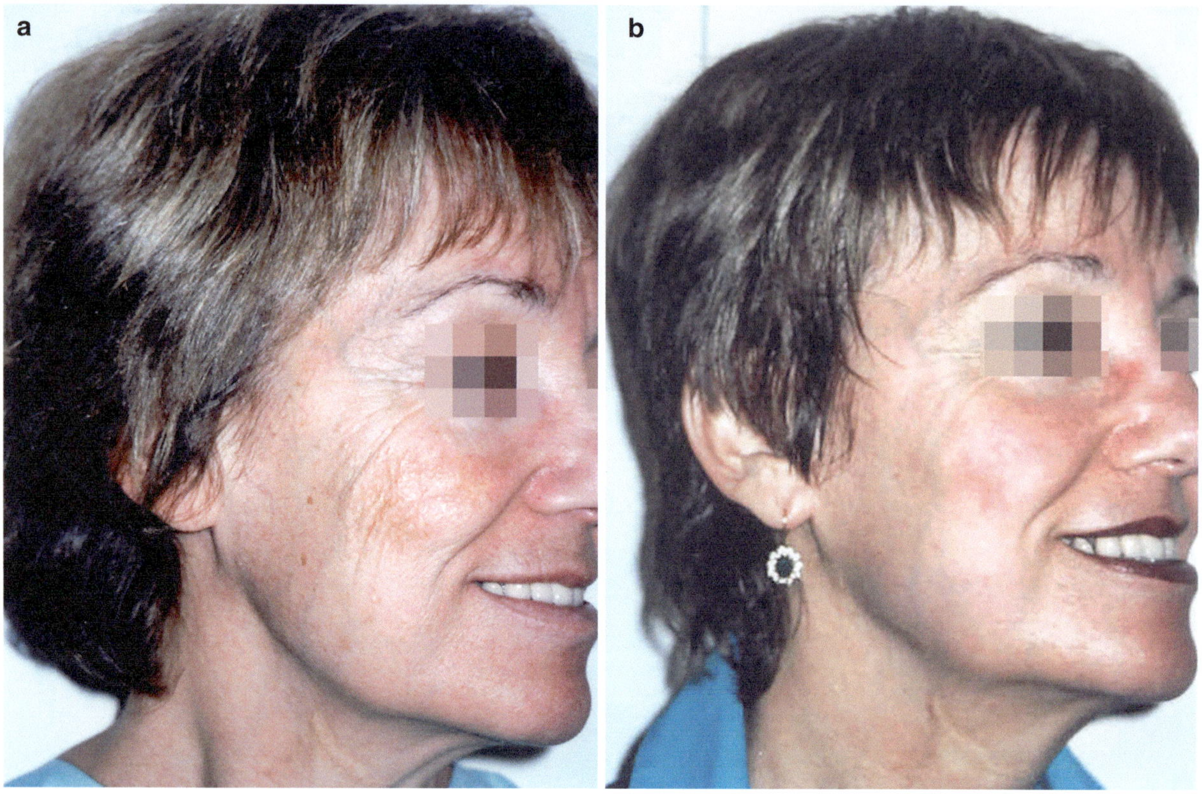

Fig. 18.15 A 56-year-old patient with wrinkles and atrophic scar due to old cutaneous leishmaniasis. (**a**) Before. (**b**) Three months after deep chemical peel

Disclaimer The authors have no financial interest in any of the products or equipment mentioned in this article.

References

1. Burton JL, Cunliffe WJ, Stafford I, Shuster S (1971) The prevalence of acne vulgaris in adolescence. Br J Dermatol 85:119–126
2. Rademaker M, Garioch JJ, Simpson NB (1989) Acne in schoolchildren: no longer a concern for dermatologists. BMJ 298:1217–1219
3. Cunliffe WJ, Gould DJ (1979) Prevalence of facial acne vulgaris in late adolescence and in adults. BMJ 1: 1109–1110
4. Layton AM, Henderson CA, Cunliffe WJ (1994) A clinical evaluation of acne scarring and its incidence. Clin Exp Dermatol 19:303–308
5. Holland DB, Jeremy AHT, Roberts SG, Seukeran DC, Layton AM (2004) Inflammation in acne scarring: a comparison of the responses in lesions from patients prone and not prone to scar. Br J Dermatol 150:72–81
6. Alam M, Dover JS (2006) Treatment of acne scarring. Skin Therapy Lett 11:7–9
7. Jacob CI, Dover JS, Kaminer MS (2001) Acne scarring: a classification system and review of treatment options. J Am Acad Dermatol 45:109–117
8. Kadunc BV, Trindade de Almeida AR (2003) Surgical treatment of facial acne scars based on morphologic classification: a Brazilian experience. Dermatol Surg 29:1200–1209
9. Goodman GJ, Baron JA (2007) The management of post-acne scarring. Dermatol Surg 33:1175–1188
10. Mackee GM, Karp FL (1952) The treatment of post acne scars with phenol. Br J Dermatol 64:456–459
11. Kurtin A (1953) Corrective surgical planning of skin: new technique for treatment of acne scars and other skin defects. AMA Arch Dermtol Syphilol 68:389–397
12. Malherbe WD, Davies DS (1971) Surgical treatment of acne scarring, by a dermatome. Plast Reconstr Surg 47:122–126
13. Orentreich N (1969) Dermabrasion. J Am Med Womens Assoc 24:331–336
14. Kurtin A (1968) Dermabrasion. Arch Dermatol 98:87
15. Rattner R, Rein CR (1955) Treatment of acne scars by dermabrasion; rotary brush method. J Am Med Assoc 159: 1299–1301
16. Knapp TR, Kaplan EN, Danieks JR (1977) Injectable collagen for soft tissue augmentation. Plast Reconstr Surg 60:398–405
17. Stegman SJ, Tromovitch TA (1980) Implantation of collagen for depressed scars. J Dermatol Surg Oncol 6:450–453

18. Varnavides CK, Forster RA, Cunliffe WJ (1987) The role of bovine collagen in the treatment of acne scars. Br J Dermatol 116:199–206
19. Thrimbke JR (1983) Dermal overgarfting in dermatology. J Dermatol Surg Oncol 9:987–993
20. Dzubow LM (1985) Scar revision by punch-graft transplants. J Dermatol Surg Oncol 11:1200–1202
21. Besecker B, Hart CG (1999) A new treatment option for acne scars: allograft dermis. Dermatol Nurs 11:111–114
22. Goodman G (1997) Laser-assisted dermal grafting for the correction of cutaneous contour defects. Dermatol Surg 23:95–99
23. Mancuso A, Farber GA (1991) The abraded punch graft for pitted facial scars. J Dermatol Surg Oncol 17:32–34
24. Sulamanidze MA, Salti G, Mascceti M, Sulamanidze GM (2000) Wire scalpel for surgical correction of soft tissue contour defects by subcutaneous dissection. Dermatol Surg 26:146–150
25. Garrett AB, Dufresne RG Jr, Ratz JL, Berlin AJ (1990) Carbon dioxide laser treatment of pitted acne scarring. J Dermatol Surg Oncol 16:737–740
26. Alster TS, West TB (1996) Resurfacing of atrophic facial acne scars with a high-energy, pulsed carbon dioxide laser. Dermatol Surg 22:151–154
27. Alster TS, McMeekin TO (1996) Improvement of facial acne scars by the 585 nm flashlamp-pumped pulsed dye laser. J Am Acad Dermatol 35:79–81
28. Kye YC (1997) Resurfacing of pitted facial scars with a pulsed Er:YAG laser. Dermatol Surg 23:880–883
29. West TB (1997) Laser resurfacing of atrophic scars. Dermatol Clin 15:449–457
30. Manusciatti W, Fitzpatrick RE, Goldman MP (2000) Treatment of facial skin using combinations of CO2, Q-switched alexandrite, flashlamp-pumped pulsed dye, and Er:YAG lasers in the same treatment session. Dermatol Surg 26:114–120
31. Jordan R, Cummins C, Burls A (2000) Laser resurfacing of the skin for the improvement of facial acne scarring: a systematic review of the evidence. Br J Dermatol 142:413–423
32. Tsai RY, Wang CN, Chan HL (1995) Aluminum oxide crystal microdermabrasion. A new technique for treating facial scarring. Dermatol Surg 21:539–542
33. Goodman GJ (2003) Post acne scarring: a review. J Cosmet Laser Ther 5:77–95
34. Fulton JE Jr (1987) Modern dermabrasion techniques: a personal appraisal. J Dermatol Surg Oncol 13:780–789
35. Solotoff SA (1986) Treatment for pitted acne scarring–postauricular punch grafts followed by dermabrasion. J Dermatol Surg Oncol 12:1079–1084
36. Grevelink JM, White VR (1998) Concurrent use of laser skin resurfacing and punch excision in the treatment of facial acne scarring. Dermatol Surg 24:527–530
37. Fulton JE Jr (1996) Dermabrasion, chemabrasion, and laserabrasion. Historical perspectives, modern dermabrasion techniques, and future trends. Dermatol Surg 22: 619–628
38. Ayhan S, Baran CN, Yavuzer R, Latifoglu O, Cenetoglu S, Baran NK (1998) Combined chemical peeling and dermabrasion for deep acne and posttraumatic scars as well as aging face. Plast Reconstr Surg 102(4):1238–1246
39. Horton CE, Sadove RC (1987) Refinements in combined chemical peel and simultaneous abrasion of the face. Ann Plast Surg 19(6):504–511
40. Fintsi Y, Kaplan H, Landau M (1999) Whether to peel or laser for acne scarring and hyperpigmentation. Int J Cosmet Surg 7:67–70
41. Fintsi Y (1998) Exoderm chemabrasion: original method for the treatment of facial acne scars. Int J Cosmet Surg 6: 111–114
42. Wang KK, Lee M (1999) The principle of a three-staged operation in the surgery of acne scars. J Am Acad Dermatol 40(1):95–97
43. Atzori L, Brundu MA, Orru A, Biggio P (1999) Glycolic acid peeling in the treatment of acne. J Eur Acad Dermatol Venereol 12:119–122
44. Monheit GD (1996) Combination medium-depth peeling: the Jessner's+TCA peel. Facial Plast Surg 12(2): 117–124
45. Lee JB, Chung WG, Kwahck H, Lee KH (2002) Focal treatment of acne scars with trichloroacetic acid: chemical reconstruction of skin scars method. Dermatol Surg 28(11): 1017–1021
46. Al-Waiz MM, Al-Sharqi AI (2002) Medium-depth chemical peels in the treatment of acne scars in dark-skinned individuals. Dermatol Surg 28(5):383–387
47. Landau M (2005) Advances in deep chemical peels. Dermatol Nurs 17:438–441
48. Park JH, Choi YD, Kim SW et al (2007) Effectiveness of modified phenol peel (Exoderm) on facial wrinkles, acne scars and other skin problems of Asian patients. J Dermatol 34:17–24
49. Bagatin E, Dos Santos Guadanhim LR, Yarak S, Kamamoto CS, De Almeida FA (2010) Dermabrasion for acne scars during treatment with oral isotretinoin. Dermatol Surg 36(4):483–489

Rosacea

19

Stefano Veraldi, Alessandra Ferla Lodigiani, and Mauro Barbareschi

19.1 Introduction

Rosacea is an inflammatory, chronic-recurring dermatitis of the face in adults of both sexes. It is characterized clinically by the presence of one or more of the following features: recurrent-persistent flushing, erythema, telangiectasia, papules, pustules, and nodules. In addition, ocular involvement can occur. Modalities of appearance of rosacea are variable; however, first manifestations usually are flushing and erythema. Many patients also complain of stinging sensation; itching is rare.

19.2 Epidemiology

Rosacea is a common disease: The prevalence ranges from 1% up to 10% of the population. It affects mainly skin phototypes I and II, between 30 and 65 years of age. Rosacea is more frequent in females than in males, but it is more severe in males. Familiarity is reported in 15–30% of patients.

S. Veraldi (✉) • A.F. Lodigiani • M. Barbareschi
Department of Anesthesiology, Intensive Care and Dermatological Sciences, University of Milan, I.R.C.C.S. Foundation, Cà Granda Ospedale Maggiore Policlinico, Milan, Italy
e-mail: stefano.veraldi@unimi.it

19.3 Etiopathogenesis

Numerous factors have been considered in the etiopathogenesis of rosacea. However, none of them has been confirmed.

19.3.1 Race

Rosacea was considered very rare in blacks [1, 2]: Ayres [1], in 1988, wrote: "I do not recall that I have treated a black for acne rosacea". Afterward, other authors [3] observed 11 patients with dark skin out of 108 patients. It is possible that rosacea characterized by flushing, erythema, and telangiectasia is, simply, less visible on dark skin.

19.3.2 Vascular Abnormalities

Some authors [3] demonstrated, by means of laser-Doppler fluxmetry, that vessels in the papillary dermis of patients with rosacea are enlarged in comparison with controls.

19.3.3 Heat

Heat induces a peripheral vessel enlargement: Therefore, it can maintain and/or worsen a pre-existing rosacea, but it does not cause the disease.

A. Tosti et al. (eds.), *Color Atlas of Chemical Peels*,
DOI 10.1007/978-3-642-20270-4_19, © Springer-Verlag Berlin Heidelberg 2012

19.3.4 Diet and Alcohol

Epidemiological studies published so far do not sustain an etiopathogenetic role of specific food, such as spicy food, or drink [4].

19.3.5 Psychological Factors

Almost all authors state that rosacea can cause depression; however, the latter is not a cause of the disease [4].

19.3.6 Drugs

The etiopathogenetic role of corticosteroids, both topical and systemic [5, 6], is well known from the 1970s, when Leyden et al. [6] described ten patients who developed a rosaceiform dermatitis on the face following a prolonged application of fluorinated corticosteroids. These authors [6] named this clinical entity "steroid rosacea." Other drugs that can uncommonly cause rosacea or rosaceiform eruptions are peripheral vasodilators, vitamins B6 and B12, amiodarone [7] and pimecrolimus [8].

19.3.7 *Demodex folliculorum*

Etiopathogenetic role of *Demodex folliculorum* was for the first time supposed by Kaufmann-Wolf in 1925 [9]. In the past, several authors stated that this mite was present only in patients with rosacea. Subsequently, the presence of *Demodex folliculorum* also in healthy subjects supported the theory according to which this mite was not specific of rosacea, but was present mainly in patients with rosacea [3, 10–13]. Afterward, some authors [10, 11, 14, 15] stated that the amount in *Demodex folliculorum* is higher in patients with rosacea. A burden higher than 5 mites/cm^2 was considered as pathologic [10]. These results were not confirmed in all studies: Some authors [15] observed that only 10 out of 38 patients with rosacea had an amount of *Demodex folliculorum* higher than 5 mites/cm^2; in addition, 5 out of 38 controls had an amount higher than 5 mites/cm^2. Also other authors [12] did not observe significant differences in the number of mites in a group of patients with rosacea in comparison with two control groups. According to several authors, *Demodex folliculorum* would be more common in papulopustular [10, 11] and steroid rosacea [5, 14]. In 1981, Rufli et al. [13] observed that mite prevalence increases with the age and that the search for the mite is positive in almost 100% of elderly healthy subjects. These results were confirmed in a study by Crawford et al. [16], who stated that "*Demodex* is found in a large number of healthy persons. In fact, with modern and sensitive techniques, the prevalence in healthy adults approaches 100%. Consequently, the simple identification of *Demodex* is by no means proof of pathogenesis." Furthermore, at least four studies [13, 14, 17, 18] clearly demonstrated that specific therapies, both topical and systemic, against *Demodex folliculorum* do not reduce the amount of the mite, but they improve the disease according to the clinical point of view. On the basis of the results of all these studies, the search for *Demodex folliculorum* in a patient with rosacea is neither necessary nor helpful for therapy.

19.3.8 *Helicobacter pylori*

Factors that support a relationship between *Helicobacter pylori* and rosacea may be summarized as follows: (a) Prevalence of *Helicobacter pylori* infection in patients with rosacea is high [19–21]; (b) these patients have high titers of anti-*Helicobacter pylori* antibodies [22–24]; and (c) eradication of *Helicobacter pylori* is sometimes associated with a clinical improvement of rosacea [24–27]. Data against this association may be summarized as follows: (a) *Helicobacter pylori* is very common in the population; (b) differences in anti-*Helicobacter pylori* antibody titers between patients with rosacea and controls are very low [28, 29]; (c) eradication of *Helicobacter pylori* in patients with rosacea and *Helicobacter pylori* sometimes induces a clinical improvement of rosacea [30]; (d) the drugs used for *Helicobacter pylori* eradication are effective also for rosacea [31, 32] ;and (e) rosacea often improves only by topical drugs. Bamford et al. [30] stated that "Treating *H pylori* infection has no short-term beneficial effect on the symptoms of rosacea to support the suggested causal association between *H pylori* infection and rosacea." Also Crawford et al. [16] wrote that "robust support for a causal association between *H pylori* and rosacea does not exist." And finally, Jones [33], "*Helicobacter pylori* in rosacea: lack of an association."

19.4 Clinical Picture

In 2002, the National Rosacea Society Expert Committee [34] suggested a clinical classification of rosacea that includes four subtypes of the disease:

(a) Subtype 1: rosacea characterized by persistent flushing and erythema in the center of the face, with or without telangiectasia.
(b) Subtype 2: papulopustular rosacea: persistent erythema with papules, papulopustules, and pustules.
(c) Subtype 3: phymatous rosacea: The area most frequently involved is the tip of the nose (Fig. 19.1). Hyperseborrhea, persistent erythema, telangiectasia, papules, pustules, and nodules are the characteristic lesions; ears, forehead, cheeks, and chin may be less frequently involved.
(d) Subtype 4: ocular rosacea: It may be characterized by foreign body sensation, burning sensation, itching, xerophthalmia, photophobia, blurred vision, periocular edema, blepharitis, and conjunctivitis.

Furthermore, some authors add a glandular variety, characterized clinically by papules, large pustules, and sometimes nodules and cysts on the cheekbones and cheeks, especially in males. In addition, a granulomatous variety has been proposed: non-inflammatory papules and nodules, yellow, brown, or reddish in color, hard in consistency, located especially in perioral and submandibular areas.

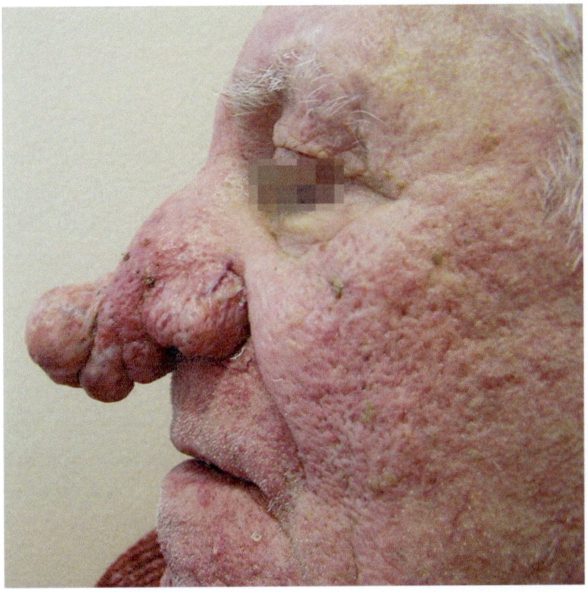

Fig. 19.1 Giant rhinophyma

19.5 Diagnosis and Differential Diagnosis

The diagnosis of rosacea is usually easy. There are no chemistry markers that can confirm a clinical diagnosis of rosacea.

Acne, folliculitis due to Gram-negative bacteria, fungi and yeasts, perioral dermatitis, and steatocystoma multiplex should be considered in differential diagnosis.

19.6 Therapy

19.6.1 Topical Therapy

19.6.1.1 Metronidazole

Metronidazole is a nitro-imidazole derivative with anti-inflammatory activity. It is mainly used in papulopustular rosacea, in which its efficacy, at a 0.75–1% concentration, is similar to that of oral tetracycline [35] as well as 15% azelaic acid [36]. Metronidazole is well tolerated: Local side effects (burning, dryness and redness) are uncommon and mild in severity [37]. Neither photoallergic nor phototoxic reactions have been reported so far [38].

19.6.1.2 Azelaic Acid

Azelaic acid is a saturated dicarboxylic acid. Its therapeutic effect in rosacea is likely based on the inhibition of the synthesis of reactive oxygen species by neutrophils. The efficacy of 15% azelaic acid gel is similar to that of 1% metronidazole gel [39, 40].

The only side effect is represented by a temporary and mild local burning sensation [41].

19.6.1.3 Topical Antibiotics

Topical antibiotics (erythromycin [42] and clindamycin [43]) are not commonly used in rosacea. They reduce neutrophil chemotaxis and oxygen-free radical synthesis [44]. These drugs are usually well tolerated: uncommon and mild side effects are erythema, dryness, and burning [45].

19.6.1.4 Benzoyl Peroxide

Used alone [46] or associated with clindamycin [47] or erythromycin [48], it showed to be effective in rosacea. Side effects are rather common (at least one-third of patients) and include erythema, dryness, scaling, and burning sensation [47].

19.6.1.5 Permethrin

Five percent permethrin significantly reduces the burden of *Demodex folliculorum* in the skin of patients with rosacea. Its efficacy is similar to that of 0.75% metronidazole gel [49, 50]. Also 10% crotamitone seems to be effective in papulopustular rosacea [51].

19.6.1.6 Sulfur

Commonly used in the past [52, 53], it is now less frequently employed. It can be used alone, at a concentration of 10% [54] or at 5% associated with 10% sodium sulfacetamide [55]. Burning, dryness, and redness are rather common side effects of sulfur-containing compounds [44].

19.6.1.7 Tretinoin

It may be used at different concentrations (from 0.01% to 0.05%, although 0.025% is the concentration most frequently used in rosacea). Its efficacy is comparable with oral isotretinoin at a daily dosage of 10 mg [56]. Side effects are much more frequent and severe than all the other topical drugs used in rosacea (burning, xerosis, redness, scaling). Because of these side effects, tretinoin is a second choice in rosacea.

19.6.1.8 Tacrolimus and Pimecrolimus

Literature data about these drugs in the treatment of rosacea are so far limited [57–59]. Some cases of rosacea induced by pimecrolimus were also reported [8]. Local side effects (burning and redness) are rather common and sometimes severe.

According to Cochrane [60], only metronidazole and azelaic acid showed to be effective in the topical treatment of rosacea.

19.6.2 Systemic Therapy

In a Cochrane study [60], 33 clinical studies on systemic therapy of rosacea were chosen, of which 8 were considered evaluable according to the methodological point of view [8]. On the basis of this study, only oral tetracyclines and metronidazole were considered effective in rosacea. Tetracyclines act as anti-inflammatory agents. In fact, they inhibit metalloproteases (MMP2, MMP9), phospholipase 2, and chemotaxis [61]. In addition, they inhibit synthesis and release of IL-1β, IL-6, and TNFα. The future of rosacea therapy may be based on the use of chemically modified tetracyclines (CMT).

Metronidazole proved to be effective by means of its anti-inflammatory activity (inhibition of ROS production by both neutrophils by xanthine–xanthine oxidase system).

Macrolides can be used in cases of intolerance, allergy, or contraindications to the use of tetracyclines (pregnancy, lactation, age <12 years). Erythromycin, clarithromycin, and azithromycin may be taken into consideration: They inhibit neutrophil chemotaxis and the synthesis of pro-inflammatory cytokines.

Oral isotretinoin can be used in patients with severe varieties of rosacea in whom only partial remissions with oral tetracyclines and metronidazole were obtained.

19.7 Peelings

Literature data about the use of peelings in rosacea are very poor. This is due to the fact that peelings can induce worsening of the disease, prolonged erythema, and delayed healing [62]. However, in very selected cases, some patients with mild varieties of papulopustular rosacea can improve by means of peelings with salicylic acid, azelaic acid, and mandelic acid [63].

Salicylic acid is an organic carboxylic acid with a hydroxyl group in position β. It can be used at concentrations ranging from 20% to 30% (rarely up to 50%).

Azelaic acid is sometimes used at a concentration of 30%, mainly in hyperseborrheic patients [64].

Mandelic acid is an α-hydroxy acid derived from almonds. It can be used alone or in combination with azelaic acid. It is considered a light peeling: Side effects (erythema, exfoliation, burning) are rare and mild in severity.

Before application, the skin should be cleaned with a solution of alcohol or ether or acetone. The application of the acid may be done with a brush, a gauze, or a cotton swab. The time in order to reach the frost varies according to the acid used: The frost period is longer for mandelic and azelaic acid. After the acid is buffered, aqueous solution at basic pH (10% sodium bicarbonate) should be applied. In following weeks, it is necessary to apply a daily photoprotection and moisturizing products. Local antibiotic therapy (2–3 applications/day for 7–10 days) after each peeling may be helpful.

References

1. Ayres S Jr (1988) Acne rosacea in blacks – were *Demodex* mites found in any patients? J Am Acad Dermatol 18:387–388
2. Rosen T, Stone MS (1987) Acne rosacea in blacks. J Am Acad Dermatol 17:70–73
3. Sibenge S, Gawkrodger DJ (1992) Rosacea: a study of clinical patterns, blood flow, and the role of *Demodex folliculorum*. J Am Acad Dermatol 26:590–593
4. Marks R (1968) Concepts in the pathogenesis of rosacea. Br J Dermatol 80:170–177
5. Basta-Juzbašić A, Šubić JS, Ljubojević S (2002) *Demodex folliculorum* in development of dermatitis rosaceiformis steroidica and rosacea-related diseases. Clin Dermatol 20:135–140
6. Leyden JJ, Thew M, Kligman AM (1974) Steroid rosacea. Arch Dermatol 110:619–622
7. Reifler DM, Verdier DD, Davy CL, Mostow ND, Wendt VE (1987) Multiple chalazia and rosacea in a patient treated with amiodarone. Am J Ophthalmol 103:594–595
8. Lübbe J, Stucky L, Saurat JH (2003) Rosaceiform dermatitis with follicular *Demodex* after treatment of facial atopic dermatitis with 1% pimecrolimus cream. Dermatology 207:205–207
9. Kaufmann-Wolf M (1925) Über regelmässiges vorkommen von *Demodex folliculorum* in den pusteln von rosacea pustulosa. Derm Wschr 81:1095–1103
10. Forton F, Seys B (1993) Density of *Demodex folliculorum* in rosacea: a case-control study using standardized skin-surface biopsy. Br J Dermatol 128:650–659
11. Georgala S, Katoulis AC, Kylafis GD, Koumantaki-Mathioudaki E, Georgala C, Aroni K (2001) Increased density of *Demodex folliculorum* and evidence of delayed hypersensitivity reaction in subjects with papulopustular rosacea. JEADV 15:441–444
12. Roihu T, Kariniemi AL (1998) *Demodex* mites in acne rosacea. J Cutan Pathol 25:550–552
13. Rufli T, Mumcuoglu Y, Cajacob A, Büchner S (1981) *Demodex folliculorum*: zur ätiopathogenese und therapie der rosazea und der perioralen dermatitis. Dermatologica 162:12–26
14. Bonnar E, Eustace P, Powell FC (1993) The *Demodex* mite population in rosacea. J Am Acad Dermatol 28:443–448
15. Erbağci Z, Özgöztaşi O (1998) The significance of *Demodex folliculorum* density in rosacea. Int J Dermatol 37:421–425
16. Crawford GH, Pelle MT, James WD (2004) Rosacea: I. Etiology, pathogenesis, and subtype classification. J Am Acad Dermatol 51:327–341
17. Persi A, Rebora A (1985) Metronidazole in the treatment of rosacea. Arch Dermatol 121:307–308
18. Robinson TWE (1965) *Demodex folliculorum* and rosacea. A clinical and histological study. Arch Dermatol 92: 542–544
19. Erel A, Öztaş M, İlter N, Senol E, Sultan N, Gürer MA (1995) *Helicobacter pylori* seroprevalence in patients with acne rosacea. JEADV 5(Suppl 1):S151
20. Rebora A, Drago F, Parodi A (1995) May *Helicobacter pylori* be important for dermatologists? Dermatology 191:6–8
21. Szlachcic A, Sliwowski Z, Karczewska E, Bielanski W, Pytko-Polonczyk J, Konturek SJ (1999) *Helicobacter pylori* and its eradication in rosacea. J Physiol Pharmacol 50:777–786
22. Argenziano G, Donnarumma G, Iovene MR, Arnese P, Baldassarre MA, Baroni A (2003) Incidence of anti-*Helicobacter pylori* and anti-CagA antibodies in rosacea patients. Int J Dermatol 42:601–604
23. Gürer MA, Erel A, Erbaş D, Çağlar K, Atahan C (2002) The seroprevalence of *Helicobacter pylori* and nitric oxide in acne rosacea. Int J Dermatol 41:768–770
24. Szlachcic A (2002) The link between *Helicobacter pylori* infection and rosacea. JEADV 16:328–333
25. Kolibášová K, Tóthová I, Baumgartner J, Filo V (1996) Eradication of *Helicobacter pylori* as the only successful treatment in rosacea. Arch Dermatol 132:1393
26. Rebora A, Drago F, Picciotto A (1994) *Helicobacter pylori* in patients with rosacea. Am J Gastroenterol 89:1603–1604
27. Utaş S, Özbakir O, Turasan A, Utaş C (1999) *Helicobacter pylori* eradication treatment reduces the severity of rosacea. J Am Acad Dermatol 40:433–435
28. Bamford J (2001) Rosacea: current thoughts on origin. Semin Cutan Med Surg 20:199–206
29. Sharma VK, Lynn A, Kaminski M, Vasudeva R, Howden CW (1998) A study of the prevalence of *Helicobacter pylori* infection and other markers of upper gastrointestinal tract disease in patients with rosacea. Am J Gastroenterol 93:220–222
30. Bamford JTM, Tilden RL, Blankush JL, Gangeness DE (1999) Effect of treatment of *Helicobacter pylori* infection on rosacea. Arch Dermatol 135:659–663
31. Bonamigo RR, Leite CS, Wagner M, Bakos L (2000) Rosacea and *Helicobacter pylori*: interference of systemic antibiotic in the study of possible association. JEADV 14:424–425
32. Mayr-Kanhauser S, Kranke B, Kaddu S, Mullegger RR (2001) Resolution of granulomatous rosacea after eradication of *Helicobacter pylori* with clarithromycin, metronidazole and pantoprazole. Eur J Gastroenterol Hepatol 13:1379–1383
33. Jones MP, Knable AL Jr, White MJ, Durning SJ (1998) *Helicobacter pylori* in rosacea: lack of an association. Arch Dermatol 134:511
34. Wilkin J, Dahl M, Detmar M, Drake L, Feinstein A, Odom R, Powell F (2002) Standard classification of rosacea: report of the National Rosacea Society Expert Committee on the classification and staging of rosacea. J Am Acad Dermatol 46:584–587
35. Sanchez J, Somolinos AL, Almodóvar PI, Webster G, Bradshaw M, Powala C (2005) A randomized, double-blind, placebo-controlled trial of the combined effect of doxycycline hyclate 20-mg tablets and metronidazole 0.75% topical lotion in the treatment of rosacea. J Am Acad Dermatol 53:791–797
36. Wolf JE Jr, Kerrouche N, Arsonnaud S (2006) Efficacy and safety of once-daily metronidazole 1% gel compared with twice-daily azelaic acid 15% gel in the treatment of rosacea. Cutis 77(Suppl 4):3–11
37. Ziel K, Yelverton CB, Balkrishnan R, Feldman SR (2005) Cumulative irritation potential of metronidazole gel compared to azelaic acid gel after repeated applications to healthy skin. J Drugs Dermatol 4:727–731
38. Beutner KR, Lemke S, Calvarese B (2006) A look at the safety of metronidazole 1% gel: cumulative irritation, contact sensitization, phototoxicity, and photoallergy potential. Cutis 77(Suppl 4):12–17

39. Elewski BE (2007) Rosacea trial comparing twice-daily azelaic acid gel 15% with once-daily metronidazole gel 1%. Cutis 79:57–58
40. Liu RH, Smith MK, Basta SA, Farmer ER (2006) Azelaic acid in the treatment of papulopustular rosacea: a systematic review of randomized controlled trials. Arch Dermatol 142:1047–1052
41. Draelos ZD (2004) Noxious sensory perceptions in patients with mild to moderate rosacea treated with azelaic acid 15% gel. Cutis 74:257–260
42. Mills OH Jr, Kligman AM (1976) Topically applied erythromycin in rosacea. Arch Dermatol 112:553–554
43. Wilkin JK, DeWitt S (1993) Treatment of rosacea: topical clindamycin versus oral tetracycline. Int J Dermatol 32:65–67
44. Shalita A, Leyden J (2004) Mechanism-based selection of pharmacologic agents for rosacea. Cutis 73(Suppl 1):15–18
45. Fisher AA (1983) Adverse reactions to topical clindamycin, erythromycin and tetracycline. Cutis 32:415, 419, 424, 428
46. Montes LF, Cordero AA, Kriner J, Loder J, Flanagan AD (1983) Topical treatment of acne rosacea with benzoyl peroxide acetone gel. Cutis 32:185–190
47. Breneman D, Savin R, VandePol C, Vamvakias G, Levy S, Leyden J (2004) Double-blind, randomized, vehicle-controlled clinical trial of once-daily benzoyl peroxide/clindamycin topical gel in the treatment of patients with moderate to severe rosacea. Int J Dermatol 43:381–387
48. Oztürkcan S, Ermertcan AT, Sahin MT, Af ar FS (2004) Efficiency of benzoyl peroxide-erythromycin gel in comparison with metronidazole gel in the treatment of acne rosacea. J Dermatol 31:610–617
49. Koçak M, Yaǧli S, Vahapoǧlu G, Ekşioǧlu M (2002) Permethrin 5% cream versus metronidazole 0.75% gel for the treatment of papulopustular rosacea. A randomized double-blind placebo-controlled study. Dermatology 205: 265–270
50. Signore RJ (1995) A pilot study of 5 percent permethrin cream versus 0.75 percent metronidazole gel in acne rosacea. Cutis 56:177–179
51. Rebora A (2002) The management of rosacea. Am J Clin Dermatol 3:489–496
52. Nally JB, Berson DS (2006) Topical therapies for rosacea. J Drugs Dermatol 5:23–26
53. Pelle MT, Crawford GH, James WD (2004) Rosacea: II. Therapy. J Am Acad Dermatol 51:499–512
54. Blom I, Hornmark AM (1984) Topical treatment with sulfur 10 per cent for rosacea. Acta Derm Venereol 64:358–359
55. Sauder DN, Miller R, Gratto D, Danby W, Griffiths C, Phillips SB (1997) The treatment of rosacea: the safety and efficacy of sodium sulfacetamide 10% and sulfur 5% lotion (Novacet) is demonstrated in a double-blind study. J Dermatol Treat 8:79–85
56. Ertl GA, Levine N, Kligman AM (1994) A comparison of the efficacy of topical tretinoin and low-dose oral isotretinoin in rosacea. Arch Dermatol 130:319–324
57. Bamford JT, Elliott BA, Haller IV (2004) Tacrolimus effect on rosacea. J Am Acad Dermatol 50:107–108
58. Cunha PR, Rossi AB (2006) Pimecrolimus cream 1% is effective in a case of granulomatous rosacea. Acta Derm Venereol 86:71–72
59. Goldman D (2001) Tacrolimus ointment for the treatment of steroid-induced rosacea: a preliminary report. J Am Acad Dermatol 44:995–998
60. Zuuren EJV, Graber MA, Hollis S, Chaudhry M, Gupta AK, Gover M (2005) Interventions for rosacea. Cochrane Database Syst Rev (3):CD003262
61. Sapadin AN, Fleischmajer R (2006) Tetracyclines: nonantibiotic properties and their clinical implications. J Am Acad Dermatol 54:258–265
62. Berson DS, Cohen JL, Rendon MI, Roberts WE, Starker I, Wang B (2009) Clinical role and application of superficial chemical peels in today's practice. J Drugs Dermatol 8:803–811
63. Lee HS, Kim IH (2003) Salicylic acid peels for the treatment of acne vulgaris in Asian patients. Dermatol Surg 29:1196–1199
64. Stinco G, Bragadin G, Trotter D, Pillon B, Patrone P (2007) Relationship between sebostatic activity, tolerability and efficacy of three topical drugs to treat mild to moderate acne. JEADV 21:320–325

Actinic Keratosis

20

Chikako Kaminaka, Yuki Yamamoto,
and Fukumi Furukawa

20.1 Definition

Actinic keratoses (AKs) are keratotic lesions occurring on chronically sun-exposed, middle-aged, and elderly skin. They represent focal areas of abnormal keratinocyte proliferation and differentiation that carry a low-risk progression to invasive squamous cell carcinoma (SCC). AK of the lip is known as actinic cheilitis, and usually affects the lower lip, which is more sun-exposed.

20.2 Epidemiology and Etiology

Evidence suggests that most AKs are the result of excessive exposure to solar ultraviolet (UV) radiation. In addition, UVB-specific p53 mutations have been observed in AKs, providing molecular evidence in support of a role for sunlight [1].

The prevalence of these lesions is high in many countries, and is influenced by the amount of ambient UV, and the proportion of susceptible individuals in the population.

They occur predominantly on chronically sun-exposed skin, such as the face and the dorsum of hands, and in fair-skinned individuals (especially Fitzpatrick's skin type 1 and 2) [2]. There is also a high prevalence among those receiving chronic immune suppression as organ transplant recipients [3]. AKs are intraepidermal skin tumors, and a risk factor for SCC development. It has been estimated that an invasive SCC develops in 8% of patients with AK [4]. When left untreated, 0.025–20% of AKs are likely to progress to invasive SCC [5, 6].

20.3 Clinical Types

AKs usually occur in middle-aged or elderly subjects on habitually sun-exposed areas such as the face, scalp, and dorsum of the hands. These lesions are usually multiple, and are comprised of either erythematous macules or papules with a rough scaly surface resulting from disorganized keratinization (Figs. 20.1–20.6). Lesions vary in size from less than 1 mm to over 2 cm, and are usually asymptomatic. In some cases, scaling may be prominent, and in time may become thick and horny.

In 2007, a clinical classification for grading AK (Grades 1, 2 and 3) was developed by Rowert-Huber J et al. Grade 1 describes slightly palpable AK (better felt than seen), Grade 2 represents moderately thick AK (easily felt and seen), and Grade 3 represents very thick, hyperkeratotic and/or obvious lesions. The clinical diagnosis between grade 3 AK and early invasive SCC is subject to variable clinical interpretation. A similar scheme for the histological grading of AK has also been established [7].

20.4 Histopathology

There is a disorderly arrangement and maturation of the epithelial cells. Multiple buds of epithelial cells may occur at the membrane zone, but no invasion is seen.

C. Kaminaka (✉) • Y. Yamamoto • F. Furukawa
Department of Dermatology, Wakayama Medical University, 811-1 Kimiidera, Wakayama 641–0012, Japan
e-mail: kamikami@wakayama-med.ac.jp

A. Tosti et al. (eds.), *Color Atlas of Chemical Peels*,
DOI 10.1007/978-3-642-20270-4_20,

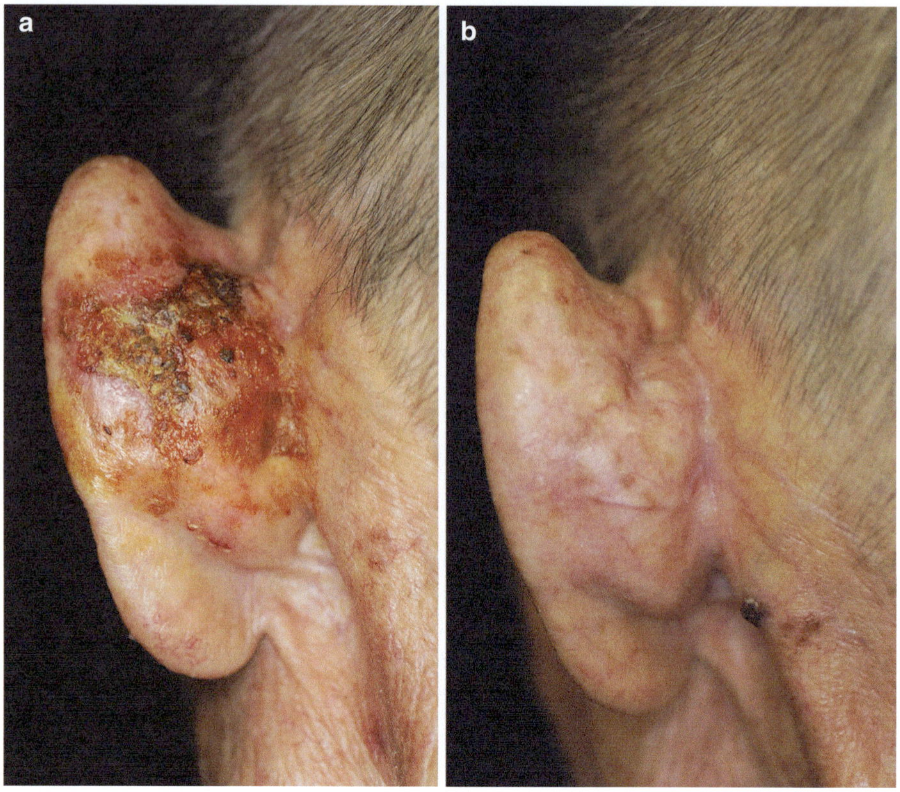

Fig. 20.1 Clinical changes in hypertrophic type actinic keratosis (AK) in a 76-year-old male. (**a, b**) AK on the ear, in which a complete response (CR) was achieved 3 years after three phenol peel sessions. (**a**) Macroscopic appearance before treatment, and (**b**) macroscopic appearance after treatment

Several histological variants of AK have been described, including hypertrophic, bowenoid, lichenoid, acantholytic, and pigmented.

20.5 Diagnostic Criteria

Most AKs are diagnosed clinically, and are rarely confirmed histologically. The diagnosis is usually based on clinical findings which take into account the morphology of the individual lesions and the clinical setting.

20.6 Differential Diagnosis

Diagnosis is frequently made on clinical appearance alone, but the differential diagnoses include superficial BCC, Bowen's disease, early SCC, and even amelanotic melanoma. A skin biopsy may be indicated in selected cases where there is clinical doubt or the suspicion of invasive malignancy. Other diagnoses that need to be considered, particularly in patients with large confluent areas of erythema and scaling, can sometimes cause AK to be mistaken for focal areas of lichen planus. When AK is pigmented, it may resemble a superficial seborrheic keratosis, but can usually be distinguished from such lesions by the lack of organization of the hyperkeratosis.

20.7 Therapy

The treatment of AK lesions commonly involves focal or multiple ablative procedures such as cryotherapy, laser, curettage/excision/shave biopsy, and chemical peel. Large area treatments include topical therapies (mainly using topical 5-fluorouracil (5-FU), imiquimod, or diclofenac 3% gel) and photodynamic therapy (PDT), which have demonstrated efficacy in the treatment of AK in evidence-based studies [8, 9].

Cryotherapy: Cryotherapy is a simple, low cost technique using liquid nitrogen that is useful for the removal of focal lesions. However, some patients find its side effects, including blistering, scarring, and pain, to be unacceptable.

Laser therapy: Carbon dioxide laser therapy is difficult and requires experience with the technique, where the skin is destroyed to a controlled depth.

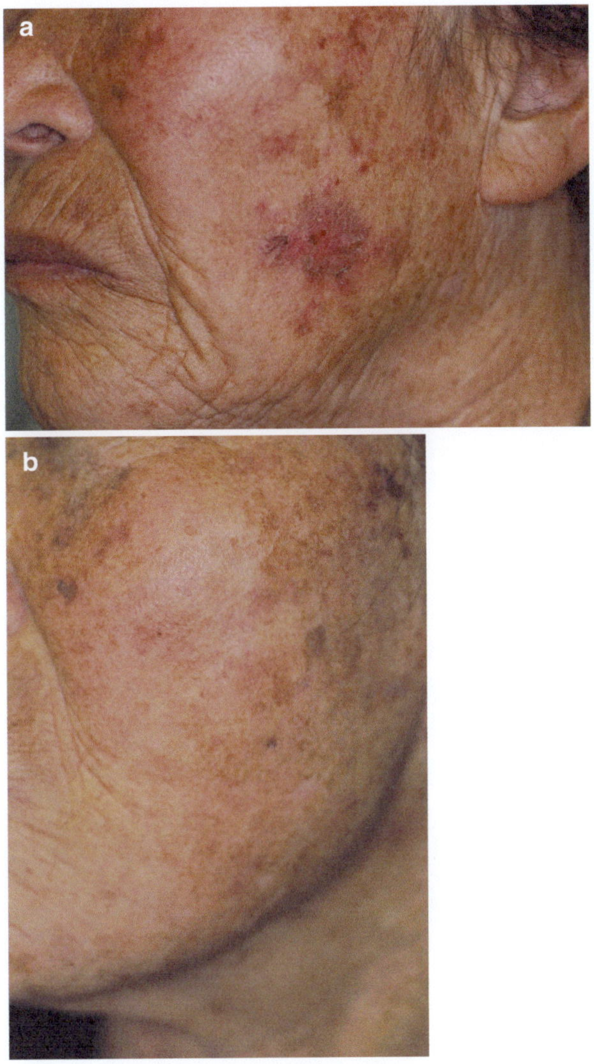

Fig. 20.2 Clinical changes in bowenoid-type actinic keratosis (AK) in an 87-year-old female. (**a, b**) AK on the lower cheek, in which a complete response (CR) was achieved 1.5 years after three phenol peel sessions. (**a**) Macroscopic appearance before treatment, and (**b**) macroscopic appearance after treatment

Although it has good cosmetic results, there is also pain associated with this technique, which may be less acceptable to patients.

Curettage/Excision/Shave biopsy: These techniques are of value in determining the exact histology of proliferative or atypical AKs unresponsive to other therapies, and where invasive SCC is suspected. However, these treatments require local anesthesia, and may result in epidermal changes and scarring.

Topical therapy: 5-FU, a chemotherapy drug, destroys AK cells by blocking essential cellular functions. Imiquimod cream is a topical immune response modifier. Imiquimod is more expensive than 5FU. Although these treatments are very effective, the marked local inflammation that commonly develops after 2–4 weeks of treatment makes it unacceptable to some patients. Diclofenac gel has moderate efficacy with low morbidity in mild AK cases.

PDT: PDT requires a dedicated light source in combination with the application of a photosensitizing cream, 5-aminolaevulinic acid (5-ALA). Although PDT is effective in up to 91% of AKs with consistently good cosmetic results, it is also costly in terms of clinical time and requires special hardware in the form of lamps [9].

20.8 Chemical Peels

20.8.1 Indications

The wounding agent application technique produces a controlled wound and reepithelialization. Medium-depth peeling refers to the application of a caustic agent or combination of agents that will routinely produce an injury that penetrates into the upper reticular dermis (depth of peel: 450 μm). These peels are usually performed as a single therapeutic procedure to treat AK, and the clinical improvements are proportionate to the depth of the agent's (or phenol) penetration. The depth of penetration depends on the strength of the wounding agent, the amount applied, the skin thickness, and the location. Before performing chemical peels, it is important to meet with the patient to discuss the various risks, benefits, alternatives, complications, and expectations of the procedure.

20.8.2 Types

Medium-depth and deep peels

This involves applying one or more chemical solutions.

1. *Phenol*: (unoccluded 100% pure phenol): (Figs. 20.1–20.4) Phenol is commonly used to treat ingrown toenails. Furthermore, deep peels using phenol are one of the most effective chemical peeling methods for elderly skin tumor patients [10–13]. Phenol injures tissues from the papillary dermis to the upper reticular dermis [10]. Our previous results suggest that phenol quickly penetrates into the skin, and induces

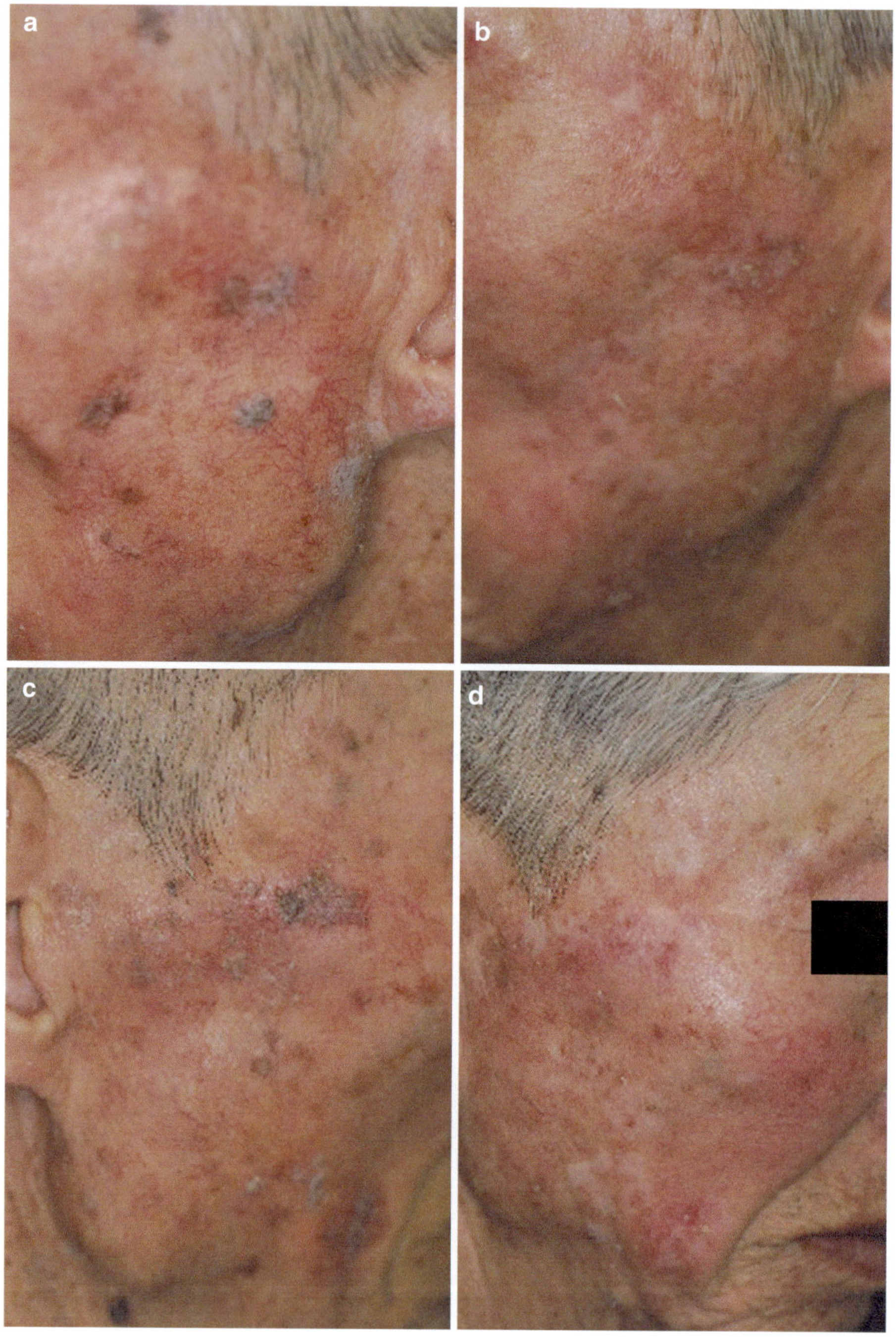

Fig. 20.3 Clinical changes in multiple actinic keratosis (AK) in an 82-year-old male. Multiple AK on the cheeks, in which a complete response (CR) was achieved 1.5 years after three phenol peel sessions. (**a, c**) Macroscopic appearance before treatment, and (**b, d**) macroscopic appearance after treatment

endothelial cell damage more rapidly than keratinocyte damage [14, 15]. It is likely that the apoptosis of endothelial cells in the dermis induces the ischemic changes, eventually resulting in epidermal necrosis [16, 17]. When absorbed systemically, phenol may cause serious side effects such as cardiac toxicity, liver and kidney damage, and respiratory depression [18]. During this procedure, systemic changes must be carefully monitored using a cardiac monitor. These side effects correlate strongly with the duration of the procedure and the peeled surface area. Actually, no arrhythmias have been reported in patients with < 50% facial peels, or in any full facial peel that lasted more than 60 min [19, 20]. Moreover, blood phenol concentrations did not reach toxic levels in patients treated with phenol peels [17].

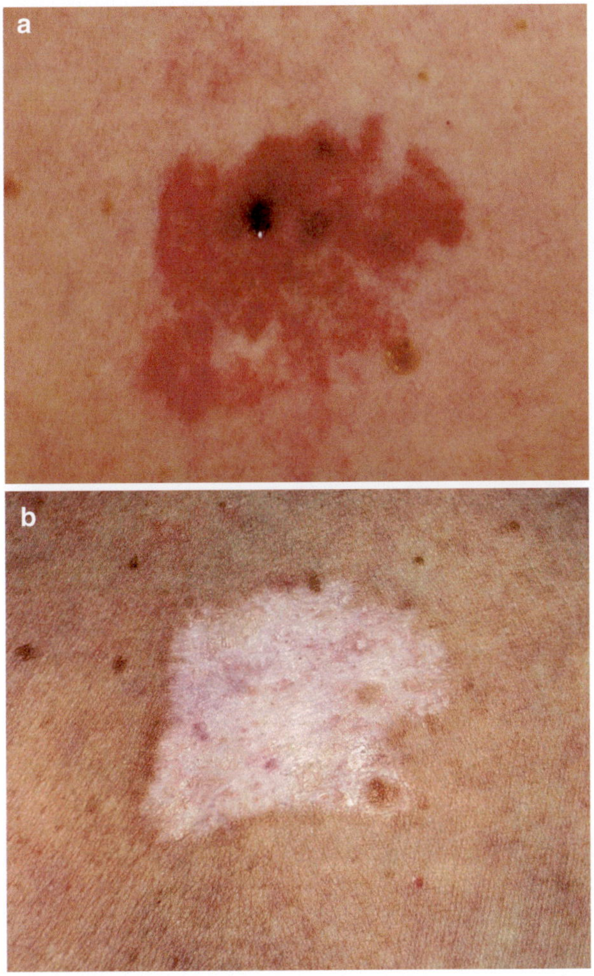

Fig. 20.4 Clinical changes in actinic keratosis (AK) in a 67-year-old female. (**a, b**) AK on the left cheek, in which a complete response (CR) was achieved 2.5 years after three phenol peel sessions. (**a**) Macroscopic appearance before treatment, and (**b**) hypopigmentation after treatment

2. *60% Trichloroacetic acid (TCA)* (Figs. 20.5 and 20.6): The 60% TCA peel has produced similar results in patients in whom phenol is contraindicated or undesired. TCA is a keratocoagulant. TCA may be applied more rapidly than phenol, but it is more likely to produce hypertrophic scarring (Fig. 20.6) [21].
3. *Combination medium-depth TCA peeling:* Since the TCA procedure tends to produce increased scarring and hypopigmentation with higher concentrations, the use of a more superficial epidermal peeling agent such as solid CO_2 [22], Jessner's solution [23], or 70% glycolic acid prior to the application of 35%TCA will produce a wound equivalent in depth to 60%TCA or pure phenol.

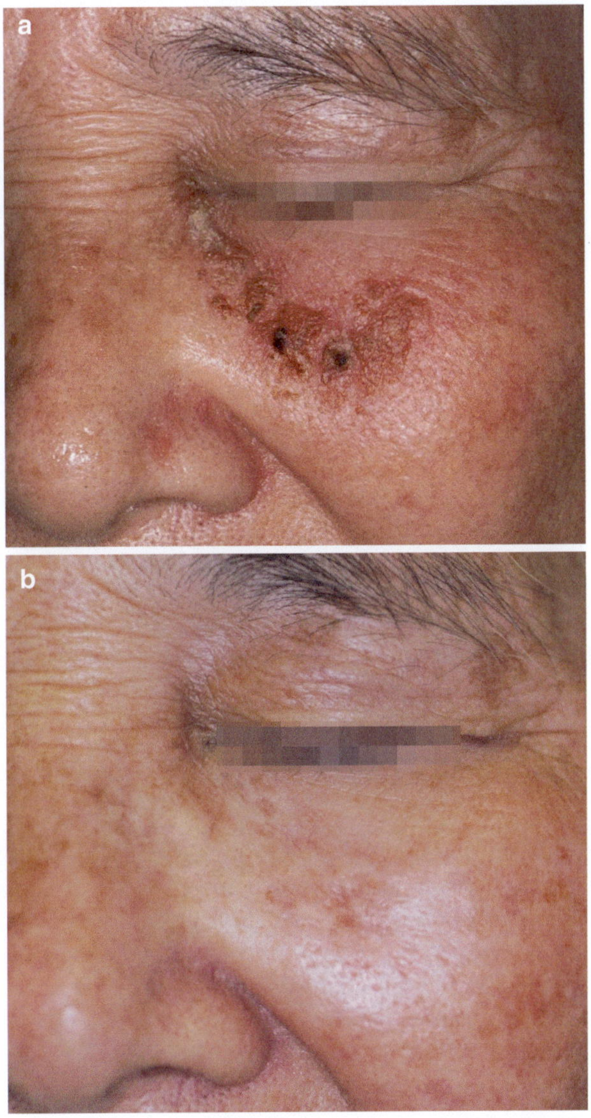

Fig. 20.5 Clinical changes in actinic keratosis (AK) in a 75-year-old female. (**a, b**) AK on the upper cheek, in which a complete response (CR) was achieved 3 years after three sessions of 60%TCA peeling. (**a**) Macroscopic appearance before treatment, and (**b**) macroscopic appearance after treatment

Recently, it was suggested that long-term, frequent peels with a low concentration of TCA might increase the risk of mutations, eventually leading to tumorigenesis [24]. Furthermore, in an ultraviolet B–irradiated mouse model, SCCs could be detected at a relatively higher incidence at peripheral sites of TCA painting [24].

Based on these histological findings and the historical safety of phenol use in medicine, patients with AK are mainly treated with phenol peels [25, 26].

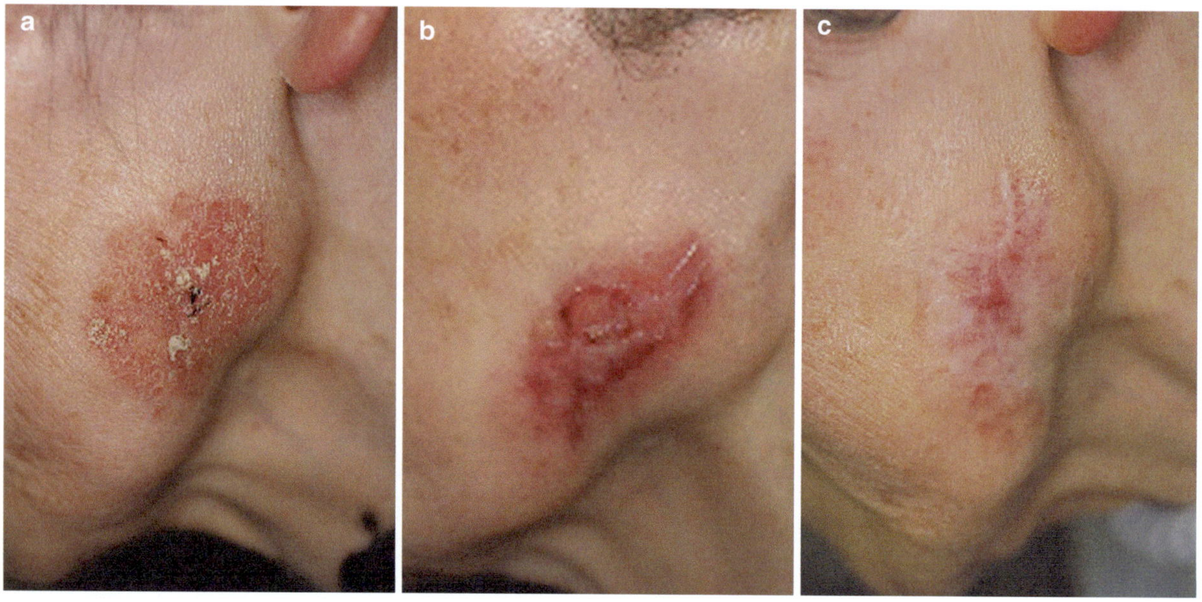

Fig. 20.6 Clinical changes in actinic keratosis (AK) in an 83-year-old female. (**a–c**) AK with thin skin on the lower jaw, in which a complete response (CR) was achieved 3 years after two sessions of 60%TCA peeling. (**a**) Macroscopic appearance before treatment, and (**b**) a hypertrophic scar with erythema occurring 3 months after treatment. (**c**) The scar remained 3 months after treatment

20.8.3 Frequency

Chemical peels are performed in accordance with established protocols, as previously described [12]. Briefly, the wounding agent is applied locally to lesions once a month up to a maximum of 8 months. After removing excess oil from the skin using acetone, the superficial crust or keratin is first removed with light curettage, and then the wounding agent is applied directly to the lesions using cotton-tipped applicators until an even white frosting appears. The subjects are examined monthly with clinical, photographic, and dermoscopic documentation by three individual clinicians.

The treatment is discontinued when a lesion achieves a complete response (CR), and the response can be maintained for at least a 1-year follow-up period. In those cases in which there is progressive disease (PD) during the follow-up period, the treatments were terminated and the lesions were surgically resected. The steps of the procedure are summarized in Fig. 20.7.

20.8.4 Advantages

When comparing noninvasive therapies with standard surgical interventions, one can easily accept that phenol peels have several advantages from the viewpoint of procedural ease, time efficiency, special equipment, therapeutic costs, pain control, and posttreatment follow-up. Moreover, chemical peels can be applied repeatedly at frequent intervals. In addition, we have reported on other possible uses of these techniques such as for neoplastic squamous (skin) lesions or superficial basal cell carcinoma [27], and stated that appropriate peeling controls and pre-peeling biopsy results are mandatory.

20.8.5 Contraindications

1. *History of cardiac and/or hepatorenal disease.* Prior to treatment, laboratory studies including blood pressure, complete blood counts, serum electrolytes, blood coagulation tests, liver function tests, urinalyses, chest X-rays, and electrocardiography are required.
2. Fitzpatrick skin types 4–5, or black skin.
3. For medium-depth and deep peels: any history of abnormal scarring or keloids.
4. Active bacterial, viral, fungal, or herpetic infections.
5. Preexisting inflammatory dermatoses such as psoriasis or atopic dermatitis.
6. Uncooperative patients (patient is careless about sun exposure or the application of medicine).
7. Patients with unrealistic expectations.

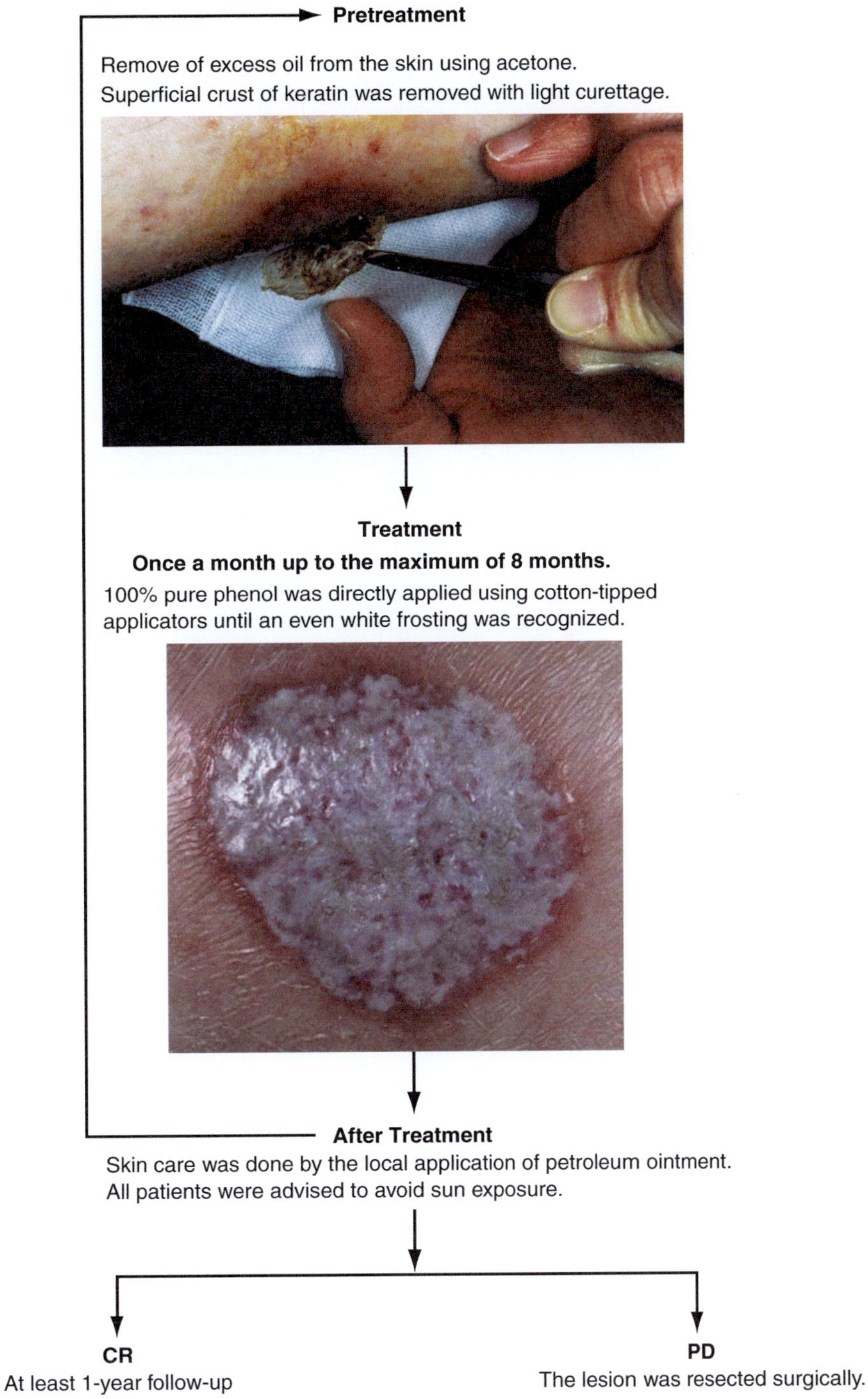

Fig. 20.7 Steps of the phenol peeling procedure

20.9 Results

We found that phenol peels caused a CR in 29 out of 32 cases (90.6%) [25]. Among those 29 cases, 28 cases (16 treated 1–2 times, 10 treated 3–5 times, 2 treated 6–8 times) showed no skin lesion recurrences for more than 1 year during the follow-up period (Figs. 20.1–20.7). However, there was only one (3.4%) recurrence following phenol treatment during the 1-year follow-up period. A medical history of other skin neoplasia would require more peeling sessions to achieve a CR. If we consider previous reports [24, 25], we can

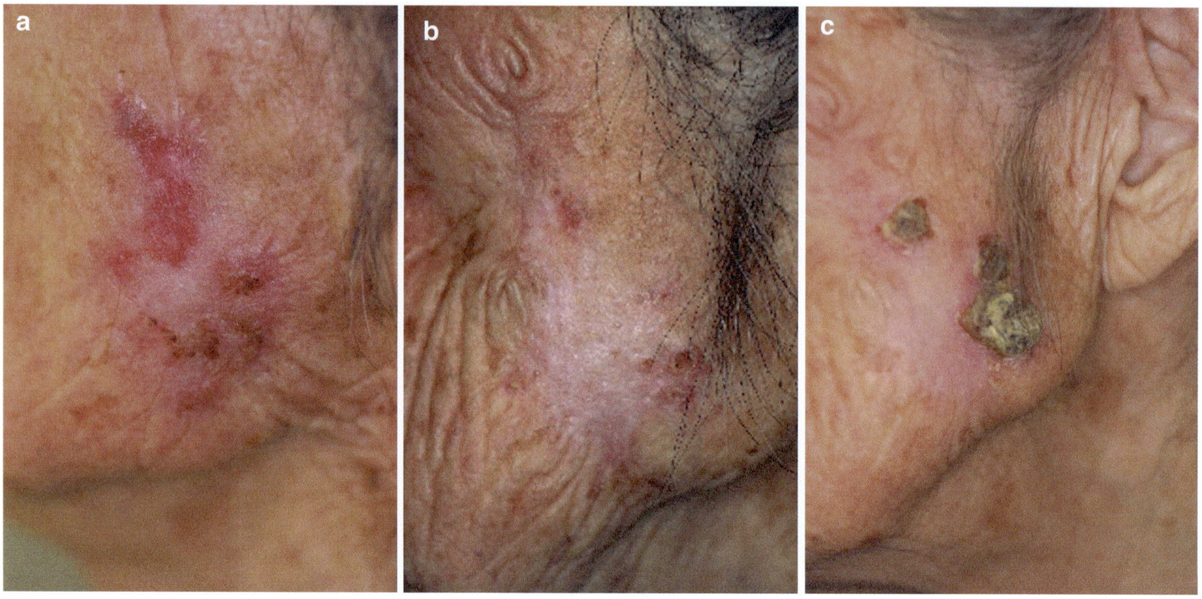

Fig. 20.8 Clinical changes in actinic keratosis (AK) in a 94-year-old female. (**a–c**) A case of AK on the face that progressed. After 7 phenol peel sessions, the lesion was surgically resected. (**a**) Macroscopic appearance before treatment, and (**b**) macroscopic appearance 9 months after treatment. (**c**) The AK which progressed 1 year after treatment

conclude that phenol peels will not cause tumorigenesis in CR cases.

Our data indicate that this clinical improvement was correlated with a decrease in the tumor thickness, and the histological depth of tumor cell injury approached a maximum of 164.2 ± 18.4 μm to 346.4 ± 43.5 μm thickness in tumor tissues. In the present study, the tumor thickness of the PD patients was 570.7 ± 164.7 μm, implying that the phenol peel might not be recommended for the treatment of >400-μm thick tumor tissues in AKs (such as grade 3 AK: Figs. 20.8 and 20.9).

20.9.1 Management of the Patient

Many options are open to patients with AKs. Ultimately, the physician should determine the treatment chosen for individual patients following a careful evaluation of the circumstances presented by the patient.

UVB radiation increases the presence of lesions, and thus, all patients should be advised to avoid sun exposure as much as possible.

In some patients, one or several AKs are persistent and/or recurred despite treatment, and thus, surgical excision should be considered.

20.9.2 Complications

1. *Toxicity:* Although rare, toxicity may occur with phenol of extensive application. When absorbed systemically, phenol may cause serious side effects such as cardiac toxicity (cardiac arrhythmias), liver and kidney damage, and respiratory depression [18].
2. *Pigment changes:* Postinflammatory hyperpigmentation and hypopigmentation may occur (Fig. 20.4). Skin reactions such as melanocyte cytotoxicity is a more serious side effect of phenol peeling in Asian patients [28, 29]. Medium-depth and deep peels are not recommended for dark skins of types 4–5 because of the high risk of prolonged pigment changes. Hypopigmentation after phenol is commonly observed, and is directly proportional to the amount of phenol applied and the degree of occlusion [28]. This pigment change can be very

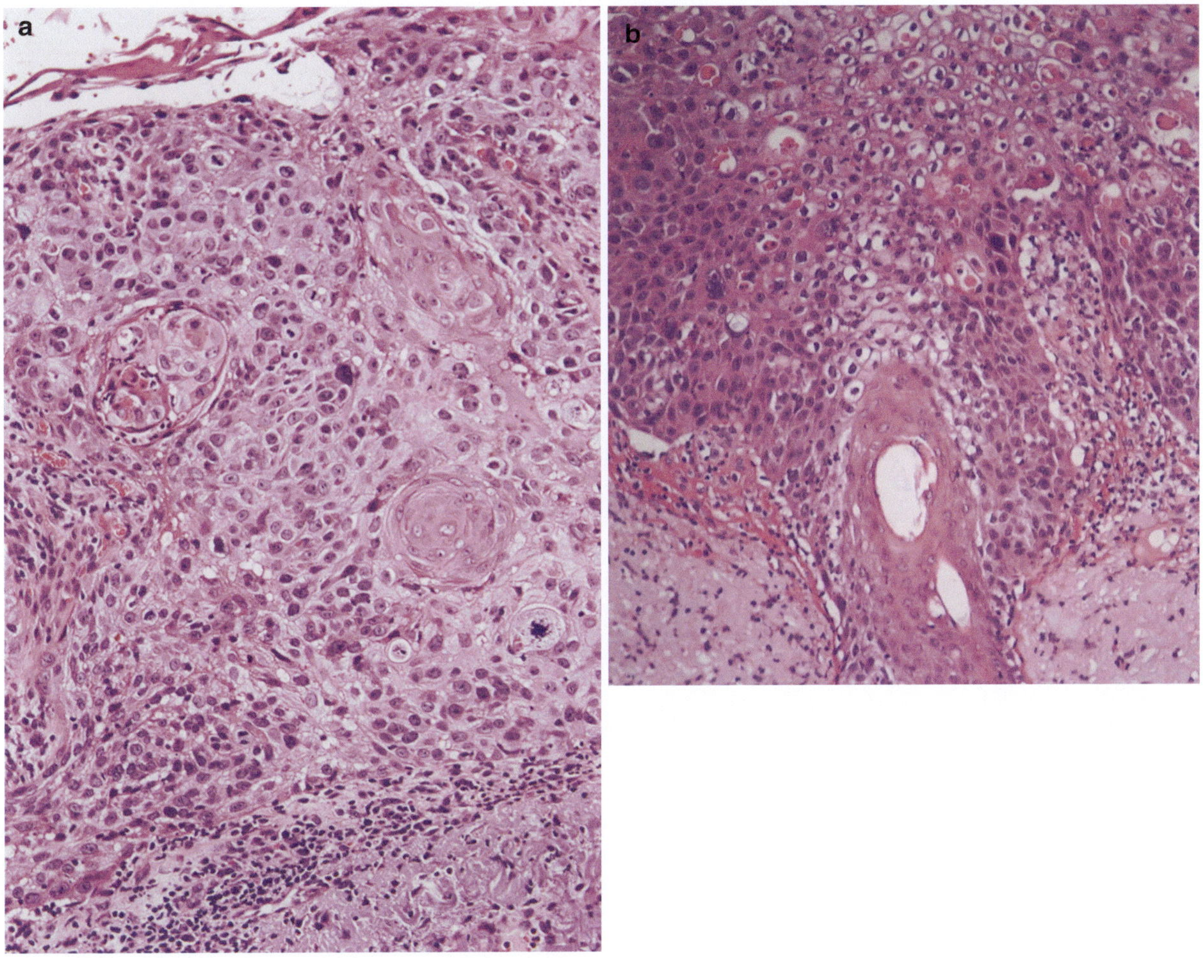

Fig. 20.9 Histological photographs of actinic keratosis (AK) (HE, original magnification: ×200). (**a, b**) The AK on the face was progressive. (**a**) Before treatment, the tumor thickness was 693 μm. (**b**) After treatment, an invasive squamous cell carcinoma was found

persistent and often difficult to treat. Although the skin reactions were tolerable, these possibilities should be explained to the patients prior to the procedure.

3. *Persistent erythema:* Erythema persisting for more than 3 weeks after a peel can occur, and should be treated with topical corticosteroids.
4. *Scarring and keloids:* Scarring remains to be the most dreadful complication of chemical peels (Fig. 20.6). The most common location of the scars is in the lower part of the face. Racially dark individuals have a higher incidence of hypertrophic scarring, and may disclose a family history of this tendency. Delayed healing and persistent erythema are important and alarming signs for forthcoming scarring.
5. *Infection: Active bacterial, viral, fungal or herpetic infection:* Bacterial and fungal complications in chemical peels are rare (Fig. 20.10). Topical antibiotics and antiviral treatment with acyclovir or valacyclovir should be introduced as soon as this diagnosis is made. Toxic shock syndrome has been reported after an occluded Baker's phenol face peel.

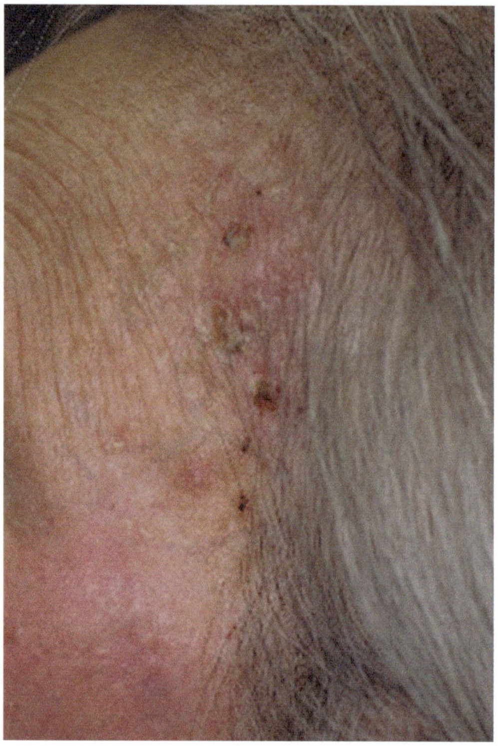

Fig. 20.10 Fungal infection following phenol peel on the forehead

Acknowledgments This work was supported by a Grant in aid from the Japanese Ministry of Education, Culture, Sports and Technology (#19659286 to FF).

References

1. Zeigler A, Jonason AS, Leffell DJ et al (1994) Sunburn and p53 in the onset of skin cancer. Nature 372:773–776
2. Freeman RG (1968) Carcinogenic effect of solar radiation and prevention measures. Cancer 21:11114–11120
3. Barr BB, Benton EC, McLaren K et al (1989) Human papillomavirus infection and skin cancer in renal allograft recipients. Lancet 2:224–225
4. Glogau RG (2000) The risk of progression to invasive disease. J Am Acad Dermatol 42:23–24
5. Collen JP, Bickers DR, Moy RL (1997) Actinic keratoses. J Am Acad Dermatol 36:650–653
6. Dodson JM, DeSpain J, Hewett JE et al (1991) Malignant potential of actinic keratoses and the controversy over treatment. A patient-oriented perspective. Arch Dermatol 127:1029–1031
7. Rowert HJ, Patel MJ, Foschner T et al (2007) Actinic keratosis is an early in situ squamous cell carcinoma: a proposal for reclassification. Br J Dermatol 156:8–12
8. Stockfleth E, Ferrandiz C, Grob J et al (2008) Development of a treatment algorithm for actinic keratoses: a European Consensus. Eur J Dermatol 18:651–659
9. de David B, Jane MM, Hughest BR (2007) Guidelines for the management of actinic keratoses. Br J Dermatol 156:222–230
10. Furukawa F, Yamamoto Y (2006) Recent advances in chemical peeling in Japan. J Dermatol 33:655–661
11. Hurwitz DJ, Pincus L, Kupper TS (2003) Imiquimod. A topically applied link between innate and acquired immunity. Arch Dermatol 139:1347–1350
12. Brody HJ (1997) Chemical peeling and resurfacing, 2nd edn. Mosby, St. Louis, Missouri, pp 29–38
13. Yamamoto Y, Ohtani T, Uede K et al (2003) Phenol and trichloroacetic acid peeling is a new tool as non-invasive therapy to the aged patients with skin cancer. J Invest Dermatol 121:1205, Abstract
14. Yamamoto Y, Uede K, Yonei N et al (2003) Expression of tenascin and human β-1 integrin in the skin peeled with phenol or trichloroacetic acid. Aesthet Dermatol 13:17–24
15. Yamamoto Y, Uede K, Ueda M et al (2002) Characterization of monoclonal anti-human skin basal cell antibody 3B 4–6 and its reactivity to the skin peeled with phenol or trichloroacetic acid (TCA). Aesthet Dermatol 12:70–76
16. Yamamoto Y, Yonei N, Kaminaka C et al (2004) Effects of phenol peeling on dermal endothelial cells. J Dermatol Sci 35:158–161
17. Yamamoto Y, Uede K, Otani T et al (2006) Different apoptotic patterns observed in tissues damaged by phenol and TCA peels. J Dermatol Sci supp. 2:75–81
18. Stuzin JM (1998) Phenol peeling and the history of phenol peeling. Clin Plast Surg 25:1–19
19. Peters W (1991) The chemical peel. Ann Plast Surg 26:564–571
20. Truppman ES, Ellenby JD (1979) Major electrocardiographic changes during chemical peeling. Plast Reconstr Surg 63:44–48
21. Brodland DG, Roenigk RK (1988) Trichloroacetic acid chemexfoliation (chemical peel) for extensive premalignant actinic damage of the face and scalp. Mayo Clin Proc 63:887–896
22. Brody HJ, Hailey CW (1986) Medium-depth chemical peeling of the skin: a variation of superficial chemosurgery. J Dermatol Surg Oncol 12:1268–1275
23. Monheit GD (1989) The Jessner's+TCA peel: a medium-depth chemical peel. J Dermatol Surg Oncol 15:945–950
24. Dainichi T, Koga T, Furue M et al (2003) Paradoxical effect of trichloroacetic acid (TCA) on ultraviolet B-induced skin tumor formation. J Dermatol Sci 31:229–231
25. Yamamoto Y, Uede K, Yonei N et al (2007) Expression patterns of proliferating cell nuclear antigen in trichloroacetic acid peeled skin. J Dermatol 34:95–98
26. Kaminaka C, Yamamoto Y, Yonei N et al (2009) Phenol peels as a novel therapeutic approach for actinic keratosis and Bowen disease: prospective pilot trial with assessment of clinical, histologic, and immunohistochemical correlations. J Am Acad Dermatol 60:615–625
27. Kaminaka C, Yamamoto Y, Furukawa F (2007) Nevoid basal cell carcinoma syndrome successfully treated with trichloroacetic acid and phenol peeling. J Dermatol 34:841–843
28. Fitzpatrick RE, Tope WD, Goldman MP et al (1996) Pulsed carbon dioxide laser, trichloroacetic acid, Baker-Gordon phenol, and dermabrasion: a comparative clinical and histologic study of cutaneous resurfacing in porcine model. Arch Dermatol 32:469–471
29. Kligman AM, Baker TJ, Gordon HL (1985) Long-term histologic follow-up of phenol face peels. Plast Reconstr Surg 75:652–659

Chemical Peels in Dark Skin

21

Pearl E. Grimes

21.1 Definition

Dark skin is a commonly used phrase to describe people of color. Other terms used to describe darker skin types include ethnic skin, brown skin, and pigmented skin. The unifying feature represented is pigmented skin (i.e., shades of tan, olive, brown, and black). Such individuals are often classified as Fitzpatrick's skin types IV through VI. These individuals represent many of the faces of North America, South America, Africa, the Caribbean, Asia, Malaysia, and Australia.

21.2 Epidemiology

The new U.S. Census data on diversity in America were reported in 2011. The U.S. Census Bureau estimated that by 2010 the total resident US population included 50.5 million Hispanic Americans (16%); 38.9 million African Americans (13%); 15.2 million Asians and Pacific Islanders (5%); and 2 million Native Americans, Eskimos, and Aleuts (0.9%). Statistical projections suggest continuing major growth of the non-white US population, with Hispanics having the most significant growth rate [1]. People of color comprise a substantial percentage of the global population. They include Africans, Hispanics, Pacific Islanders, Asians, East Indians, Aleuts, Eskimos, Middle Easterners, Caribbeans, Arabs, and Malaysians.

21.3 Morphologic and Physiologic Skin Differences in Dark Skin

Myriad morphologic and physiologic features define pigmented skin (Table 21.1). Although there are no quantitative differences in melanocytes among various racial/ethnic groups, the melanocytes of darker-skinned individuals, in particular black skin, produce more epidermal melanin. Melanosomes are often large and singly dispersed within melanocytes and keratinocytes [2–4]. Melanosomes are distributed throughout the epidermis in black skin, whereas in whites, they are limited to the basal and lower malpighian layer of the epidermis. Melanosomes in whites and Asians are smaller and often aggregated and membrane bound, whereas in black skin, they are most often singly dispersed within melanocytes and keratinocytes. Dark skin (i.e., black skin) has more stage IV melanosomes. The transmission of ultraviolet radiation (UVA and UVB) through white and black skin has been assessed [5]. On an average, five times as much ultraviolet light reached the upper dermis of whites than in blacks. Differences in transmission between the stratum corneum of blacks and whites were less striking. The increased epidermal melanin content of black skin serves as a significant filter for blocking ultraviolet light transmission. In addition, other reported differences include increased stratum corneum cell layers, increased desquamation, increased lipid content,

P.E. Grimes
Division of Dermatology, Department of Medicine, David Geffen School of Medicine, University of California—Los Angeles, Vitiligo and Pigmentation Institute of Southern California, 5670 Wilshire Blvd., Suite 650, Los Angeles, CA 90036, USA
e-mail: pegrimesmd@earthlink.net

A. Tosti et al. (eds.), *Color Atlas of Chemical Peels*,
DOI 10.1007/978-3-642-20270-4_21, © Springer-Verlag Berlin Heidelberg 2012

Table 21.1 Morphological features of deeply pigmented skin

Increased stratum corneum layers
Often individually dispersed melanosomes
Decreased Vitamin D production
Thick compact dermis
Large and numerous fibroblasts

decreased ceramide content, and increased recovery time after tape stripping [6].

Dark skin demonstrates significantly greater intrinsic photoprotection because of the increased content of epidermal melanin. Clinical photodamage, actinic keratoses, rhytides, and skin malignancies are less common problems in deeply pigmented skin. However, darker skin types are frequently plagued with dyschromias because of the labile responses of cutaneous melanocytes [7]. In a survey of 2000 black patients seeking dermatologic care in a private practice in Washington, DC, the third most commonly cited skin disorders following acne and eczema were pigmentary problems other than vitiligo [8]. Of these patients, the majority had a diagnosis of postinflammatory hyperpigmentation, followed in frequency by melasma. In a survey of 100 women of color assessing issues of cosmetic concerns for darker skin types, the most commonly cited problems were dark spots or blotchy skin, texturally rough skin, and increased sensitivity to topical products [9]. Patients surveyed also complained of oily skin. Wrinkles and photodamage were significantly less frequent issues of cosmetic concern when the data was compared to an age-matched Caucasian population of 141 women.

21.4 Peeling Indications in Dark Skin

Given the basic morphologic and physiologic differences in light compared to darker skin types, peel indications differ. Key indications in Fitzpatrick's skin types I, II, and III include photodamage, rhytides, acne, scarring, and the dyschromias characterized by hyperpigmentation. In contrast, survey data suggest that key indications in darker skin types include disorders of hyperpigmentation such as melasma and postinflammatory hyperpigmentation, acne, pseudofolliculitis barbae, textural charges, oily skin and wrinkles, and photodamage.

Despite major concerns regarding peel complications such as postinflammatory hyperpigmentation, hypopigmentation, and scarring in darker racial/ethnic groups, recent studies suggest that peeling procedures, particularly superficial procedures, can be performed safely in darker racial/ethnic groups [10]. These peels induce epidermal and papillary dermal wounding (Fig. 21.1).

21.5 Histology of Peeling Agents

Grimes [11] compared the histologic alterations induced by a variety of chemical peels in 17 patients with skin types IV, V, and VI, including glycolic acid 70%, salicylic acid 30%, Jessner's solution, and 25% and 30% TCA. Peels were applied to 4 × 4 cm areas of the back and 2 × 2 cm postauricular sites. Biopsies were performed at 24 h (Fig. 21.2a–d). Glycolic acid induced the most significant stratum corneum necrosis. Compared to the other tested peels, salicylic acid and Jessner's peels caused mild lymphohistiocytic der-

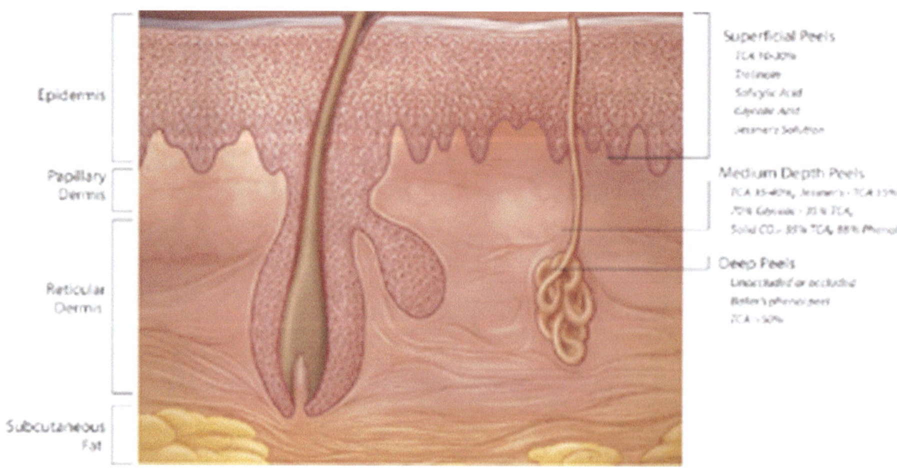

Fig. 21.1 Illustration of the depth of wounding caused by peeling agents

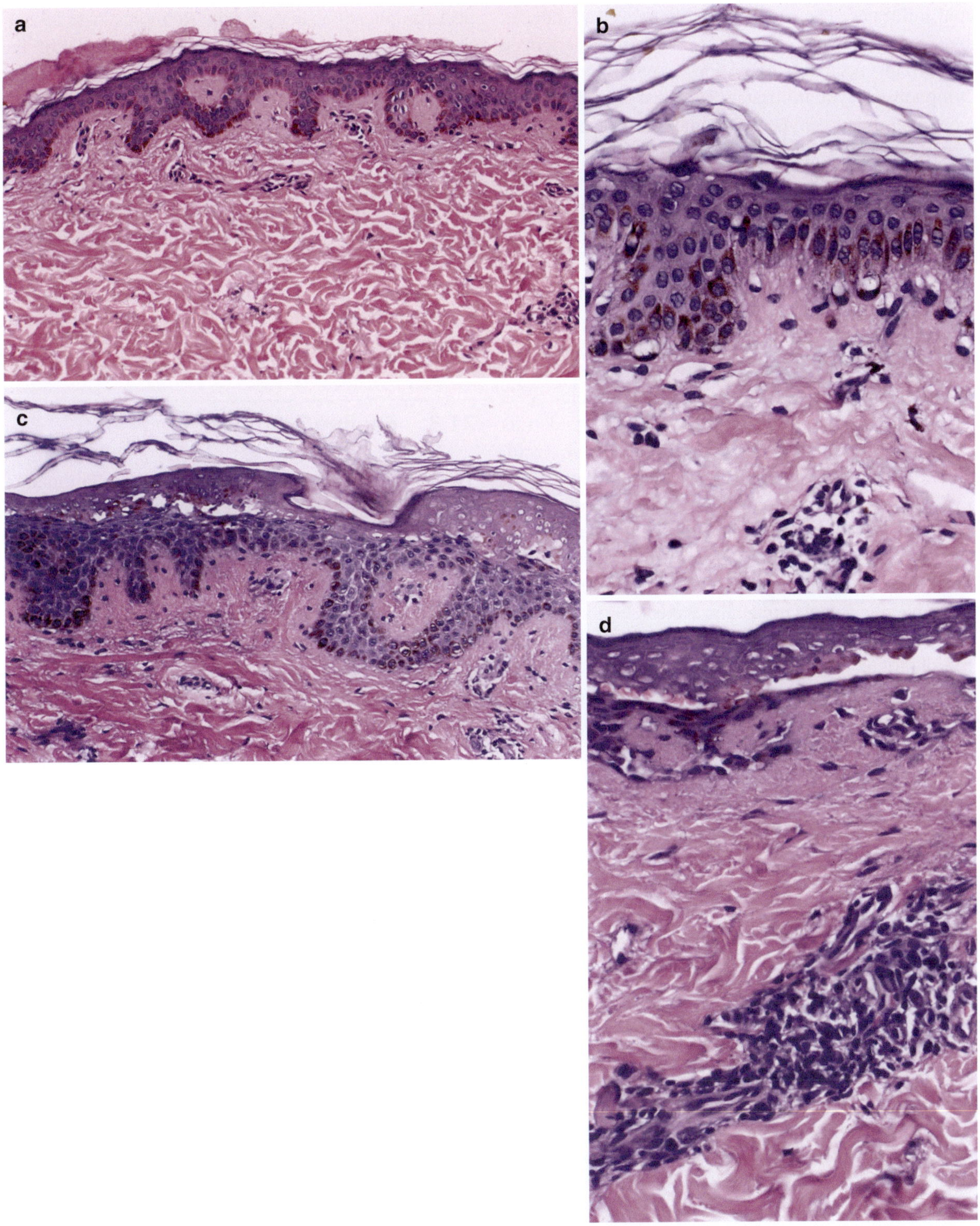

Fig. 21.2 (**a–d**) Hematoxylin/eosin stains of biopsies of back skin taken 24 h post chemical peeling. (**a**) Glycolic acid peel 70%. Note stratum corneum necrosis. (**b**) Salicylic acid 230%. Note mild lymphohistiocytic infiltrate. (**c**) 35% TCA-induced mid-epidermal wounding/separation. (**d**) 30% TCA peel caused deep epidermal separation

mal infiltrates. The most severe damage was induced by 25% TCA and 30% TCA, which caused deep epidermal necrosis and dense papillary dermal lymphohistiocytic infiltrates. TCA test sites developed postinflammatory hyperpigmentation. These findings corroborate our clinical experience using these agents. In general, glycolic, salicylic acid, and Jessner's peels induce a lower frequency of postpeeling complications compared to 25% and 30% superficial TCA peels.

21.6 Peel Selection

Chemical peeling agents are classified as superficial, medium-depth, or deep peels [13]. Superficial peels target the stratum corneum to the papillary dermis (Fig. 21.1). They include glycolic acid, salicylic acid, Jessner's solution, tretinoin, and trichloroacetic acid (TCA) in concentrations of 10–30%. Medium-depth peels penetrate to the upper reticular dermis and include TCA (35–50%) combination glycolic acid 70%/TCA 35%, Jessner's/TCA 35%, and phenol 88%. Deep chemical peels utilize the Baker-Gordon formula and penetrate to the midreticular dermis. Analyses of morphologic, physiologic, and clinical data (see introduction) suggest that the benefits of chemical peeling in dark skin can be maximally achieved utilizing superficial peels while simultaneously minimizing risks.

21.7 Peeling Preparation

Despite some general predictable outcomes, there is tremendous variability in the reactivity and responses to chemical peels. Even superficial chemical peeling can cause hyperpigmentation and scarring in susceptible individuals. Therefore, the author always performs the initial peel with the lowest concentration of the peeling agent to assess the patient's sensitivity and reactivity. The author's standard protocol involves initial pretreatment for 2–4 weeks with 4% hydroquinone formulations. Higher strength formulations (5–10%) can be compounded for recalcitrant hyperpigmentation. Azelaic acid or kojic acid formulations are used if patients are experiencing irritation or hypersensitivity to hydroquinone. Tretinoin, tazarotene, or retinol is often used to treat acne, hyperpigmentation, or photodamage in darker skin types. However, these agents should be discontinued 1–2 weeks prior to peeling to avoid postpeel complications in dark skin. Retinoids increase epidermal turnover, and they increase the depth of the peeling agent. This may be a desired effect in skin types I–III; however, in dark skin, increasing the depth of the peel may result in excessive erythema, crusting, desquamation, and postinflammatory hyperpigmentation. Topical bleaching agents which do not contain retinoids and lower-strength alpha-hydroxy acids, polyhydroxy acids, and beta-hydroxy acids can be continued up to 1 or 2 days prior to peeling. These are less aggressive agents compared to retinoids. Superficial peels are performed at 2- to 4-week intervals and a series of three to six superficial peels are routinely performed.

21.8 Peeling Techniques

The author has observed significant postinflammatory hyperpigmentation with even low concentrations of superficial peeling agents. Hence, cautious titration is appropriate in darker skin types. Glycolic acid peels are titrated from 20% to 35%, 50%, and finally 70%. Similar titration methods are used for salicylic acid and TCA. Salicylic acid peels should be titrated from 20% to 30%. Despite the use of higher concentrations of TCA in some studies [12, 13], it is best to initiate TCA peeling in dark skin with low concentrations (i.e., 10–15%). Postpeel care includes the use of bland cleansers and emollients until irritation and peeling subsides. The patient then resumes the use of topical skin care products and bleaching agents. Postpeel reactions such as excessive erythema, desquamation, and irritation are treated with low- to high-potency topical steroids. Clearing usually occurs on 5–7 days.

21.9 Superficial Peeling Agents

21.9.1 Glycolic Acid

Glycolic acid, an alpha-hydroxy acid (AHA), has become the most widely used organic carboxylic acid for skin peeling. Glycolic acid formulations include buffered, partially neutralized, and esterified products. Concentrations for peeling range from 20% to 70%. Several published studies have assessed the efficacy of glycolic acid peels in darker-skinned racial/ethnic groups. A series of ten Asian women with melasma and fine wrinkles were treated with 2% hydroquinone and 10% glycolic acid applied to both sides of the face [14]. A series of 20–70% glycolic peels were performed on one side for comparison. Greater improvement with minimal side effects was noted on the side treated with the series of glycolic acid peels. Forty Asian patients with moderate to moderately severe acne were treated with a series of 35–70% glycolic acid peels [15]. The investigators noted significant improvement in skin texture and acne. Side effects were reported in 5.6% of patients.

Nineteen black patients with postinflammatory hyperpigmentation were treated with glycolic acid peeling [16]. The control group was treated with 2% hydroquinone/10% glycolic acid twice a day and tretinoin 0.05% at bedtime, whereas the active peel group received the same topical regimen plus a series of six serial glycolic acid peels. Although not statistically significant, greater improvement was noted in the chemical peel group.

The safety and efficacy of a series of glycolic acid facial peels were investigated in 25 Indian women with melasma [17]. Patients were treated with 50% glycolic acid peels monthly for 3 months. Improvement was noted in 91% of patients with maximal clearing occurring in patients classified with epidermal melasma. Side effects were observed in one patient who developed brow hyperpigmentation.

In a separate study, the combination of glycolic acid peels with a topical regimen for the treatment of melasma was assessed in a series of dark-skinned patients with melasma [18]. The authors compared the efficacy of serial glycolic acid peeling with a series 3–30% glycolic peels and 3–40% peels in combination with a modified Kligman bleaching regimen (hydroquinone 5%, hydrocortisone acetate 1% and tretinoin 0.05%) to the use of the modified Kligman formulation alone. Forty women were included in each group. Both groups showed a statistically significant improvement in the Melasma Area Severity Index (MASI) score at 21 weeks. However, maximal improvement occurred in the group treated with the series of glycolic acid peels in combination with the topical bleaching regimen.

Glycolic acid peels are well tolerated in darker-skinned racial/ethnic groups (Figs. 21.3a, b and 21.4a, b). Side effects are substantially minimized when concentrations are gradually titrated from the lower concentrations of 20–35% to the full-strength 70% peel. Glycolic acid peels are most advantageous when treating darker skin types with sensitive skin.

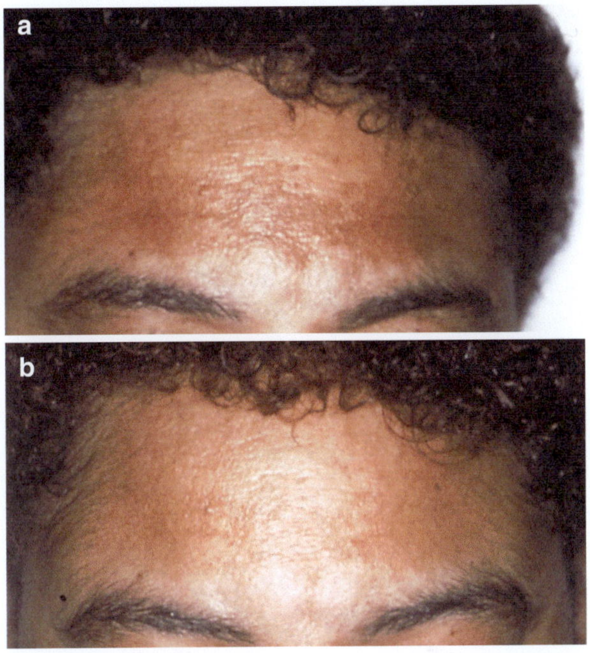

Fig. 21.3 (**a**) Forehead postinflammatory hyperpigmentation. (**b**) Significant improvement in forehead hyperpigmentation following a series of glycolic acid 20–50% peels

21.9.2 Salicylic Acid

Salicylic acid has been formulated in a hydroethanolic vehicle at concentrations of 20% and 30% for use as a superficial peeling agent [19]. It is a lipophilic agent that produces desquamation of the upper lipophilic layers of the stratum corneum. Grimes [20] treated 25 patients with skin types V and VI with salicylic acid peels. Conditions treated included acne vulgaris, postinflammatory hyperpigmentation, rough, oily skin with textural changes, and melasma (Figs. 21.5a, b and 21.6a, b). Patients were pretreated for 2 weeks with hydroquinone 4%, followed by a series of two 20% and three 30% salicylic acid peels. Peels were performed biweekly. Moderate to significant improvement was observed in 88% of the patients treated. Minimal to mild side effects occurred in 16%. Three patients experienced hyperpigmentation that resolved in 7–14 days. Thirty-five Korean patients with facial acne were treated biweekly for 12 weeks with 30% salicylic acid peels [21]. Both inflammatory and non-inflammatory lesions were significantly improved. In general, the peel was well tolerated with few side effects.

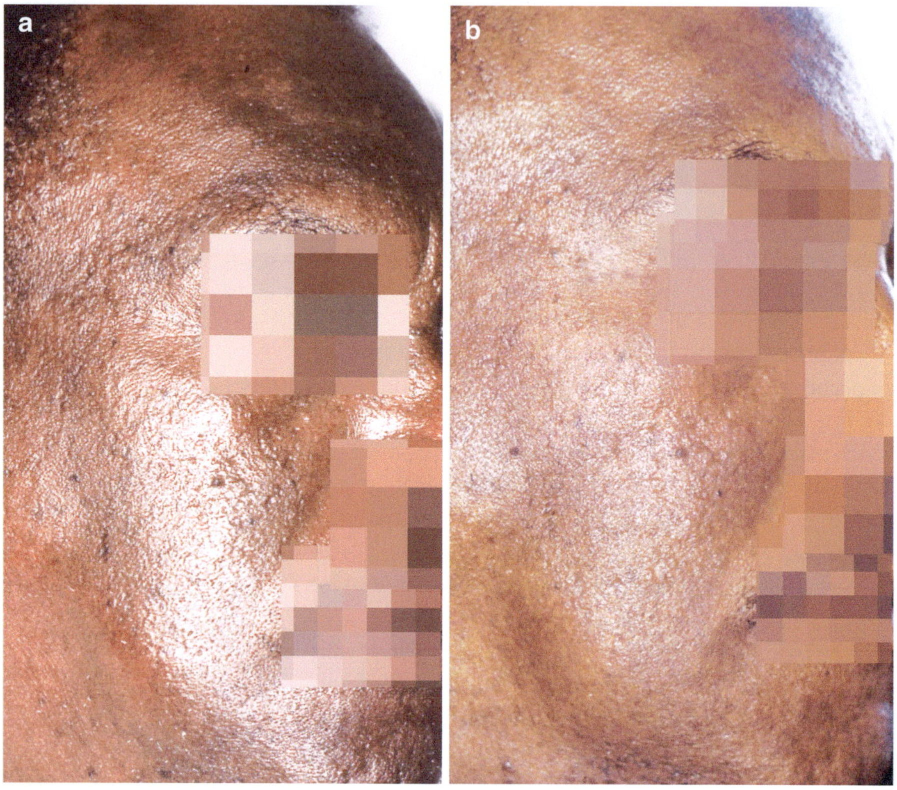

Fig. 21.4 (**a**, **b**) Significant improvement after a series of five glycolic acid 20–70% peels

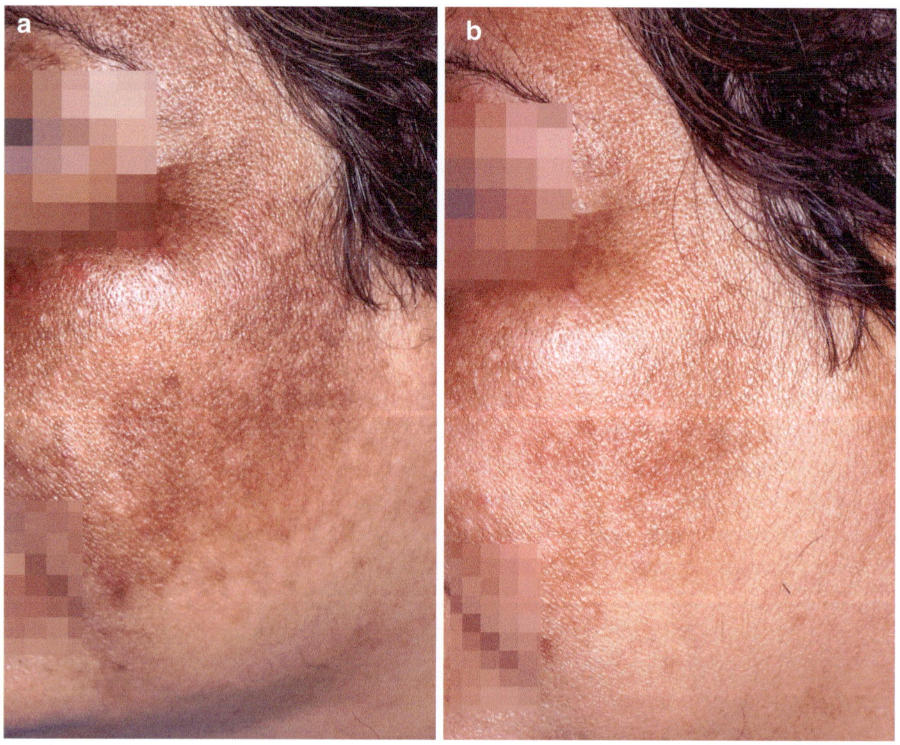

Fig. 21.5 (**a**, **b**) Moderate improvement in melasma after a series of two 15% TCA peels plus hydroquinone 6%

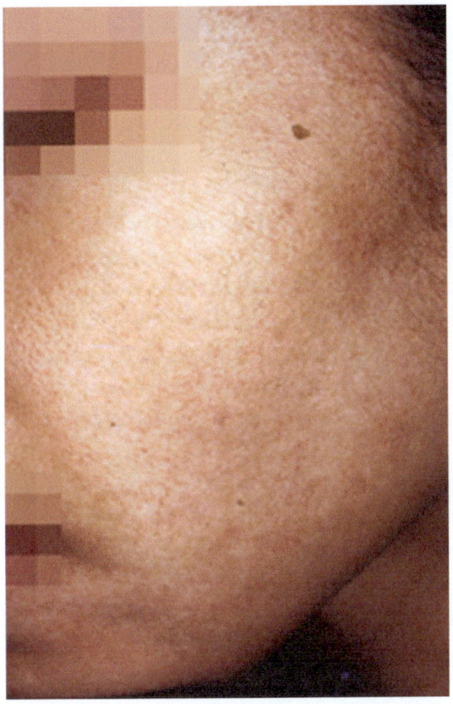

Fig. 21.6 Postpeel persistent hypopigmentation following a 35% TCA peel

The author has observed enhanced improvement of oily skin, enlarged pores, and acne vulgaris and with salicylic acid peels compared to glycolic acid peels. Possible mechanisms for this observation include salicylic acid's effect on lipid solubility and microcomedone formation.

21.9.3 Jessner's Solution

Jessner's solution contains 14% resorcinol, 14% salicylic acid, and 14% lactic acid. Jessner's solution has been used alone for superficial peeling, or in combination with TCA 35% to achieve a medium-depth peel. Increasing the number of coats applied to the treated area increases the depth and reaction induced by the Jessner's peel. These peels are well tolerated with minimal side effects in the author's practice. As with glycolic acid and salicylic peels, Jessner's peels are most commonly used as adjunctive therapy for moderate to severe facial dyschromias, acne, oily skin, texturally rough skin, fine wrinkles, and pseudofolliculitis barbae.

Lawrence et al. [22] compared the efficacy of Jessner's solution and 70% glycolic acid in a split-face study of 16 patients. Of the total group, five were skin type IV, three were skin type V, and one was skin type VI. There was no statistically significant difference in improvement between the two groups. The investigator did not report an increased frequency of side effects in patients of skin types IV–VI.

21.9.4 Tretinoin Peeling

Tretinoin 1% has also been used as a chemical peeling agent [23, 24]. The efficacy of tretinoin peels was compared to glycolic acid peels in the treatment of melasma in dark-skinned patients [24]. In a split-face study of ten Indian women, 1% tretinoin was applied to one half of the face, while 70% glycolic acid was applied to the opposite side. Peels were performed weekly. Significant improvement occurred on both sides as assessed by photographs and a Modified Melasma Area and Severity Index Score. However, there were no significant differences between the tretinoin-peeled side and the glycolic acid–treated areas. Side effects despite the weekly frequency of peel applications were minimal throughout the 12-week study.

21.9.5 Trichloroacetic Acid

TCA peels were first described by Roberts in 1926. Many consider TCA the gold standard by which other peels are measured. Concentrations of 10–30% are used for superficial peeling. TCA precipitates epidermal proteins, causing sloughing and necrosis of the treated area. The extent of damage is concentration dependent. In contrast to glycolic acid, Jessner's solution, and salicylic acid, there is a substantially smaller window of safety when TCA peels are applied to skin types IV–VI. The frequency of postpeel hyperpigmentation is significantly more common in dark skin. Therefore, the author only uses TCA peels in patients recalcitrant to glycolic acid, salicylic acid, or Jessner's peels. TCA peels are cautiously used in darker-skinned patients. Indications include wrinkles, photodamage, stubborn pigmentation, and scarring.

In a histometric, immunohistochemical and ultrastructural study, TCA peeling in concentrations of

10%, 20%, and 30% was compared to dermabrasion in nine dark-skinned patients (Fitzpatrick's IV and V) with photodamage [25]. Both procedures induced increasing amounts of Types I and III collagen. However, the most prominent changes were observed in the group treated with dermabrasion.

There is minimal published data on the use of combination peeling protocols in deeply pigmented skin (Fitzpatrick skin types IV through VI). The author has reported the efficacy of combination peeling with salicylic acid 20% and 30% in combination with 10% TCA for recalcitrant melasma patients. This peeling regimen was well tolerated with minimal side effects in darker racial/ethnic groups (see Salicylic Acid/TCA section).

21.9.6 Medium and Deep Peels

Medium-depth and deep peels utilize TCA concentrations of 40% or greater or phenol combinations. Medium-depth peels also utilize glycolic acid 70% or Jessner's solution in combination with 35% TCA. Combination medium-depth peels are often used to treat moderate to severe photodamage. Fifteen Middle Eastern patients with atrophic or pitted acne scars were treated with a combination of Jessner's solution and 35% TCA peeling [11]. All patients were of light brown to dark brown complexion. Six percent had excellent improvement, 53% moderate improvement. Mild improvement was noted in 27%. Nine patients (73.4%) developed transient postinflammatory hyperpigmentation which resolved after 3 months. Patients with light brown complexions did not develop hyperpigmentation. In the author's experience, aggressive peels of this nature have a substantially greater likelihood of inducing persistent hyperpigmentation and hypopigmentation in darker skin types.

Clinicians should be acutely aware that deeper peels carry substantial risks of inducing scarring and hypopigmentation in darker-skinned racial/ethnic groups (Fig. 21.6).

21.10 Summary

In contrast to the previous decade, chemical peels are commonly performed in darker racial/ethnic groups, individuals comprising skin types IV–VI (Asians, Hispanics, Blacks, and Native Americans). Serial superficial glycolic acid, salicylic acid, Jessner's solution, and TCA peels (when appropriate) offer substantial benefits for postinflammatory hyperpigmentation, melasma, acne, pseudofolliculitis barbae, oily skin, and texturally rough skin. When selecting a peeling agent, the benefits of the procedure should always substantially outweigh any associated risks or complications. Superficial peels with appropriate titration of concentrations are generally safe and efficacious for darker-skinned patients. However, given the labile nature of melanocytes of darker complexioned individuals, medium-depth and deep peels are more likely to induce substantial complications and side effects.

Disclaimer The author has no financial interest in any of the products or equipment mentioned in this chapter.

References

1. U.S. Census Bureau News, 2010 Census shows American diversity, March 24, 2011
2. Montagna W, Prota G, Kenney JA (1993) Black skin structure and function. Academic, San Diego, pp 42–45
3. Szabo G, Gerald AB, Patnak MA, Fitzpatrick TB (1969) Racial differences in the fate of melanosomes in human epidermis. Nature 222:1081–1082
4. Olson RL, Gaynor J, Everett MA (1973) Skin color, melanin, and erythema. Arch Dermatol 108:541–544
5. Kaidbey KH, Agin PP, Sayre RM, Kligman A (1979) Photoprotection by melanin – a comparison of black and Caucasian skin. J Am Acad Dermatol 1:249–260
6. Berardesca E, Maibach H (1996) Racial differences in skin pathophysiology. J Am Acad Dermatol 34:667–672
7. Grimes PE, David LT (1991) Cosmetics in blacks. Dermatol Clin 9:53–63
8. Halder RM, Grimes PE, McLauren C, Kress MA, Kenney JA Jr (1983) Incidence of common dermatoses in predominantly black dermatologic practice. Cutis 32:388–390
9. Grimes PE (2000) Skin and hair cosmetic issues in women of color. Dermatol Clin 15(4):659–665
10. Grimes PE, Hunt SG (1993) Considerations for cosmetic surgery in the black population. Clin Plast Surg 20:27–34
11. Grimes PE (2000) Agents for ethnic skin peeling. Dermatol Ther 13:159–164
12. Pierce HE, Brown LA (1986) Laminar dermal reticulotomy and chemical face peeling in the black patient. J Dermatol Surg Oncol 12:69–73
13. Al-Waiz MM, Al-Sharqi AI (2002) Medium-depth chemical peels in the treatment of acne scars in dark-skinned individuals. Dermatol Surg 28:383–387
14. Lim JT, Tham SN (1997) Glycolic acid peels in the treatment of melasma in Asian women. Dermatol Surg 20:27–34
15. Wang CM, Huang CL, Hu CT, Chan HL (1997) The effects of glycolic acid on the treatment of melasma among Asian skin. Dermatol Surg 23:23–29

16. Burns RI, Provost-Blank PC, Lawry MA et al (1997) Glycolic acid peels for post inflammatory hyperpigmentation in black patients: a comparative study. Dermatol Surg 23:171–174
17. Javaheri SM, Handa S, Kaur I et al (2001) Safety and efficacy of glycolic acid facial peel in Indian women with melasma. Int J Dermatol 40:354–357
18. Sarkar R, Kaur C, Bhalla M et al (2002) The combination of glycolic acid peels with a topical regimen in the treatment of melasma in dark-skinned patients: a comparative study. Dermatol Surg 28:828–832
19. Kligman D, Kligman AM (1998) Salicylic acid peels for the treatment of photoaging. Dermatol Surg 24:325–328
20. Grimes PE (1999) The safety and efficacy of salicylic acid chemical peels in darker racial-ethnic groups. Dermatol Surg 25:18–22
21. Lee Ho-S, Kim IH (2003) Salicylic acid peels for the treatment of acne vulgaris in Asian patients. Dermatol Surg 29:1196–1199
22. Lawrence NL, Cox SE, Brady HJ (1977) Treatment of melasma with Jessner's solution verses glycolic acid: a comparison of clinical efficacy and evaluation of the predictive ability of Wood's light examination. J Am Acad Dermatol 36:589–593
23. Cuce LC, Bertino MCM, Scattone L, Birkenhauer MC (2001) Tretinoin peeling. Dermatol Surg 25:12–14
24. Khunger N, Sarkar R, Jain RK (2004) Tretinoin peels verses glycolic acid peels in the treatment of melasma in dark-skinned patients. Dermatol Surg 25:270–273
25. El-Domyati MB, Attia SK, Saleh FY, Ahmad HM, Uitto JJ (2004) Trichloroacetic acid peeling versus dermabrasion: a histometric, immunohistochemical, and ultrastructural comparison. Dermatol Surg 30(2 Pt 1):179–188

22 How to Choose the Best Peeling Agent for the Patient: Asian Skin

Rashmi Sarkar

22.1 Introduction

Chemical peeling is a common dermatosurgical procedure, which is basically an accelerated form of exfoliation induced by the use of a chemical cauterant or escharotic agent on the skin. It has been known since ancient times and modified by different workers over several decades. But, it was only in 1980, when Stegman's benchmark work on the histological changes of wound injury after chemical peeling provided scientific basis for the classification of peels [1].

Superficial peeling is a painless office procedure performed without any surgical instruments but revolves around the scientific knowledge of healing pattern of chemical skin burns. Very light peeling agents induce faster sloughing of the cells in the stratum corneum, whereas deeper peeling agents work by creating necrosis and inflammation of the epidermis, papillary dermis, or reticular dermis. The process of exfoliation is followed by subsequent resurfacing of epidermis, as well as, remodeling of collagen and elastic fibers and deposition of glycosaminoglycans in the dermis [2].

R. Sarkar
Department of Dermatology,
Maulana Azad Medical College,
318, Ashirwad Enclave,
Plot No. 104, Indraprastha Extension, Patparganj,
New Delhi 110092, India
e-mail: rashmisarkar@yahoo.com

22.2 Indications for Peeling in Patients of Asian Origin

The clinical manifestation of photoaging may differ in Caucasian skin as compared to darker skin types. South Asians are of Caucasian ethnic background but have brown to dark brown skin [3]. Advanced and severe photodamage is less common in Asians [4]. Skin cancers and telangiectasias are also less frequent. They also develop thicker, deeper wrinkles on the forehead, periorbital, and crow's feet area when compared with finer wrinkles in these regions in fair-skinned patients. Moreover, in Asian patients having Fitzpatrick's skin phototypes IV to V, overall photoaging is delayed and may not be apparent till the fifth or sixth decade of life [3].

In patients of Indian origin, photodamage is characterized by fine wrinkles, texturally rough skin, and pigmentation changes including mottled facial pigmentation, lentigines, actinic keratosis as well as larger pores.

The chief indications of chemical peeling in Asian patients are:

- Disorders of hyperpigmentation like melasma and postinflammatory hyperigmentation
- Acne
- Oily skin, textural skin
- Photoaging, especially fine wrinkles

Very superficial and superficial depth peels are useful in Asian patients as they have lower postpeel complications. Medium-depth peels are done only in selected patients by experienced dermatologists as they can potentially cause postinflammatory hyperpigmentation. However, in dark-skinned individuals, deep chemical

A. Tosti et al. (eds.), *Color Atlas of Chemical Peels*,
DOI 10.1007/978-3-642-20270-4_22, © Springer-Verlag Berlin Heidelberg 2012

peels are better avoided as they can cause severe complications such as postinflammatory hyperpigmentation, hypopigmentation, uneven skin pigmentation, and scarring [5].They also have a longer period of recovery or downtime.

22.3 Prepeel Preparation/Priming with Topical Agents

Preparing the skin for a peel, or priming, is one of the most important components in chemical peeling. The prepeeling agents are used for at least 2–4 weeks prior to chemical peeling.

22.3.1 Advantages of Prepeel or Adjunct Topical Agents

- They allow more rapid penetration of the peel.
- Accelerate re-epithelization.
- Reduces wound healing time.
- They cause a skin lightening effect due to dispersion of melanin granules, hence decreasing the risk of postinflammatory hyperpigmentation.
- They enforce the concept of maintenance regime.

The agents used as prepeel agents or adjunct topical agents in dark-skinned patients of Asian origin are:

1. Hydroquinone – 2–4% is used in Asians, concentrations up to 8% are used in persons with lighter skin. Hydroquinone blocks the tyrosine activity and reduces melanin production. Thus, it helps in maintaining the results obtained by chemical peel in the postpeel period and decreases the risk of postinflammatory hyperpigmentation. Two percent hydroquinone is found to be more effective than 0.025% tretinoin for this purpose in reducing postpeel hyperpigmentation both with trichloroacetic acid and glycolic acid in Indian patients with melasma [6, 7].
2. Broad-spectrum sunscreens – decrease the UV damage to the skin and decrease the darkening of the skin.
3. Tretinoin – 0.025–0.05% is found useful for darker Asian skin whereas 0.1% is used in lighter skin types. It decreases corneocyte adhesion, decreases stratum corneum thickness, redistributes the melanin pigment, affects new collagen production, and causes mild peeling of the skin.
4. Glycolic acid 8–12% is used for its exfoliating action.
5. Others: salicylic acid and lactic acid.

22.4 Commonly Used Peeling Agents for the Asian Skin

22.4.1 Alpha-Hydroxy Acids

Alpha-hydroxy acids or fruit acids are: glycolic acid derived from sugar cane, lactic acid from sour milk, citric acid from citrus fruits, malic acid from apples, and tartaric acid from grapes.

22.4.2 Advantages

Glycolic acid (GA) is the most commonly used agent in Asian patients and is considered the most versatile of all due to: good penetration of the skin due to its low molecular weight; increased bioavailability as the pH decreases; it can be easily neutralized; its effect is mostly superficial (considered safe); and has very few postpeel complications. Also used as "lunch time peels" and its results are time dependent [8, 9].

22.4.3 Indications

Its indications are in treating melasma, fine wrinkles, benign keratoses, and mild inflammatory acne. Studies of glycolic acid peels done in India and Asia show that it is efficacious and well tolerated in various indications [9–11] (Fig. 22.1a, b).

22.4.4 Formulations

In India, it is mostly available in 70% solution in 100-ml bottles prepared from crystals or readymade Neostrata peels. The 70% solution can be easily diluted using distilled water, alcohol, or propylene glycol. It has to be stored in tightly capped bottles but is not light sensitive. It can be diluted to different strengths ranging from 20% to 65%. The higher the concentration used, the deeper is the penetration and the level of destruction. Further, the nearer the pH of resulting solution to 5.5 (acid mantle of the skin), the less is the

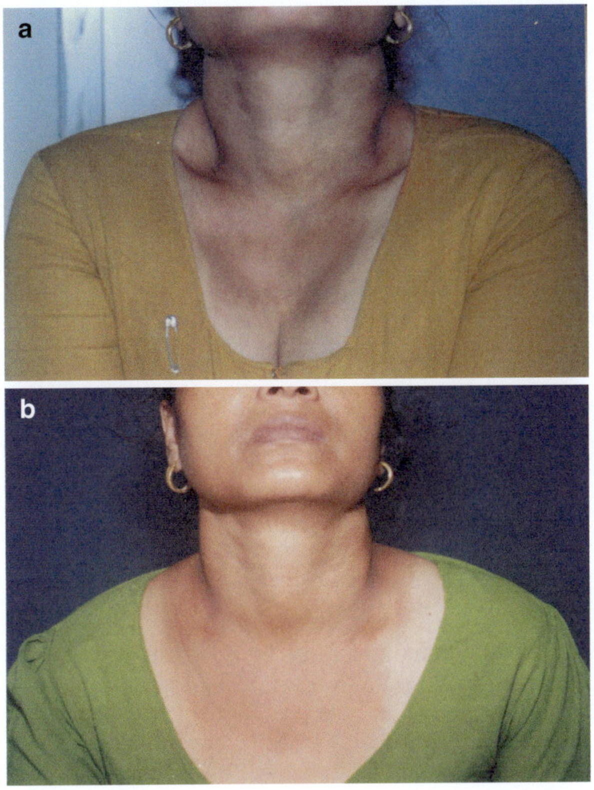

Fig. 22.1 (**a**) Improvement in melasma and postinflammatory hyperpigmentation after glycolic acid peeling (**b**) Melasma before and after trichloroacetic acid peeling

stinging and more uniform the peeling. However, for chemical peeling, availability of free glycolic acid in the solution is very important, for it to be effective. It is available as buffered, esterified, partially neutralized, and free glycolic acid. Good results are obtained with lower pH of the acid and higher concentration of the free glycolic acid. The free, non-neutralized glycolic acid (pH 0.6–1.7 in aqueous vehicle) is generally used by experienced dermatologists, as it works better than partially neutralized GA in dark-complexioned patients, although it must be used cautiously as it can cause extensive epidermolysis.

The time of application depends on the indication for treatment and the skin type. Weekly, once in 2 or 3 weeks, or monthly applications are used to obtain optimum results. The acid is neutralized with cold water or 5% sodium bicarbonate after a few minutes. The glycolic acid peels are well tolerated, and postpeel erythema and burning may be accompanied by peeling and exfoliation for 1–3 days.

Sarkar et al. conducted a controlled study of 40 Indian women with melasma, divided into two groups in which they compared the efficacy of serial glycolic acid peels, three each 30% and 40% glycolic acid peels in combination with a topical bleaching agent, the modified Kligman's regime (hydroquinone 5%, hydrocortisone acetate 1%, and tretinoin 0.05%) and with the topical bleaching agent alone. Although both groups showed a statistically significant decrease in the Melasma Area and Severity Index (MASI) score at 21 weeks, the combination side being treated with glycolic acid peels had a greater improvement [9]. In another Indian study of 25 patients with melasma, a prepeel program of daily application of sunscreens and 10% glycolic acid lotion followed by 50% glycolic acid peels monthly for 3 months was found to be effective and well tolerated [12]. Lim and Tham treated a series of ten Asian women from Singapore with melasma and fine wrinkles with 2% hydroquinone and 10% glycolic acid on both sides of the face. A series of 20–70% glycolic peels were applied on one side of the face for comparison. The side treated with glycolic acid peels had greater improvement [10]. In another study, 40 Taiwanese women with moderate to severe acne were treated with 35–50% glycolic acid peels resulting in significant improvement in skin texture and acne; the glycolic acid peels appeared to be an ideal adjunctive treatment of acne [13].

22.5 Trichloroacetic Acid (TCA)

Trichloroacetic acid has been considered the gold standard of chemical peeling agents due to its long history of usage, chemical stability, and versatility as a peeling agent.

22.5.1 Indications

1. As a superficial peel in melasma
2. Medium-depth peels for actinic damage and acne scars
3. As a deep peel (70% and above) for acne scars

As a superficial depth peel, it is used to treat dyschromias and, as a medium-depth peel for actinic damage, wrinkles, and acne scars.

22.5.2 Advantages

- It is safe and inexpensive.
- Lack of systemic toxicity.
- Stability.
- Has an easily visualized end point-frosting.
- Does not need to be neutralized.
- The peel depth correlates with intensity of skin frost.
- In higher concentrations, TCA is most commonly used in combination with other peeling agents, such as CO_2, Jessner's solution, or 70% glycolic acid.

22.5.3 Formulations

TCA is usually prepared by a weight-to-volume aqueous solution. TCA 100% is available in crystal form. Commercial and ready to use such as Ogablue, Accupeel, and Easy TCA peel kit (Skintech), which are colorless and ready to be diluted with water. The solution has to be prepared afresh every 6 months. In order to get 30% concentration, 30 g of TCA crystals are added in distilled water to get a total volume of 100 ml. In this manner, various other concentrations can also be prepared. The crystals are hygroscopic and have to be stored in tightly capped, acid-resistant plastic or glass bottles. Once prepared, TCA solution is no longer hygroscopic but light sensitive and has to be stored in amber-colored bottles away from sunlight. In order to avoid contamination, the solution should ideally be poured, from a master bottle into a separate container, for each peel procedure.

There are hardly any studies on trichloroacetic acid alone for chemical peeling in Asian patients. In a study of 15 patients from Iraq, a medium-depth chemical peel using a combination of Jessner's solution followed by the application of 35% trichloroacetic acid was performed for up to three sessions for acne scars. This medium-depth chemical peel was found to be a safe and effective way of treating patients of dark complexion. The side effects noted were transient postinflammatory hyperpigmentation [14].

22.5.4 Disadvantages

In darkly pigmented skin, such as Asian skin, concentrations above 25% can cause hyperpigmentation, hypopigmentation, and scarring. Unlike GA peels, its effect is not contact time dependent and, once frosting is achieved, the changes cannot be reversed.

22.6 Salicylic Acid Peels

Salicylic acid is a lipophilic beta-hydroxy acid which is used as a peeling agent, compounded as 20–40% solution with ethanol. It is a hydroxyl derivative of benzoic acid and represents a carboxylic acid attached to an aromatic alcohol, phenol. It is a white crystalline powder derived from willow bark, winter green leaves, and sweet birch [15].

22.6.1 Formulations

Salicylic acid paste (salicylic powder USP 50%, methyl salicylate 16 drops, aquaphor 11.2 g), 20–30% on weight-to-volume basis in a hydro-ethanolic solution, salicylic acid peel kits (Skinceuticals salicylic acid peel kits).

22.6.2 Indications

Acne vulgaris, enlarged pores, rough and oily skin, melasma, postinflammatory hyperpigmentation, and photoaging (Fig. 22.2a, b).

22.6.3 Advantages

It is a superficial chemical agent which has been found to be safe and effective in darker-skinned races including Asians, as well as due to its predictable response, less downtime, and efficacy compared with glycolic acid peels [16]. As the white "pseudofrost" occurs, uniformity of application is easily achieved.

In a study from Korea, by Lee and Kim, 35 patients with facial acne were treated with 30% salicylic acid peels biweekly for 12 weeks. Lesion counts and Dr. Cunliffe's scores revealed a decrease in both inflammatory and noninflammatory acne lesions. The peels were also well tolerated [17]. In another prospective, noncomparative study of 268 Asian patients who underwent 30% salicylic acid peels weekly for 8 weeks for various indications including melasma, acne vulgaris, freckles, postinflammatory scars/pigmentation, the peels were tolerated well. Mild discomfort, burn-

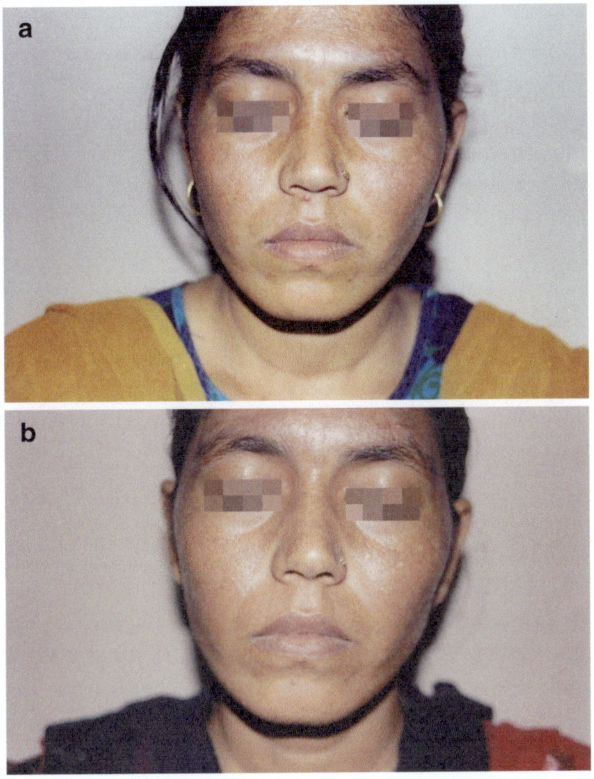

Fig. 22.2 (**a**, **b**) Melasma and photodamage before and after salicylic acid peeling

ing, irritation, and erythema were quite common, but the incidence of major side effects was low and easily manageable [18]. In another study from Korea, 24 patients underwent 30% salicylic acid peels biweekly for 3 months for acne. The salicylic acid peels were found beneficial in reducing both acne lesions and postinflammatory hyperpigmentation [19].

22.6.4 Disadvantages

It is contraindicated in patients allergic to aspirin and those who are pregnant or lactating.

The peel only has a limited depth of peeling and less efficacy in patients with significant photodamage.

22.7 Tretinoin Peels

Although tretinoin is classified as a superficial peel, it has a superficial peeling action, only after repeated use. Hence, according to Mark Rubin, it should not be referred as a true peeling agent [2].

22.7.1 Formulation

One percent tretinoin peel consists of 1% tretinoin in 95% isopropyl alcohol base and 5% chloroform with antioxidant 1-butylated hydroxytoluene [20]. It is stored in amber-colored bottles, in the dark, to prevent photodegradation. On application to the skin, there is a yellowish coloration, which makes it easy to visualize the agent [20, 21].

22.7.2 Advantage

It is a superficial peel which is quite well tolerated in Asian skin, although it has not been tried sufficiently in large number of patients.

22.7.3 Indications

Only recently, 1% tretinoin peel has been tried by Cuce et al., in the treatment of photoaged skins I and II, melasma, ephelis, and acne grade I, and found to be a practical and quick agent which does not have significant side effects as compared to glycolic acid peels [21]. It can be applied once or twice a week, and the peel solution is left in contact with the skin for about 4 h. It is applied just like any other peeling agent, and appears to be promising. A subsequent study from India compared the efficacy of 1% tretinoin peels to 70% glycolic acid peels in a split-face trial in patients of melasma. A significant reduction was seen in the modified MASI score and by photographic assessment on both the sides of the face, with no significant difference between the two sides of the face. Thus, tretinoin peels were well tolerated in patients with dark skin [20]. However, larger controlled trials may be undertaken to reconfirm its usefulness.

22.7.4 Disadvantage

Tretinoin has to be left in contact with the skin for 4–6 h, the "yellow discoloration" may be difficult to tolerate.

22.8 Lactic Acid Peels

This is another member of the alpha-hydroxy acid family which has been used in the treatment of melasma in Asians.

22.8.1 Formulations

Pure lactic acid, full-strength (92%; pH 3.5), ready-made lactic acid peels.

22.8.2 Advantages

It has similar activity as glycolic acid but is cheaper and more available.

22.8.3 Indication

Sharquie et al. conducted six peeling sessions with pure lactic acid on 20 patients of Asian origin with melasma and found it to be safe and effective. An erythematous response started after 2–3 min. The lactic acid peel was left in contact with the skin for 10 min and then washed off with water [22].

22.9 Jessner's Solution

Jessner's solution has been used over several years as a superficial peeling agent.

22.9.1 Formulations

The standard formulation of Jessner's solution contains resorcinol (14 g), salicylic acid (14 g), and lactic acid (85%, 14 g) mixed in a sufficient quantity of ethanol to make 100 ml. Modified Jessner's solution contains 17% lactic acid, 17% salicylic acid, and 8% citric acid mixed in a sufficient quantity of ethanol to make 100 ml. Solutions are available (Delasco, Pubmed).

22.9.2 Advantages

Jessner's peels are well tolerated in Asian skin, although there is paucity of literature on the same. It has a good safety profile and enhances the penetration of TCA.

22.9.3 Indications

It is used to treat acne, melasma, postinflammatory hyperpigmentation, lentigines, freckles, and photodamages. Kim et al. conducted a comparative study on the effectiveness of treatment and side effects in the treatment of facial acne in 26 Korean patients by two agents, 70% glycolic acid and Jessner's solution. Acne improved after three treatment sessions with both agents. However, a greater degree of exfoliation was observed with Jessner's solution [23].

22.9.4 Disadvantages

Instability on exposure to light and air, manufacturing variations, and resorcinol toxicity are concerns. Excessive exfoliation is another concern.

22.10 Combination Peels

A large number of combination peels are in the market which combine various alpha-hydroxy acids and also with beta-hydroxy acids. There are other proprietary peels, the exact composition of which is not known. There are hardly any randomized controlled studies on these in Asian patients. There are concerns about their stability and efficacy. Some are made for home use. A comparative study on 44 Indian patients with acne which had two groups, one receiving 35% glycolic acid peels and the other 20% salicylic acid–10% mandelic acid peels for six sessions at 2-weekly intervals, found salicylic–mandelic peel more efficacious for active acne and postacne hyperpigmentation [24]. Mandelic acid penetrates less but in the combination with salicylic acid has a beneficial role in postinflammatory hyperpigmentation.

22.11 Contraindications for Chemical Peels

- Inflamed acne lesions
- Open cuts on scratches on the face
- Any facial surgery within 3 months
- Active herpes simplex
- Uncooperative patient
- Unrealistic expectations
- A mentally unstable patient
- Photosensitivity
- A patient sensitive to components of the peel

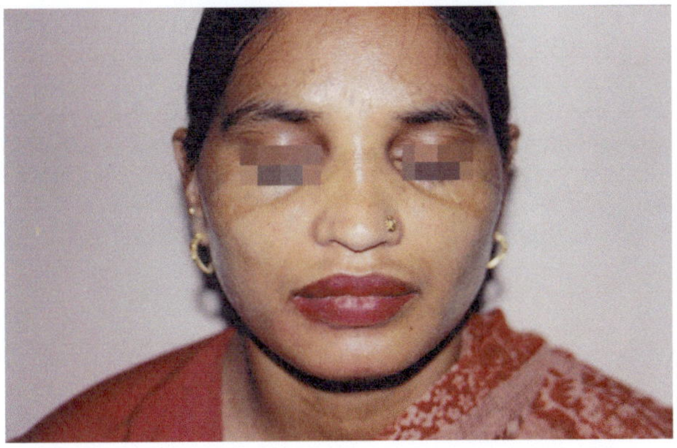

Fig. 22.3 Postinflammatory hypopigmentation with trichloroacetic acid peel

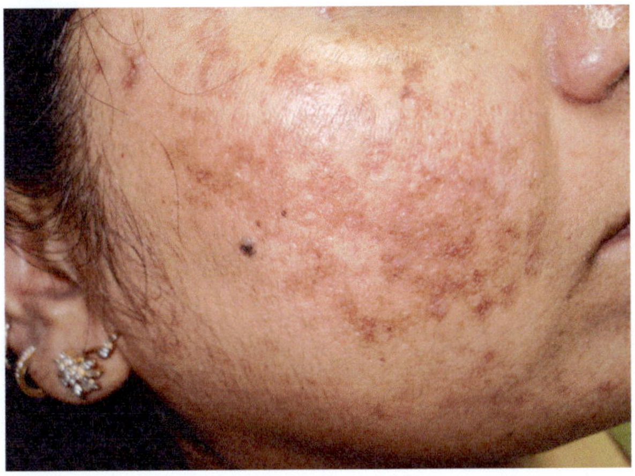

Fig. 22.4 Postinflammatory hyperpigmentation in an acne patient treated with glycolic acid peels (Courtesy: Dr. M.K. Shetty, Bangalore, India)

- Use of isotretinoin within the past year
- Abnormal scarring
- History of delayed wound healing
- Immunosuppression
- History of radiation

22.12 Complications of Chemical Peels

- Postinflammatory hyperpigmentation (Fig. 22.4)
- Postinflammatory hypopigmentation (Fig. 22.3)
- Persistent erythema
- Scarring
- Atrophy of the skin and textural changes
- Allergic reaction to the chemicals
- Milia

References

1. Stegman SJ (1982) A comparative histologic study of the effects of the three peeling agents and dermbrasion on normal and sun damaged skin. Aesthetic Plast Surg 6:123
2. Rubin MG (1995) What are skin peels? In: Winters SR, James M, Caputo GR (eds) Manual of chemical peels: superficial and medium depth, 1st edn. JB Lippincott Co, Philadelphia, pp 17–25
3. Elsaie ML, Lloyd HW (2008) Latest laser and light based advances for ethic skin rejuvenation. Indian J Dermatol Venereol Leprol 23(3):49–53
4. Grimes PE, Hexsel DM, Rutowitsch M (2008) The aging face in darker racial ethnic groups. In: Grimes PE (ed) Aesthetics and cosmetic surgery for darker skin types. Lippincott William and Wilkins, Philadelphia, pp 27–36
5. Savant SS, Mehta N (1998) Superficial and medium depth chemical peeling. In: Savant SS, Atal-Shah R, Gore D (eds) Textbook and atlas of dermatosurgery and cosmetology, 1st edn. Association of Scientific Cosmetologists and Dermatologists, Mumbai, pp 136–144
6. Nanda S, Grover C, Reddy BSN (2004) Efficacy of hydroquinone (2%) versus tretinoin (0.025%) as adjunct topical agents for chemical peeling in patients of melasma. Dermatol Surg 30:385–389
7. Garg VK, Sarkar R, Agarwal R (2008) Comparative evaluation of beneficiary effects of riming agents (2% hydroquinone versus 0.025% retinoic acid) in the treatment of melasma with glycolic acid peels. Dermatol Surg 34:1032–1039
8. Clark CP (1996) Alpha hydroxy acids in skin care. Clin Plast Surg 23:49–56
9. Sarkar R, Kaur C, Bhalla M, Kanwar AJ (2002) The combination of glycolic acid peels with a topical regimen in the treatment of melasma in dark-skinned patients: a comparative study. Dermatol Surg 28:828–832
10. Lim JT, Tham SN (1997) Glycolic acid peels in the treatment of melasma among Asian women. Dermatol Surg 23: 177–179
11. Sehgal VN, Luthra A, Aggarwal AK (2003) Evaluation of graded strength glycolic acid (GA) facial peal: an Indian experience. J Dermatol 30:758–761
12. Javaheri SM, Handa S, Kaur I, Kumar B (2001) Safety and efficacy of glycolic acid facial peel in Indian women with melasma. Int J Dermatol 40:354–357
13. Wang CM, Huang CL, Sindy CT, Chan HL (1997) The effect of glycolic acid on the treatment of acne in Asian skin. Dermatol Surg 23:23–29
14. Al-Waiz MM, Al-Sharqi AI (2002) Medium – depth chemical peels in the treatment of acne in dark-skinned individuals. Dermatol Surg 28:383–387
15. Monheit GD, Kayal JD (2004) Chemical peeling. In: Nouri K, Leal Khouri S (eds) Techniques in dermatologic surgery, 1st edn. Mosby, St. Louis, pp 233–244
16. Vedamurthy M (2004) Salicylic acid peels. Indian J Dermatol Venereol Leprol 70:136–138
17. Lee HS, Kim IH (2003) Salicylic acid peels for the treatment of acne vulgaris in Asian patients. Dermatol Surg 29:1196–1199
18. Bari AU, Iqbal Z, Rahman SB (2005) Tolerance and safety of superficial chemical peeling with salicylic acid in various facial dermatoses. Indian J Dermatol Venereol Leprol 71(2):87–90
19. Ahn HH, Kim IH (2006) Whitening effect of salicylic acid peels in Asian patients. Dermatol Surg 32:372–375

20. Khunger N, Sarkar R, Jain RK (2004) Tretinoin peels versus glycolic acid peels in the treatment of melasma in dark skinned patients. Dermatol Surg 30:756–760
21. Cuce LC, Bertino MCM, Scattone L, Birkenhauer MC (2001) Tretinoin peeling. Dermatol Surg 25:12–14
22. Sharquie KE, Al-Tikreety MM, Al-Mashhadani SA (2005) Lactic acid as a new therapeutic peeling agent in melasma. Dermatol Surg 31:149–154
23. Kim SW, Moon SE, Kim JA, Eun HC (1999) Glycolic acid versus Jessner's solution: which is better for facial acne patients? Dermatol Surg 25:270–273
24. Garg VK, Sinha S, Sarkar R (2009) Glycolic acid peels versus salicylic-mandelic acid peels in active acne vulgaris and post-acne scarring and hyperpigmentation: a comparative study. Dermatol Surg 35:59–65

Part IV

Management of Complications

Adverse Reactions and Complications

23

Antonella Tosti and Maria Pia De Padova

Complications can be due to doctor or patient's responsibilities.

Doctor's possible mistakes include

- Choice of excessive concentrations
  In case of overpeeling, prescribe a systemic steroid (Methylprednisolone 8 mg/day) for a few days and monitor strictly the patient in the postpeeling period. Prescribe a moisturizer to be applied four to five times a day and explain the necessity of complete avoidance of sun exposure.
- Inadequate evaluation of patient's phototype
  Dark phototypes are more susceptible to develop hypo/hyperpigmentation (Fig. 23.1a, b). This is already evident 2–3 weeks after peeling and can be treated with regular application of bleaching agents, tretinoin and topical steroids, and absolute sun avoidance.
- Inadequate modality of application resulting in dishomogeneous penetration
  You can retreat the skin areas that do not develop erythema or frosting. Be careful not to overpeel the other areas.
- Accidental dropping of the peeling solution into the eyes, mouth, or other sensitive regions (Fig. 23.2)
  Rinse immediately with tap water that dilutes the concentration. Refer to ophthalmologist in case of eye involvement.

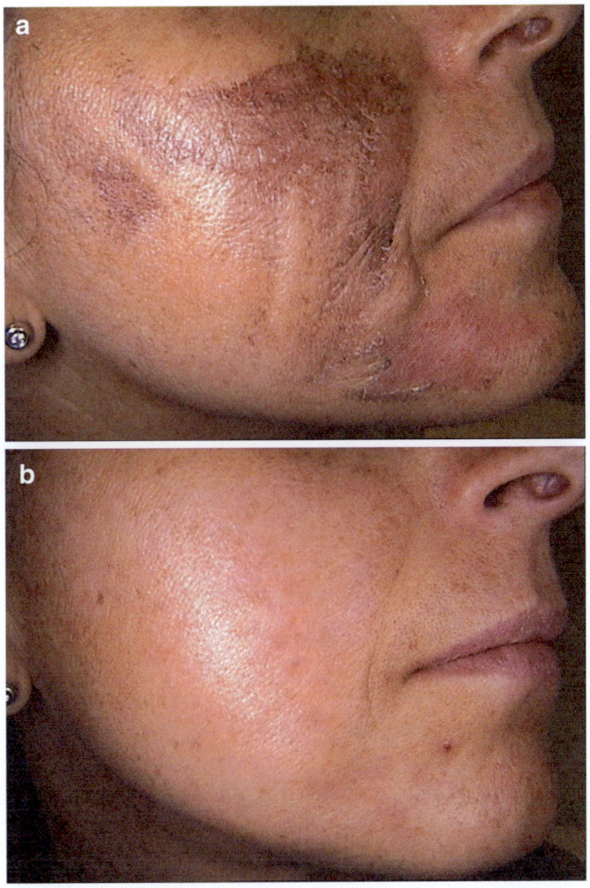

Fig. 23.1 (**a**, **b**) This patient was treated with 30% TCA for melasma. Note severe crusting (**a**) followed by hypopigmented spots (**b**) 4 weeks after the procedure

- Herpes simplex reactivation may occur if prophylaxis has not been prescribed
  Treat with systemic antivirals (acyclovir, penciclovir, and famciclovir) for 5 days.

A. Tosti (✉)
Department of Dermatology and Cutaneous Surgery, Miller School of Medicine, University of Miami, US
e-mail: atosti@med.miami.edu

M.P. De Padova
Ospedale Privato Nigrisoli, Bologna, Italy
e-mail: mdepadova@gmail.com

A. Tosti et al. (eds.), *Color Atlas of Chemical Peels*,
DOI 10.1007/978-3-642-20270-4_23, © Springer-Verlag Berlin Heidelberg 2012

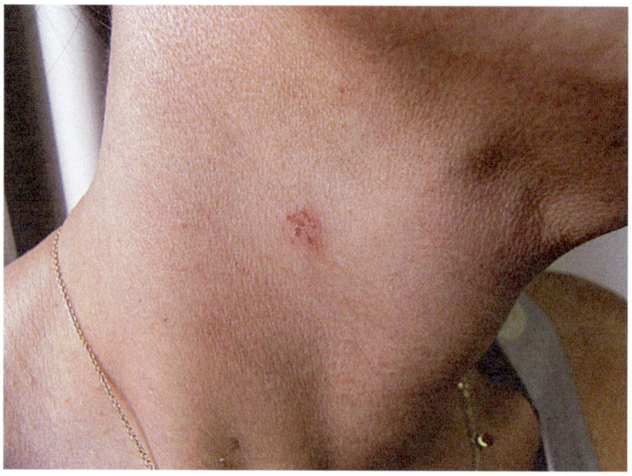

Fig. 23.2 Skin erosion due to accidental dropping of 50% pyruvic acid on the neck

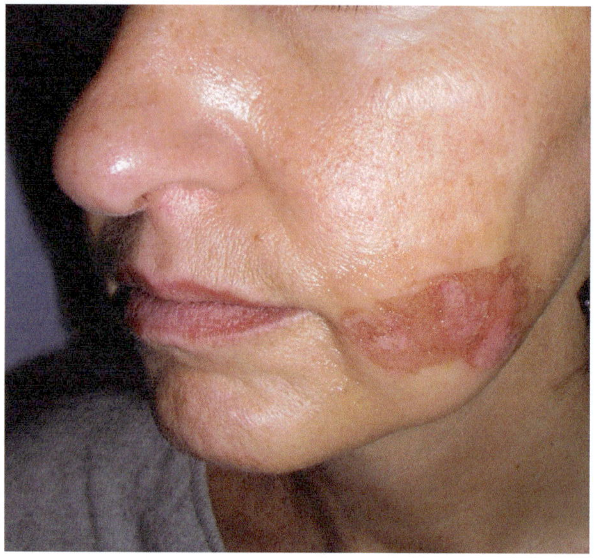

Fig. 23.3 Skin erosions due to mechanical removal of crusts after peeling

Patient's responsibilities include

- Application of inadequate topical products (scrubs, exfoliating agents) before complete reepithelization
  This results in severe irritation with intense erythema and edema. Prescribe topical and systemic steroids for a few days. Prescribe bleaching agents (hydroquinone 3–4%, kojic acid, arbutin, azelaic) acid after reepithelization as the risk of hyperpigmentation is increased.
- Removal of scales and crust
  This results in exudative erosions (Fig. 23.3). In exudative phase, apply 3% boric acid solution. Then prescribe a moisturizer to be applied every 3 h and a topical preparation containing an antibiotic in association with a steroid. Explain the necessity of complete avoidance of sun exposure.
- Sun exposure
  In case of hyperpigmented spots due to inadequate sun avoidance (Fig. 23.4), prescribe bleaching agents, topical tretinoin, and topical steroids. A soft peeling with 25% salicylic acid or 40% pyruvic acid can reduce the pigmentation.

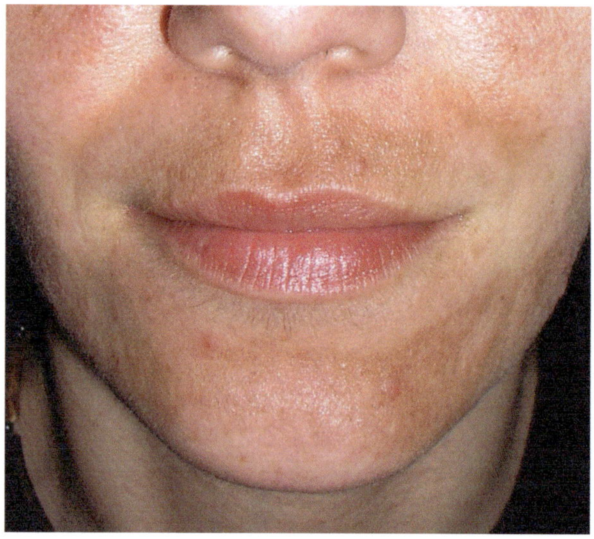

Fig. 23.4 Hyperpigmentation following 20% TCA for melasma. The patient went on vacation and did not strictly avoid sun exposure

23.1 Minor Local Adverse Reactions

Most minor reactions resolve spontaneously.

- Intense swelling
  Prescribe systemic steroids (Methylprednisolone 8 mg/day) for 1 week.
- Eye irritation
  Prescribe eyedrops containing low-potency steroids for a few days.
- Nose and oral irritation
  Explain that this is transitory, and does not require treatment.
- Prolonged erythema: In some patients, erythema persists after 3 week from the procedure (Fig. 23.5)
  Prescribe systemic steroids (Methylprednisolone 8 mg/day) for 2–3 weeks.
- Dishomogeneous skin color: This is due to irregular penetration of the peeling agent

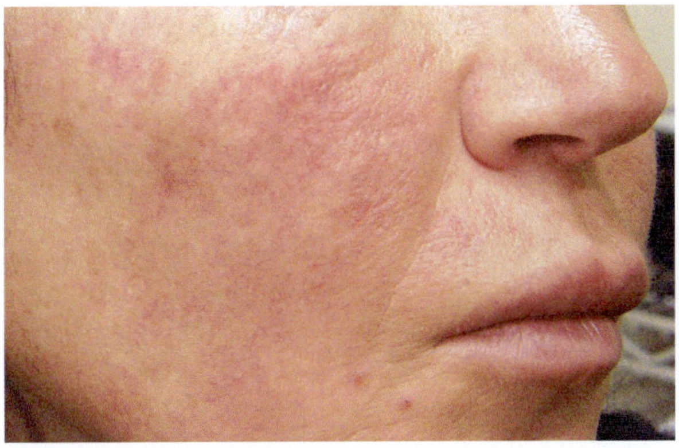

Fig. 23.5 Prolonged erythema after 30% TCA for the treatment of photoaging

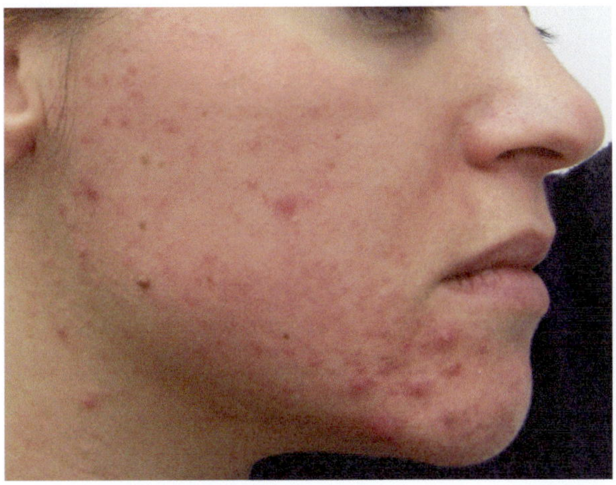

Fig. 23.6 Acneiform eruption after 50% pyruvic acid for the treatment of active acne

Prescribe 3–4% Hydrochinone and topical tretinoin for 2 months.

- Persistent itching/burning sensation
  Prescribe low-potency topical steroid for a few days.
- Skin hypersensitivity
  Prescribe preservative and fragrance-free moisturizers. Avoid overcleaning.
- Localized skin infections: herpes simplex, impetigo
  Prescribe systemic antivirals/antibiotics.
- Acneiform eruptions: These usually develop a few days after peeling and may persist for 1 month (Fig. 23.6)
  Prescribe oral tetracyclines as for the treatment of acne.

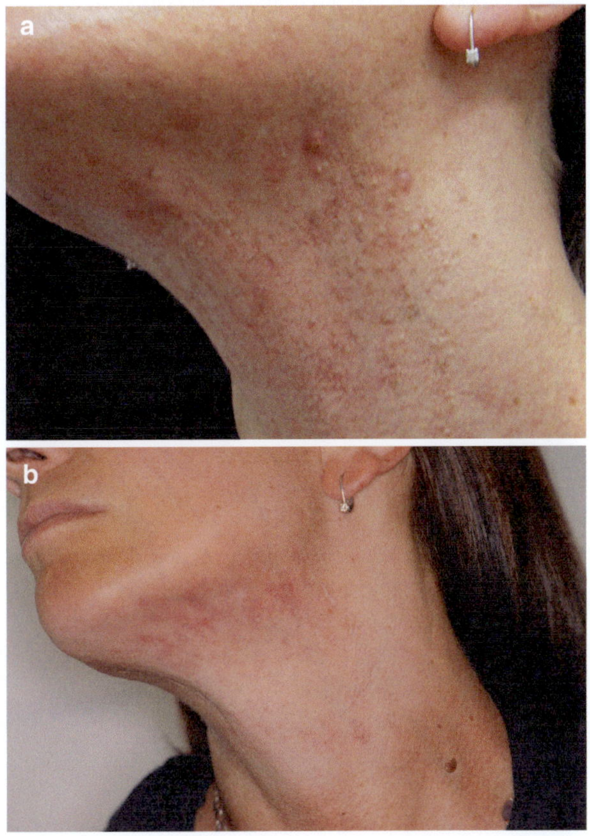

Fig. 23.7 (**a**, **b**) Milia after 30% TCA for the treatment of acne scars (**a**). Note considerable improvement after 3 months of tretinoin 0.05% treatment (**b**)

- Milia: These are uncommon after peeling and may be caused by use of occlusive postpeeling topical product (Fig. 23.7a)
  Prescribe topical tretinoin (Fig. 23.7b).
- Allergic reactions: These may be due to the peeling agent or to the topical products applied in the prepeeling or postpeeling period. Allergic contact dermatitis to peeling agents is rare and occurs most frequently with resorcinol. Patch testing is necessary
  Prescribe systemic and topical steroids.

23.2 Major Local Adverse Reactions

- Corneal damage
  Eye bandage and ophthalmologic referral.
- Textural changes: These are most often seen after deep peeling and produce a porcelain skin appearance
  The only treatment is camouflage.

- Atrophic scars
  Wait for 2 months after peeling before treating. Possible treatments include skin needling, injections of hyaluronic acid /collagen fillers, TCA cross.
- Hypertrophic scars
  Hypertrophic scars should be treated immediately. Prescribe silicone gel sheets for 6 months. Then treat with intralesional injections of triamcinolone acetonide 10–40 mg/mL at 4- to 6-week intervals.
- Diffuse or spotted hypopigmentation
  This is usually persistent. Skin needling sometimes induces repigmentation. Camouflaging maybe necessary.
- Diffuse or spotted hyperpigmentation
  Prescribe 3–4% Hydrochinon, topical tretinoin, and topical steroids.
  A soft peeling with 25% salicylic acid or 40% pyruvic acid or 5% retinoic acid *can reduce the pigmentation. Absolute sun avoidance.*
- Ochronosis
  This is a complication of prolonged utilization of high concentration of hydroquinone and is more commonly observed in patients with dark phototypes. The skin presents a bluish black discoloration; treatment is usually unsuccessful.

23.3 Systemic Adverse Reactions

- Cardiac arrhythmia: This may occur with phenol and resorcinol peelings. Death following a serious cardiac adverse reaction has been reported.
  Cardiac monitoring and anesthesiological support is mandatory with this procedures.
- Laryngeal edema and toxic shock syndrome have been reported with phenol.
- Salicylism.
  Salicylism is characterized by rapid breathing, tinnitus, abdominal cramps, and neurological symptoms. It has been reported after application of 20% salicylic acid on extensive body areas (50%) or after application of 50% salicylic acid. We never observed this complication despite our large experience with salicylic acid peels.
- Hypothyroidism is a very uncommon side effect of very high concentration resorcinol.

Part V

Management of the Patient

Management of the Patient

24

Aurora Tedeschi, Doriana Massimino, Lee E. West, and Giuseppe Micali

24.1 Patient Selection and Evaluation

Before performing any peeling procedure, an accurate evaluation of the patient is very important. In order to assure a satisfactory outcome and to minimize the risk of scarring and delayed reepithelialization, the appropriate peeling agent for a patient needs to be determined and a period of pretreatment is required [1, 2]. Considerations for the individual choice of peeling agent include: lifestyle, including avoidance of sun exposure and appropriate use of sunscreen, history of perioral herpes simplex virus (HSV) infection, previous or concomitant treatments (oral isotretinoin, contraceptives and other photosensitizing medications such as radiation and laser skin resurfacing), and positive history for abnormal or keloid scarring. For example, patients susceptible to facial herpes simplex virus infection may be treated with antiviral drugs from the pre-peel period until reepithelialization is complete, especially when medium-depth or deep peeling is performed [3–8].

Moreover, some skin-related factors, such as skin phototype, anatomic site, sex, age, degree of photoaging and concurrent skin disorders, as well as any psychological discomfort, must all be considered in the choice of peeling agent.

Skin phototype should be evaluated to minimize the risk of abnormal pigmentation occurring post treatment. Skin types IV–VI, according to Fitzpatrick's classification, should typically not undergo medium and deep peeling because of the high risk for pigmentary dyschromias (hyperpigmentation or hypopigmentation). Therefore, it is recommended that patients with skin types IV–VI receive very superficial to superficial peeling procedures [3, 6].

Anatomic site for chemical peeling is important since reepithelialization occurs from the epithelium of the adnexal skin structures (sebaceous glands, hair follicles, and sweat glands). As a result, areas where adnexae are more represented, such as the face, have a faster reepithelialization compared to other sites such as the upper chest. Stratum corneum thickness should also be considered, since it varies according to anatomic region and gender (thicker in men compared to women). For these reasons, thinner or more sensitive areas, such as the periorbital region, require lighter treatments compared to the forehead and glabella, while thicker and/or sebaceous oily skin is more resistant to peeling penetration and requires deeper treatment than other skin types.

Age, skin aging, and photoaging should all be considered as well. Glogau's classification describes four types of skin damage due to photoaging, evaluating both epidermal and dermal degenerative effects (Table 24.1). According to this classification, patients with mild photoaging can be treated successfully with light/superficial chemical peeling, whereas those with moderate, advanced, or severe photoaging may better benefit from medium-depth and deep peeling [3, 4, 6, 8, 9].

Finally, concomitant skin disorders, such as atopic dermatitis, seborrheic dermatitis, psoriasis, contact dermatitis, and rosacea, must be carefully considered for potential exacerbation of the preexisting disorder in the post-peeling period. Also, these skin disorders may be responsible for prolonged healing time, post-peel erythema syndrome, or contact sensitivity during

A. Tedeschi • D. Massimino • G. Micali
Dermatology Clinic, University of Catania, Catania, Italy

L.E. West (✉)
Northwestern Memorial Hospital, Chicago, IL, USA
email: lwest@nmh.org

A. Tosti et al. (eds.), *Color Atlas of Chemical Peels*,
DOI 10.1007/978-3-642-20270-4_24, © Springer-Verlag Berlin Heidelberg 2012

Table 24.1 Glogau classification of photoaging

Type I: *Mild photoaging*
1. Mild pigmentary changes
2. No keratoses
3. Minimal wrinkles and/or acne scarring
4. Patient age: 28–35 years
5. Little or no makeup
Type II: *Mild to moderate photoaging*
1. Minimal dyschromias (senile lentigines)
2. Early actinic keratoses
3. Slight lines near the eyes and mouth; mild acne scarring
4. Patient age: 35–50 years
5. Need for some makeup
Type III: *Advanced photoaging*
1. Discoloration with telangiectasia
2. Visible actinic keratoses
3. Persistent wrinkles; moderate acne scarring
4. Patient age: 50–65 years
5. Need for heavy makeup
Type IV: *Severe photoaging*
1. Yellow or gray skin
2. Actinic keratoses with or without skin malignancies
3. Wrinkles throughout; severe acne scarring
4. Patient age: 60–75 years
5. Makeup cakes and cracks with poor coverage

the postoperative period [6]. Patients with significant history or current evidence of psychological disorders, immunocompromising disease, or allergies should generally not be treated.

Patients eligible for a peeling procedure must be informed about both risks and benefits of chemical peeling and about the need to use sun protection for a period varying from 15 days, after a superficial peel, to 6 months after a medium-depth peel [3, 4].

24.2 Photographs

All patients undergoing chemical peeling should also undergo signed informed consent concerning the potential side effects, complications, discomfort, and skin changes that may occur during and/or after the procedure. Also, skin appearance of the patient should be assessed at baseline and during each peeling session using digital photography in order to assess outcomes.

24.3 Pre-peeling Treatment

Skin priming is necessary to improve peel results and reduce risks of complications. Priming allows an easier and more uniform penetration of the peeling agent, reduces the duration of reepithelialization, minimizes the risk for post-treatment hyperpigmentation, and helps evaluate the patient's skin tolerance [3, 10, 11].

Skin priming consists of topical application of compounds, such as retinoic acid 0.05%, glycolic acid 10%, pyruvic acid 7%, and hydroquinone 2–4%, used alone or in combination, for at least 2 weeks before the peel procedure. These agents used in the pre-peel period cause a superficial exfoliation due to keratinocyte discohesion, and allow a more uniform, rapid, and deeper penetration [11].

24.4 Post-peeling Treatment

Post-peeling treatments are suggested after reepithelialization is complete and are necessary to skin maintenance post-peeling as well as for preparation of the skin if the patient will be undergoing another peeling procedure. The compounds used in the post-peel period are usually the same or similar to those used for skin priming [3, 4]. In order to avoid post-treatment complications such as hyperpigmentation, the regular and frequent use of sun protection is recommended [4].

24.5 Management of Patient with Peeling's Complications

Pigmentary changes represent the most frequent complication following a peeling procedure. Usually hyperpigmentation is more frequently observed, but hypopigmentation is not uncommon, especially when a deep peel is performed. Patients undergoing medium-depth peeling and/or who are IV–VI skin phototype are more prone to pigmentary changes [3, 8]. Also, sun exposure and use of oral contraceptives enhance the risk for hyperpigmentation [7]. Daily use of total sun blockers, alone or together with a combination of hydroquinone 2–4% and retinoic acid 0.1% used before and after the peeling procedure, minimizes the risk of this side effect [9, 12].

Scarring, including atrophic scars, hypertrophic scars, and keloids, represents another side effect that may occur, especially after a deep peel [7]. History of poor healing or keloid formation should be carefully evaluated before performing peel procedures. Skin pigment must also be carefully considered since patients with skin phototype IV–VI are at a higher risk for scarring after chemical peels. The lower part of the face and the perioral region represent the most frequently involved sites for scarring side effects, probably due to mechanical stretching occurring during eating and speaking. Lower eyelid ectropion has been reported to occur 3–6 months after phenol peeling [13].

Herpes simplex infection outbreak is the most frequent complication in patients with a history of recurrent HSV, especially after medium-depth peeling. To minimize the risk of this complication, prophylaxis with 400 mg of oral acyclovir, from 1 to 2 days before peeling to 4–5 days after peeling, is suggested. If HSV outbreak occurs, 800-mg oral acyclovir three to five times daily and valacyclovir or famciclovir 500 mg orally twice daily are recommended as treatment approaches until reepithelialization is complete [3, 8]. Among common bacterial infections, *Pseudomonas* represents the most problematic, may especially occur after a deep peel, and can be responsible for pigmentary changes [14]. *Staphylococcus*, *Streptococcus*, and *Candida* infections are also reported post-peel procedures.

Persistent erythema, due to angiogenic factors stimulating vasodilatation, is considered a physiological event if it occurs within 3 weeks after the peel procedure [6]. If erythema associated with pruritus persists for more than 3 weeks, treatment with potent topical corticosteroids, systemic corticosteroids, and/or intralesional corticosteroids should be administered. Silicone sheets or pulsating dye laser treatments may be also adopted, especially when evident thickening or scarring has occurred [6, 15].

Milia may also be observed 8–16 weeks after a peeling procedure, possibly due to occlusive post-peeling treatments.

Acne-prone skin, as well as use of occlusive products during the reepithelialization phase or immediately after, may result in an acneiform eruption in a small percentage of patients [15]. Administration of systemic antibiotics may be necessary.

Allergic reactions are relatively rare and most frequently described in cases utilizing resorcinol peeling [15]. Allergic reactions are often misdiagnosed because the normal clinical post-peeling presentation is characterized by erythema, pruritus, and edema. Administration of antihistamines together with corticosteroids may be used to reduce the intensity of these clinical symptoms.

Finally, cardiotoxicity is a well-known, serious, and potentially life-threatening complication after phenol peeling. Cardiac toxicity, post phenol chemical peel, includes arrhythmias such as premature ventricular beats, bigeminy, and atrial and ventricular tachycardia [9, 16], along with the potential for liver and kidney toxicity [14]. For these reasons, a phenol peel requires a physician with experience as well as cardiopulmonary monitoring of the patient in an operating room environment [9].

References

1. Tosti A, De Padova MP, Iorizzo M (2006) Types of chimica peels: advantages/disadvantages. In: Tosti A, Grimes PE, De Padova MP (eds) Color atlas of chemical peels. Springer, Berlin, pp 3–10
2. Furukawa F, Yamamoto Y (2006) Recent advances in chemical peeling in Japan. J Dermatol 33:655–661
3. Tedeschi A, Massimino D, Fabbrocini G, West EL, De Padova MP, Micali G. Chemical peeling. In: Scuderi N, Toth B (eds) International textbook of aesthetic surgery, Verduci Editore, Roma (in press)
4. Bennett ML, Henderson RL (2003) Introduction to cosmetic dermatology. Curr Probl Dermatol 15:43–83
5. Coleman WP III, Brody HJ (1997) Advances in chemical peeling. Dermatol Clin 15:19–26
6. Monheit GD (2001) Chemical peels. Curr Probl Dermatol 13:65–79
7. Clark E, Scerri L (2008) Superficial and medium-depth chemical peels. Clin Dermatol 26:209–218
8. Bernstein EF (2002) Chemical peels. Semin Cutan Med Surg 21:27–45
9. Landau M (2008) Chemical peels. Clin Dermatol 26: 200–208
10. Khunger N, IADVL Task Force (2008) Standard guidelines of care for chemical peels. Indian J Dermatol Venereol Leprol 74:5–12
11. Zakopoulou N, Kontochristopoulos G (2006) Superficial chemical peels. J Cosmet Dermatol 5:246–253
12. Lawrence N, Cox SE, Brody HJ (1997) Treatment of melasma with Jessner's solution versus glycolic acid: a comparison of clinical efficacy and evaluation of the predictive ability of Wood's light examination. J Am Acad Dermatol 36:589–593
13. Stuzin JM (1998) Phenol peeling and the history of phenol peeling. Clin Plast Surg 25:1–19
14. Monti M (1995) Il peeling chimico. In: Caputo R, Monti M (eds) Manuale di dermocosmetologia medica. Raffaello Cortina Editore, Milano, pp 919–945
15. Ghersetich I, Teofoli P, Gantcheva M, Ribuffo M, Puddu P (1997) Chemical peeling: how, when, why? J Eur Acad Dermatol Venereol 8:1–11
16. Park JH, Choi YD, Kim SW, Kim YC, Park SW (2007) Effectiveness of modified phenol peel (Exoderm) on facial wrinkles, acne scars and other skin problems of Asian patients. J Dermatol 34:17–24

Index

A. Tosti et al. (eds.), *Color Atlas of Chemical Peels*,
DOI 10.1007/978-3-642-20270-4,

MIX
Papier aus verantwortungsvollen Quellen
Paper from responsible sources
FSC® C105338

If you have any concerns about our products,
you can contact us on
ProductSafety@springernature.com

In case Publisher is established outside the EU,
the EU authorized representative is:
Springer Nature Customer Service Center GmbH
Europaplatz 3, 69115 Heidelberg, Germany

Printed by Libri Plureos GmbH
in Hamburg, Germany